DIGITAL HEALTH INFORMATION FOR THE CONSUMER

Digital Health Information for the Consumer
Evidence and Policy Implications

DAVID NICHOLAS, PAUL HUNTINGTON and HAMID JAMALI
with PETER WILLIAMS
University College London, UK

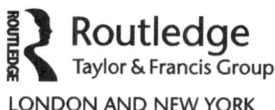

Routledge
Taylor & Francis Group

LONDON AND NEW YORK

First published 2007 by Ashgate Publishing

Published 2016 by Routledge
4 Park Square, Milton Park, Abingdon, Oxon OX14 4RN
605 Third Avenue, New York, NY 10017

First issued in paperback 2017

Routledge is an imprint of the Taylor & Francis Group, an informa business

British Library Cataloguing in Publication Data
Nicholas, David
   Digital health information for the consumer : evidence and
   policy implications
   1. Health - Great Britain - Electronic information
   resources 2. Medicine - Great Britain - Electronic
   information resources 3. Telecommunication in medicine -
   Great Britain 4. Medical informatics - Great Britain
   I. Title II. Huntington, Paul III. Jamali, Hamid
   IV. Williams, Peter
   025'.0661'0941

Library of Congress Cataloging-in-Publication Data
Digital health information for the consumer : evidence and policy implications / by David Nicholas ... [et al.].
     p. cm.
   Includes bibliographical references and index.
   ISBN 978-07546-4803-1
  1. Health education--Great Britain--Computer-assisted instruction. 2. Television in health education--Great Britain. 3. Internet in medicine--Great Britain. 4. Interactive television--Great Britain. 5. Digital television--Great Britain. 6. Touch screens--Great Britain. 7. Market surveys--Great Britain. 8. Health surveys--Great Britain. I. Nicholas, David, 1947-

   RA440.57.D54 2007
   610.2850941--dc22

                             2007009693
ISBN 13: 978-0-8153-9946-9 (pbk)
ISBN 13: 978-0-7546-4803-1 (hbk)

Contents

List of Figures

List of Tables

Preface

The aim of *Digital Health Information for the Consumer* is to provide a detailed understanding of the use and impact of key digital heath platforms and services offered to the general public in the UK during the period 2000-2005, many of which are still running. We believe this to be the largest, most exhaustive and detailed account of the use and impact of digital consumer health services ever provided. A user-orientated evaluation covering hundreds of thousands of people is provided employing robust evidence based techniques, which means that it sits very well in the general health field, where such techniques are widely employed. The origins of this book are to be found in what is, arguably, the biggest consumer information health research project ever conducted in Europe. The five year-long investigation was funded by the Department of Health (DoH) during the period 2000-2005 and undertaken by the research group, CIBER,[1] now based at University College London (UCL).

The book provides an extensive reference source on how health consumers behave when online, whether this differs according to digital platform or type of user, how they perceive digital health services and what health benefits these services deliver. The data are of particular relevance to policy makers and health professionals who are typically in the dark as to how the digital health consumer behaves and, as a consequence, make many mistakes when rolling digital services out to the general public, as even a cursory glance of any newspaper will soon reveal. The data provided in the book are unique. While the services covered were largely located in the UK in the case of the Internet services covered the audience is, of course, international.

The opening chapter, Introduction, describes the aims, objectives and scope of the book (and the research investigation that underpins it). It also provides an explanation of the innovative methods employed to study the digital health information consumer on an unheard of scale. Specifically, it covers the methodology developed specially for the purpose of studying the digital consumer, deep log analysis. Chapter 2 provides an overview of the published literature on the digital health consumer and provides a context for the detailed investigations described later in the book.

The following chapters provide evaluations of a range of digital information health services. Chapter 3 covers touchscreen kiosks, majoring on those of InTouch with Health and NHS Direct. Chapter 4 concerns itself with health websites, specifically SurgeryDoor, NHS Direct Online and Medicdirect. Digital Interactive television (DiTV) is the subject of Chapter 5, and four programmes are featured.

Chapter 6 is where the main digital platform comparisons are made. The chapter features five cross platform studies regarding: 1) usage comparisons between the three platforms (kiosks, internet and DiTV); 2) comparisons of the health content of

---

1   Centre for Information Behaviour and the Evaluation of Research.

the three platforms; 3) the impact of platform location on health information seeking behaviour, 4) consumer characteristics of health information seeking behaviour in a digital environment, and; 5) characterising users according to types of health information sources used/preferred. Chapter 7 discuses the barriers to the general public accessing electronic health information systems, and the way they could be overcome. It also describes health inequalities that arose as a result of widespread digital information provision.

The last chapter of the book (Chapter 8: Conclusions) presents the main findings of the study and present recommendations for health policy makers and health information providers.

Nicholas, Huntington and Jamali
Bloomsbury, London, February 2007

Acknowledgements

A large number of people helped us in the preparation and writing and we would like to pay most thanks to Barrie Gunter, a consultant and co-researcher on the DiTV pilot evaluations who contributed to the digital interactive health television section. Special thanks also to: Paul Blackburn of InTouch with Health who provided the early inspiration for the project and supplied us so willingly with data and advice regarding the kiosks and website his company produces; others, who deserve our thanks include: Matt Jordan; Neil Sellors and Julius Weinberg. The following research students were also involved in contributing information to the project: Mary Last, Kyriaki Kasnesi, Debbie Thompson, Xiang Yin, Karen Dennis, Janet Homewood and Panayiota Polydoratou.

Chapter 1

Introduction

This book provides a comprehensive and detailed evaluation of the roll-out of digital consumer health services in the UK during the period 2000-2005. It was a roll-out partly instigated by the Government and was conducted on a grand-scale. Not only was the scale of the roll-out unprecedented but, very unusually, the scale and detail of the evaluation was similarly unprecedented. There are many lessons to be learnt from this roll-out for health service professionals in countries all around the world.

In 2000 the Department of Health (DoH), aware of the recent, rapid, uneven and largely unregulated developments that were occurring in regard to the UK consumer being provided with widespread and accessible digital health information and advice services, decided there was a need to find out how the general public was reacting to these developments, to determine what impact this was having on the National Health Service (NHS) and what role there was for Government in driving digital health developments. Clearly the very provision of so much information to a public that had been generally short of information was likely to have many repercussions, but nobody really had any data to say what they would be. Whether, for instance, it would lead to a decrease in use of hospitals and surgeries or whether it would actually lead to increases in use. In consequence, the Centre for Information Behaviour and the Evaluation of Research (CIBER) was commissioned to undertake a national evaluation, leading on an innovative methodology (deep log analysis), particularly suitable for providing evaluations of digital roll-outs to very large and heterogeneous populations, where the outcomes were uncertain – as they clearly where in this case. The findings of this work are the subject of this book. The foresight of the DoH in detecting early the need for detailed evaluation has meant that, after five years of intensive research, it was to the health field that policy makers in other fields have turned, to obtain an understanding of the impact of digital roll-outs in their areas (e.g. publishing, newspapers).

More specifically, what we describe here is the take-up and impact of consumer digital health services on a variety of platforms (internet, touchscreen kiosk and digital interactive television), and consider the implications for health professionals, providers and policy makers.

The rapid march of so many expensive, strategic health information systems is examined in the book to determine whether these systems benefited the public's health in some way. The field is so new, the knowledge vacuum so large and the task so important – there are not many matters more important than health   that it was vital to ensure that information systems are subject to user evaluation. This is what we have undertaken to do in this book; to present and represent the users' voices (hundreds of thousands of them) through our innovative and triangulated research methods (deep log analysis). Given the size of the task – the sheer number of platforms, services and users involved – a 'grip' on this digital phenomenon could only be provided through a 'big picture', multi-method approach, with deep log analysis at its heart.

The book is built upon the findings of a large number of individual (and linking) studies. These studies variously covered: different health platforms; a range of digital health services; a variety of user groups; different aspects of information seeking; health impacts of digital information seeking; and comparisons between different platforms and services.

The book is data-rich and we make no apology for this as this is what is missing from the whole digital health debate. It should be used as a resource to support decision making and innovation.

Aims and objectives

The broad purpose of the book is then to provide an evidence-based evaluation of the potential demand for, and take-up of, health information delivery to consumers through the newly and rapidly emerging Information and Communication Technologies (ICTs) – specifically, in regard to touchscreen kiosks, DiTV and the Internet.

More specifically the aims are to:

1. Develop a new framework for understanding the wider issues connected with ICT delivery of healthcare information: e.g. the impact on healthcare professions, their training needs, the possibilities for addressing health inequalities and the role of brand/importance of authority.
2. Assess and compare consumer attitudes to healthcare information delivery from various ICTs and other sources, regarding, for instance, satisfaction, authority, health outcomes;
3. Identify the constraints and limitations of the various health information systems.

Scope/coverage

The book is concerned primarily with digital information and advice services (mostly the former) provided for the general public, the patient etc. and not those specifically provided for health or medical professionals. In recognition of the massive digital choice that the general public now has in the health field, their opportunity to 'shop' around for information and the pro-active nature of many of these services, the term 'digital information health consumers' is used throughout this book to more aptly describe them. The alternative terms patient, customer or user were all felt to be inadequate to describe the individual's new found information (and shopping) powers. Of course, everyone can be considered to be a potential digital health information consumer and, as indicated by the numbers reported in this book, their numbers are very large and growing fast. The book fills a vacuum as our knowledge of the use of digital health services largely comes from studies of services provided for health professionals.

The information platforms and services

Three digital platforms – touchscreen kiosk, Internet and DiTV, were the subject of evaluation (plus a hybrid – the web-enabled kiosk), but, plainly, not all output/ services from these platforms could be monitored. Only UK based services were covered, although, of course, in the case of the Internet, even for such an avowedly British service as NHS Direct Online, which was covered, the audience was inevitably international. In the case of kiosks, coverage was very comprehensive, certainly the most comprehensive analysis of kiosk usage produced to date in the UK, and, probably, the world. Kiosks from InTouch with Health and NHS Direct were covered. In all, use at nearly two hundred and fifty kiosk locations was monitored and evaluated.

With regard to the Internet, two of the most popular (and contrasting) sites were studied in some depth – SurgeryDoor, a commercial site run by InTouch with Health, the producers of the kiosks mentioned above, and the Government funded NHS Direct Online website. In addition, a smaller investigation of Medicdirect, a consumer health website run by practising medical doctors, was also undertaken because of the specialist services it offered.

DiTV is represented by four pilot services funded by the Department of Health (DoH) for a period ranging from four-six months during 2001. The four DiTV pilots offered distinctive services. Although there were some overlapping features, each had many special qualities. These included the type of platform on which the service was transmitted, the amount and nature of content, the presentation formats used, and the degree of interactivity offered. The four consortia were: Flextech Living Health, Communicopia, Channel Health and dktv (A Different Kind of Television). Living Health transmitted a largely text-based health information service to Telewest cable television subscribers in Birmingham, together with an experimental GP appointments booking service, and InVision – a video nurse from an NHS Direct call-centre who appeared on the caller's TV screen as they spoke to each other over the telephone. Communicopia presented a mixed text-based and video-on-demand health information service branded as NHS Direct Digital and transmitted over a broadband telephone network operated by Kingston Interactive Television (KIT) in Hull. The operator also provided users with an interactive online medical records-keeping service, which focused on immunisation records. Channel Health presented a text-based information service linked to special broadcasts in its regular schedule on the Sky Digital platform. It majored on the theme of maternity issues and experimented, on a local basis, with a package of other interactive services for pregnant women comprising mainly e-mail support links between users and health professionals. dktv, via a broadband service, offered interactive links to community health services together with videos on health issues accessible through the TV set.

Time period

In all, the research reported in the book covered a period of five years (2000–2005), probably the longest continuous period over which digital health information services of any kind – consumer or otherwise, have been studied. The length of the study enabled data to be collated over a significant period of time to detect changes in use and perception, and this was undertaken particularly in the case of kiosks. However, inevitably, given the restraints of funding and personnel, different platforms, services and information seeking behavioural traits were studied at various times throughout the period of the investigation as priorities emerged and new lines of investigation pursued.

Methodology

A wide range of methods were used to evaluate digital health services, which were, in some cases, specially developed by the authors. This is particularly true of the kinds of log analyses we have conducted throughout the book. Indeed, as a result of more than four years of trialling, the authors have developed a unique set of methodologies, which provide the most efficient and effective method for monitoring use and satisfaction of digital information services, This methodological mix is called 'deep log analysis' in recognition of the lead role log analysis plays, but it is not a purely quantitative methodology, a range of supporting qualitative methods (e.g. surveys and observation) are utilised too.

The precise blend of methods that constitute deep log analysis was determined by: 1) the need to produce a big-picture analysis for the DoH and health policy makers; 2) the requirements of an investigation of a large, disparate, dynamic population who were being confronted with something extremely new, and about which they had minimal grasp/knowledge and, as a result, might have difficulties telling us what they thought or what they would do.

The individual methodological components used as part of the deep log analysis approach were as follows:

- Server transaction log analysis
- Survey (quantitative) methods, including
  - Postal questionnaires (open and closed)
  - Online questionnaires
  - Exit questionnaires
- Qualitative exploratory work, including:
  - Focus groups
  - In-depth interviews
  - Participant observation
  - Non-participant observation
- Action research

The great advantages of the digital logs are not simply their size and reach, although the dividend here is indeed a rich and unparalleled one. Just as important is the fact that they are a direct and immediately available record of what people have done: not what they say they might, or would, do; not what they were prompted to say; not what they thought they did (the traditional domain of questionnaires and focus groups). This is especially important in an area such as digital information use where issues are complex and people are all too easily shoe horned into answers manufactured by researchers.

The log data are placed and explained through the use of questionnaires, interviews and observation. Logs map the digital environment and raise the questions that really need to be asked by questionnaire, interview and observation. This method produces a powerful triangulation of the data. For more details about log analysis see Nicholas *et al* (2000).

It must be remembered that what is being discussed throughout the book is not the use of a limited choice/option bibliographic system by intermediaries or digital libraries by health professionals, but the use of information and advisory consumer systems, which offer massive choice and high levels of interactivity, by end-users of every possible ilk. The really pressing challenge for the methods was to determine what people did when they were given so much digital freedom and choice in the health field and how this manifested itself in information seeking terms.

Methodological stages

The investigation of each platform was undertaken in the following stages:

Stage 1 A comprehensive literature review was conducted to provide context, information on current developments, research issues and questions.

Stage 2 A transaction log analysis study and report was undertaken. The aim here was to get a big picture of what all users were doing online. This stage sometimes involved pilot work. All transaction logs were analysed using the SPSS (Statistical Package for Social Sciences).

Stage 3 Questionnaire surveys of users and, where possible, non-users were conducted. The aim here was to get a richer profile of users, analyse differences between users and non-users, assess outcomes, examine ease of use and to ask specific questions (or check data) that arose from the literature review (Stage 1) and the transaction log study and report (Stage 2). All questionnaires were analysed using SPSS.

Stage 4 Finally, there was the qualitative analysis, which explored the issues identified above at a deeper level.

It is important to note that, although there is a logical progression in the methods outlined above, the steps are not necessarily chronological – each dataset informs and is informed by the others. User studies, for example, (Stages 3 and 4) both fed off and fed into log analyses. Unexpected patterns of use, as revealed by logs, prompted questions that that may not have been anticipated. In the study of touchscreens, for example, the low number of pages accessed by elderly users (many of whom did not progress past the menu hierarchy) prompted us to examine issues such as the level of navigational understanding, hand-eye co-ordination and whether the necessity to stand when using the system inhibited use.

Methodological limitations

Each method comes with its problems and limitations. Those associated with log analysis are probably not well known and are therefore reviewed here.

Essentially, deep log analysis maps and monitors, in a seamless and continuous manner, user behaviour on each digital platform. The attraction of logs is that they provide abundant and fairly robust evidence of use. Logs however are not problem-free. Problems arise from the identification of the user, how to handle unrecorded page views (caching), what to do with electronic agents or robots who visit the site for indexing purposes and determining when users log-off (for the problems associated with log analysis see Jamali, Nicholas and Huntington 2005).

User identification To really make the most of logs we need to identify individual users and obtain some personal and background characteristics about them.

Kiosks are located in public places and in consequence their logs do not identify individual users, just the separate search sessions conducted. Web logs, on the other hand, provide a user trace, but not real user identification. All we have is an Internet Protocol (IP) number for identity purposes. However, the IP number cannot be traced back to an individual, only to a computer. Also, the use of proxy servers mean that the IP address cannot be assumed to relate to use on a specific machine and use might also relate to a group of users, rather than an individual. Furthermore, access to a site may be via a multiple user machine or the IP number might have been allocated temporarily to a client's machine. Cookie technology, which sits on the client's machine and is recognised by the server as an identification tag, can be employed to help overcome these problems. However, web users are typically very sensitive to having cookies placed on their machines. They certainly would be sensitive to their use in the health field.

User identification on DiTV depends on the routing and access by the provider. In most cases however, DiTV subscriber households can be identified by a numerical code. Because of data protection concerns this number cannot be easily used to enrich usage logs with subscriber details. Furthermore, television sets are multiple user machines. So although a user can be identified, once hub caching is defeated, the user may in fact be a family of users – parent, child etc.

Caching Caching, a facility used to speed up searching, undermines a number of key evaluation metrics. Caching is an Internet browser feature, switched on at the client's machine, whereby pages once viewed are stored and available from the terminal being used. Thus, any pages re-viewed do not have to be downloaded again from the server, obviously saving considerable time. From the point of view of recording logs, however, this practice creates a serious problem. Views of previously seen pages are made from the cache and are, therefore, not recorded by the server access log file as files that have been used. Caching can result in the significant under recording of the number of pages viewed, especially where single HTML pages contains information on a number of topics with a menu structured as internal links at the top of the page. Here users would have cached a multiple topic information page and a menu page by downloading just one page. The user could then access the cached information and menu page 'exploring' a number of related topics without requesting further pages from the server. Caching creates a false picture in that it negatively impacts on two key evaluation metrics: it underreports the number of pages viewed and provides incorrect page view times. Fortunately, caching only concerns web logs and are not an issue with Kiosk and DiTV logs.

Robots Robots are electronic agents used by search engines and organisations to log and index pages into a searchable database. Robots may account for a third of the use of a web site. Robots raise the issue of whether the pages they view should be counted as 'hits'. The question that needs asking, although seldom is, is whether robots constitute 'real' users. Robot activity is recorded as a use in Internet log files. Robots are identified by their visit to the 'Robot.txt' file located on the server and their use was excluded from the analysis of all the log studies reported here. Importantly, robots do not affect DiTV and kiosks.

Logging off There are differences between platforms with regard to how users log off and this impacts on time metrics. Kiosk logs record the log-off time of the user, either as a result of a user generated termination request or the automatic log off that occurs after two minutes of inactivity. DiTV and Internet logs do not have a user generated termination request, though in theory a cookie could pick up this information. As far as the logs are concerned nobody logs off on the web or DiTV – they depart quite anonymously. Typically then, to estimate a log off – or a session end – a time lapse of inactivity has to be assumed. The web industry normally assumes a 30-minute inactivity to constitute a termination signal. This is probably too generous (and therefore inaccurate) given a typical page reading time of a minute. As a consequence, we have not adopted this convention.

Chapter 2

Literature Review

This chapter, through an analysis of the work of others in the consumer health field, provides a historical context for the results of the field research that follow, especially in regard to the information needs of health consumers.

Health information needs

Evaluations of the use and impact of an information system or service should be conducted with full knowledge of the information needs of the potential or actual user group. Various researchers have examined information needs with regard to medical or health information provision. Kai (1996), for example, examined 'disadvantaged' parents' difficulties and information needs in coping with acute illnesses in their pre-school children. They proved to be:

- How to gauge the severity of illness
- How doctors assess illness
- When to seek advice
- How over the counter medicines and antibiotics work
- The nature of rashes, viral diseases etc. and
- Learning about other parents' experiences.

It could be argued that all of these requirements could be met, at least in general terms, by well produced cross-referenced web pages or similar digital content. Subjects of the study stressed the need for more information on these topics, and 'emphasised the importance of the information being accessible' in terms of ease of understanding. They learned more about specific illnesses, from 'the media, parenting magazines, television dramas and publicity campaigns' than from doctors or medical literature.

James *et al* (1999) similarly found that their sample of cancer patients also clamoured for information (74% said they wanted as much as possible) and used television as a source of both general and cancer specific health information. Beresford and Slopper (2000) looked at the issue of the information needs of both the chronically ill and physically disabled children and adolescents. They found that psycho-social information that enabled the management of 'the emotional, social, educational and future aspects' of their lives with the condition was as important as medical information. As with findings of other studies, there was a fundamental need for contact with those suffering similar conditions, for self-help, mutual support, and to compare experiences, and as the authors acknowledged, the Internet 'may well play a role in meeting medical and psycho-social needs'. Clearly, this could also apply to kiosk terminals, assuming the incorporation of interactive facilities, as is the case with web-enabled types.

While there have been many studies on the information needs of different patient groups, especially cancer patients (James *et al* 1999; Ankem 2006), there have been very few studies on the information needs of the general public. One has to readily admit that it is harder to assess the information needs of those not immediately affected by illness – i.e. members of the public who may require health information for general uses unrelated to specific conditions. This is both because they do not constitute a closely defined user group and also because any definition of 'health information' would have to be so broad to be considered in a generalist sense as to render it difficult to examine. Of course, these people are the target of many of the digital services that are being developed and are the subject of the book.

It is, of course, possible to infer generalist needs from the information that is used by the public, and to determine the needs of large numbers of the public this is what has to be done, and is something that this book seeks to do. The following section looks at such information take-up (and subsequent use) from studies of access to digital, remote systems.

Information use and users of electronic systems

Just as the literature seems to suggest that people affected either directly or indirectly, from a medical complaint have extensive information needs, there are myriad statistics to show an ever-increasing consumption generally of electronic health information. To give one example, less than one year after Medline, a medical information service largely intended for doctors, became freely available to all on the web, the number of searches increased tenfold, with no less than 30% of users being members of the general public (Lindberg 1998). In another manifestation of the thirst for information, London (1999) pointed to a consumer phenomenon he coined as 'if it's there, they'll find it'. London was instrumental in the design of the academic cancer website, Kimmel Cancer Center (at www.kcc.tju.edu), which has pages for healthcare professionals and general scientific researchers, as well as those targeted at the lay public. He quickly found that 'our database listings of currently open clinical trials, targeted at cancer physicians, were frequently accessed by members of the lay public'. Following this discovery, the site developers began to include lay descriptions in their trial listings. Similarly, Eysenbach *et al* (1999) found that, even a dermatology website intended for medical practitioners, was accessed more by lay consumers than healthcare workers. Of course, this all results from the public being given huge digital choice and easy access to the data. In these circumstances they plainly availed themselves of the data, no matter for whom it was intended. Morahan-Martin (2004) reported that about 4.5% of all Internet searches worldwide were for health-related information.

Some evidence on the type of information which people search online services for is available. The Internet health organisation Health on the Net Foundation's 'Evolution of Internet use for health purposes' survey (HoNF 2001) found that the vast majority searched for medical literature (83%), with 67% looking for the 'description of a disease', and 38% for clinical trial information. This suggests a traditional approach to health information seeking, even when conducted in a digital environment.

Apart from retrieving information electronically, it appears people are becoming ever more involved in generating and exchanging information, bearing out the information needs studies described earlier, which identified contact with co-sufferers as being an important source of information and help. Quick (1999) studied the role of online support groups for those suffering from kidney disease. Results did not yield clear evidence to support the view that they offered real support benefits, although the subjects did participate in discussions and remained members of the group throughout the duration of the fieldwork.

Online support groups

Some work has been carried out on the impact of the Internet on various specialist groups, principally with regard to online support groups. Gann (1998) found, for example, that participation in these fora was particularly heavy in the field of HIV/ AIDS, with 'peer support and sharing of information on treatment advances, clinical trials etc.' Bacon (1999) described an Internet self help group for widows with dependent children. Eighty-six percent of the widows reported that having contact with and receiving mutual support from their peers enhanced coping with their grief, although this is hardly surprising given the nature of the group. The major weakness of online self-help, reported by 57% of the sample, was the amount of time required to read and answer email. Thirty-three percent also noted that occasional technical problems limited their participation. A study by Rodgers and Chen (2005) revealed a positive correlation between the amount of participation in an Internet community group and the psycho-social well-being of women with breast cancer. The information posted on support groups by participants tended to be mostly accurate. A study by Rimer *et al* (2005) concluded that cancer-related online mailing lists appeared to be an important resource, especially for information seeking, but also for support of cancer survivors. Esquivel, Meric-Bernstam and Bernstam (2006) found just 0.2% inaccurate postings on a breast cancer support group site, which mostly were rapidly corrected by participants in subsequent postings. Finn (1999) found, again unsurprisingly, that a disability group's communication exhibited many of the same features as face-to-face self-help and mutual aid groups, with an emphasis on problem solving, information sharing, expression of feelings, and mutual support and empathy. Other studies have shown the importance of the World Wide Web in providing social support, particularly to groups with chronic health problems such as diabetes, HIV or cancer (Reeves 2000; Zrebiec and Jacobson 2001).

The literature shows that an increasing number of people engage in online support group discussions, either as active participants or silent observers ('lurkers'). Studies (Cummings *et al* 2002; Davison *et al* 2000; Han and Belcher 2001; Klemm *et al* 2003; White and Dorman 2000) disclosed that groups that support people suffering from the so-called stigmatising illnesses (HIV/Aids, cancer, mental health problems, addictions) showed the greatest increase in numbers. Ferguson (1997) identified three types of self-support groups in cyberspace: those addressing physical health concerns, mental health concerns and those dealing with recovery/problems of living.

There are a number of reasons why people participate in online support groups (Cline and Haynes 2001; White and Dorman 2001) and the most important of these are: 24 hour access to information; anonymity; mutual support from similar sufferers; that they are not discriminatory; and the ease with which second opinions may be obtained. Problems associated with online support groups (Ferguson 1997) include the dissemination of inaccurate and misleading information. However, as we have seen, users have been found to correct misleading information (White and Dorman 2001). Further problems relate to respondents having to wait for a response to their query, and the fact that the process might have an impact on the users' behaviour, in that the participation in online support groups could become addictive and have an adverse impact on social life. Access is also an issue. The chief barrier to the use of online support groups has to be accessibility as not everybody owns a computer and has an Internet connection. Computer literacy and language are also barriers (White and Dorman 2001; Klemm *et al* 2003). Language is a particular barrier as the majority of the online support groups conduct their affairs in English.

Socio-demographic factors such as age, gender, racial or ethnic identity, income and social status have not been found to be significant in determining whether people use support groups or not (White and Dorman 2001). Geographic location was also not found to be significant in determining who uses support groups. Klemm *et al* (1999) conducted a content analysis across 3 online support groups lists and did find significant, but unsurprising, patterns in user characteristics. The research found that the breast cancer list was accessed mainly by women while the prostate list mainly by men. Owen *et al* (2003) in a study of 167 undergraduate psychology students with a friend or family member suffering from cancer found no differences between genders in terms of the content of communication. They also found out that preparation for participation in an online group was not associated with greater emotional disclosure.

Klemm *et al* (1999) identified four categories of use: information giving/ seeking; encouragement/support; personal opinion; and personal experience. The four categories accounted for approximately 80% of responses across the groups. Information giving/seeking was ranked first in the prostate group, and personal experience took priority in the breast group. Interestingly, men were more than twice as likely to give information and women more than twice as likely to give encouragement and support.

Health information exchange between peers is not restricted to online discussion boards. Baker *et al* (2003) surveyed 4,764 US Internet users and found that just over a quarter had used email or the Internet to communicate with family or friends about health. However, by its nature, such material is not as accessible to research as online discussion messages. In addition to these mushrooming networks of online mutual support groups and communication, there is a growing movement within the medical profession for promoting partnerships between patients and doctors. *The Times* (Rumbelow 1999), for example, reported as early as 1999 that research had shown that families were using the Internet to negotiate treatment from doctors.

Jadad and Gagliardi (1998) suggested that the Internet 'will have a profound effect on the way that patients and clinicians interact'. The 'new level of knowledge' fostered by information available on the Internet will enable patients to 'participate in active partnerships with many groups of decision makers such as clinicians, policymakers and clinicians'. It has to be said that, in the light of the work reported here, we probably still have along way to go before these (eight-year old) suggestions actually bear fruit, but no doubt they eventually will.

Usefulness/satisfaction

A paucity of literature exists with regard to patient and public satisfaction with information found by electronic means – hence the importance of this book. In a rare example, Tucker (2000) sought to discover why women from the UK used the Internet for health information and their levels of satisfaction with the information obtained. UK women were identified through an established information website (www.womens-health.co.uk) and asked to complete an anonymous questionnaire relating to their Internet usage. Nearly a half of the respondents had used the Internet for one to three hours, either daily or every few days. Eighty seven percent described Internet-acquired information as high or good quality, though a small percentage (14%) felt it was too detailed. Forty three percent of users found consistent and relevant information, a further 47% finding useful, but, sometimes, contradictory information. In a survey conducted by Tassone *et al* (2004) it was found that of the 344 studied patients with access to the Internet, 18% had searched the Web for medical information prior to their consultation and ninety-five per cent planned to use the Internet again.

Echoing Tuckers' findings, the Health on the Net Foundation surveys (HoNF 1999a; 1999b) have found that consumers increasingly perceived medical and health information on the World Wide Web as 'useful'. HoNF's fifth survey (HoNF 1999b) confirmed persistently high levels of user satisfaction. Ninety eight percent of over 3,000 respondents agreed with the statement 'I have found useful medical and health information on the Internet' (95% for the fourth survey and 93% in the case of the third). In the fourth survey, 82% of those for whom English was not a first language said they found information in their mother-tongue. However, despite growing familiarity with the medium, 'more users than ever' according to HoNF (1999b) said that information quality was insufficient, as the following extended extract confirms: 'A record 71% of all HON survey respondents either agree or strongly agree with the statement "The quality of medical/health information on the Internet needs to improve". This number was 53% in our third survey (May-June 1998) and 69% in the fourth (March-April 1999)'. It has to be said, however, that the question is rather leading in tone and is likely to encourage such a response. In a later survey (HoNF 2001) the researchers included a section on the 'shortcomings' of the Internet. Results indicated that the accuracy (or lack of it) was the major problem with 83% of respondents citing it. Seventy nine percent said 'trustworthiness', 76% 'Availability of information', and 72% 'Findings things' as other problems. The most recent survey by NoHF (2005) showed that the criteria perceived as the most important indicators of quality and usefulness for health Websites were the same as in 2002. However, by 2005, their order of importance was identical for non-professional and professional groups of users: (1) availability of information, (2) ease of finding information/navigation, (3) trustworthiness/credibility and (4) accuracy of information. The survey also showed that patients were not only using the Internet to better educates themselves, but many were also using it to assist in discussion with their physicians.

More research is available regarding patient satisfaction in regard to telemedicine. Mair and Whitten (2000) undertook a systematic review of studies of patient satisfaction with telemedicine. The studies mainly used simple survey instruments to ascertain patient satisfaction. Firm conclusions were limited by methodological difficulties, but it would seem that the patients found tele-consultations acceptable; noted definite advantages, particularly the increased accessibility of specialist expertise, less travel required, and reduced waiting times; but also voiced some disquiet about this mode of healthcare delivery, particularly relating to communication between provider and client via this medium. Several problems with the studies, however, were found, that affected their reliability and validity. There tended, in addition, to be no clear definition of what constituted 'satisfaction'.

Studies have been carried out that do not seek to measure 'satisfaction' per se, but concentrate on the qualities of the information system which may make it appealing, and the benefits which may accrue by using the systems. Fox and Rainie (2000), for example, reported that users valued the convenience, anonymity, and volume of online information.

Ease of use/usability

Digital data, especially in the case of DiTV are often held to be accessible, easy to use, the panacea etc, but clearly this cannot be taken as read. A number of studies have looked at issues of usability of websites, and of those that have, this has generally been as part of a wider study. Thus the Centre for Information Research at the University of Central England, for instance, investigated public use of the National Electronic Library for Health (NeLH), which is primarily (but not exclusively) aimed at the medical profession. The study included an examination of the possible barriers to usage. The researchers found several usability problems with the website. These were:

Visual appearance: where the 'home' page was considered to 'cluttered' and difficult to read: this resulted in, for example, the search facility being hard to find,

The search facility: here the fact that only one basic search option was available was cited as inappropriate for users of varying degrees of Information Technology (IT) ability, and the search results were not ranked very well,

Mis-spellings: medical terminology may not be easy for lay users, and a system for dealing with mis-spellings and common names for conditions was recommended.

Williams *et al* (2004) looked at the usability of a pilot National Electronic Library for Communicable Diseases (NeLCD) branch for the NeLH as part of a wider study of public understanding of the health information posted on the NeLH. Several points emerged. Firstly, as has been found with other websites (e.g. Williams *et al* 2002a; 2002b), interviews and observation showed there were possibly too many main menu items. Secondly, there were question marks about hyperlinks, with complaints from users that there were too many and that some of the links were 'dead'. In observations conducted by the researchers, some searchers were seen to attempt to activate what they thought were hyperlinks but were, in fact, simply bold text. An issue that has arisen previously in usability studies by Williams and Nicholas (e.g. 2001b) is that of new browser windows opening. This happened on the NeLCD site, which users found a little disconcerting. Many people did not know how to close a window, and some were confused by the 'back' button being greyed out (when a new window opens, its 'history' starts from the moment it appears). Previous pages are recorded by the original browser, from where one can 'back-navigate'.

In addition to hyperlinks and contents or 'menu' items, site navigational aids include a search engine, site map and glossary. However, observed navigation consisted virtually solely of using the main menu and the back button of the web browser. By contrast, few people were seen to be using the search facility, and one of those did so only because he asked the researcher what the options there were for finding information. Although this lack of use might be in part due to the comprehensive menu list, it may well also be due to people simply not noticing these facilities, as noted by McNicol and Nankivell (2002).

Cumbo *et al* (2002) converted two patient education CD-ROMs to a web-based environment, and asked subscribers to a web newsletter to view one of the two programmes (Colorectal Cancer Program and Chemotherapy Program) and to complete a survey. Three hundred and one surveys were completed. Sixty-eight percent of Colorectal Cancer Program respondents and 50% of Chemotherapy Program respondents considered the program to be more useful or much more useful than any other source of information on the topic. A majority of users for both programmes preferred to view the information on the Internet rather than on CD-ROM. Many users reported trouble accessing certain sections of the material presented. This included the inability to open video or audio clips and the length of time needed for each page to load, despite a high-speed Internet connection. Although the authors did not state this in their article, it may be that for maximum usability simpler formats – such as text and images only, may be appropriate, at least in the short term, until the technology improves and users also become more sophisticated.

Readability/Understandability of information

An issue related to usability is the readability and understandability of information retrieved or, more generally, the issue of health literacy (McCray 2005). Readability tests have been carried out on consumer health information resources for many years, the majority of studies involving hard-copy information resources. It has been recognised that literacy skills do not correlate with intelligence or level of education

(Mayberry and Mayberry 1996). Many studies have shown that consumer health information resources are written at very high readability levels (Mumford 1997). One study, however, recognised that there was little known about the readability of consumer information on the Internet (Graber *et al* 1999). Graber *et al* (1999), with exactly this problem in mind, surveyed the Internet to assess the readability of lay-targeted medical information on the web. Text from 50 such websites was rated for readability using the Flesch reading score and Flesch-Kinkaid reading level. Most information was written at a '10th grade, 2nd month' (i.e. 15 year old) reading level. The authors claim that 'much of the medical information targeted for the general public on the web is written at a reading level higher than is easily understood by much of the patient population'.

Echoing this finding, Smith (1998) pointed out that a US Adult Literacy Survey in 1992 showed that about half of adults read at or below the 'Standard' eighth grade (13 years) level. Smith also claimed that this reflected other research findings that most adults read three to five grades below their years of school completed, and that average educational achievement is that which should have been completed at the age of 11.6 years.

Alternative methods of measuring the readability of information resources have included assessing writing style and layout. For example, it has been found that information written in an active voice and simple language aids understanding. Similarly, a consistent layout and careful use of colour is also beneficial (Serxner 2000). Those, admittedly dated, studies that have assessed the content of health information have found that many resources use unclear terminology, include inaccurate information, and omit important facts (Impicciatore *et al* 1997; Meredith *et al* 1995).

Information quality

The rise of the Internet as a consumer source of information has stimulated much research into the quality of information itself, and how this can be assured. The reason for the great interest is that the tremendous growth of the Internet has meant that there are thousands of unregulated, unsourced and, possibly, unscrupulous sites and documents accessible at one's fingertips through the World Wide Web. Something not really faced before on this scale. The authority of these sites has come under much scrutiny. Impicciatore *et al* (1997), for example, assessed the quality of Internet sites, which focused on one particular medical condition. The researchers undertook Internet searches for 'parent oriented web pages relating to home management of feverish children'. The information given on the 41 sites retrieved was checked by comparison with published guidelines. Only four sites 'adhered closely' to official recommendations the largest deviations being in sponging procedures and how to take a child's temperature. Their most worrying finding was that two sites recommended practices that may actually induce coma. Disturbingly, complete and accurate information for the condition was 'almost universally lacking'. Worryingly, too, Ekman *et al* (2005) investigated the quality of interactive cancer risk sites on the Internet and concluded that overall quality of the documentation on the cancer risk sites was poor.

Similarly, Griffiths and Christensen (2000) surveyed 21 websites that provided information about depression, and assessed the quality of information against a number of criteria. They classified sites according to their stated purpose, ownership, involvement with major drug companies, and whether they had a professional editorial board or similar. They also scored site information against US federal best practice guidelines embodied in the code published by the Agency for Health Care Policy and Research. They also assessed the identification, affiliations and credentials of authors associated with the sites. Findings indicated that the quality of content varied and was often poor in terms of these criteria. Furthermore, accountability criteria as indicated by the reported credentials of content authors might in fact be poor quality guarantees. Instead, evidence of ownership and the existence of an independent editorial board were more useful quality indicators.

Ways of ensuring the quality – and therefore, the authority – of Internet information, it is claimed (e.g. Impicciatore *et al* 1997), are badly needed, and not just to enhance the public's view of the authority of the provider. Wrongly diagnosed ailments or other manifestations of poor information provision could have fatal consequences. It is no surprise, therefore, that a number of health bodies and information providers (e.g. HoNF 1997; BHIA 1996) have attempted to formulate policy statements, guidelines and principles regarding web based health information. Kim *et al* (1999) have surveyed these in order to identify concerns, recommendations and areas of consensus. The authority and reputability of the site was fourth in their 'top ten' of issues cited in commentators' lists of quality criteria.

Concern has been expressed, somewhat ironically, about the quality of quality rating bodies and systems themselves. For example, Hernández-Borges *et al* (1999), in a study looking at the rating criteria of a number of systems, found that only three gave information about their own editorial boards – despite attribution, authority and openness generally being stated criteria for evaluating medical sites. Jadad and Gagliardi (1998) analysed sources that reviewed and rated health information sites, and concluded that the evaluation instruments were not comprehensive and many did not actually measure what they claimed. Their presence, therefore, was not necessarily as informative as desired. Not surprisingly then when we look at the results of the research reported in this report we find that the public often shop around for information and on the basis of comparisons take decisions for themselves on what they perceive to be 'good' information.

The issue of branding, brand recognition and advertising has taken on a new dimension on the web. Simon (2001) considered that the surfeit of choice online produced 'a concomitant change in consumer attitudes' moving them from what he described as 'receptive space' to 'sceptical space'. It may be that with such a glut of information – including that concerned with health – users feel they do not have to tolerate advertising. They can move effortlessly from one brand to another. Travis (2000) suggested from a number of usability studies undertaken by Forrester Research that fewer than 20% of website visitors looked for a favourite brand – in keeping with the finding that the attribution of information and, therefore, authority was not important for the users studied. This leads us to the concept of the 'promiscuous user', which we will return to later.

Perceptions of the authority of information

Despite the attention given by commentators to the quality issues, outlined above, the perceptions and attitudes of the information users appear to have been neglected. Whilst this might be natural, given the importance of authoritative and accurate information in the health field, the apparent lack of interest in public perception is a serious omission. This is particularly true when one considers the importance of targeting different groups with different messages, e.g. with information about influenza vaccinations, giving up smoking etc., and the array of platforms available to information providers.

Of particular interest is the degree to which people invest authority in the National Health Service. Despite well publicised scandals, such as the conviction of 'serial killer' Harold Shipman, researchers have found that trust in the NHS remains high. Mulligan (2000) cited a poll carried out for the British Medical Association shortly after the Shipman trial, indicating that the public still rated doctors the trustworthiest of a number of professions listed. Eighty seven percent said they would generally trust doctors to tell them the truth; doctors were followed by teachers (85%), the clergy (78%), and judges (77%). The British Medical Association also cited the poll in a news roundup (BMA 2000). It mentioned the fact that, when asked how well or badly doctors were doing their jobs and reminded of recent medical reports about the inquiry into the deaths of babies in Bristol (Bristol Inquiry Unit 2000) and stories about doctors helping people to die, 89% said that doctors were doing very or fairly well.

Ferriman (2001) cited a poll, by the independent research agency MORI, which also showed that the public trusted doctors to tell the truth more than any other group. Eighty nine percent of the respondents thought that doctors told the truth, compared with 86% for teachers, 78% for judges and clergymen, 18% for journalists, and 17% for politicians. Similarly, satisfaction with doctors was high. The same proportion of the public (89%) said they were either very satisfied (36%) or fairly satisfied (53%) with the way doctors did their jobs. Only nurses scored more highly, with 95% of respondents saying that they were either very satisfied (54%) or fairly satisfied (41%). A study by Hesse *et al* (2006) showed that, although the use of the internet as a source of health information continues to rise, patients were still more likely to both trust and desire information from their physician; however, younger age-groups were increasingly turning to the internet as a primary information source.

Health information impacts and outcomes

Only a few studies have attempted to measure actual health outcomes or impacts in terms of behaviour or attitude change resulting from using health information acquired from electronic sources, although, of course, there is a body of literature on the effectiveness of information in hardcopy form. For example, studies have shown that, as an aide memoire, written information can increase patient compliance with their General Practitioners' instructions and so help the healing process (Arthur 1995; Ley 1982). It has also been shown that information leaflets contribute to better health outcomes, for example, in improving blood sugar control and having fewer functional limitations in diabetics (Greenfield *et al* 1985; 1988).

There is other evidence that information can, result in clinical improvements. Clark *et al* (1997), for example, found that patients with hyperlipidemia who received computer-based, diet-mediated counselling were just as likely to succeed in reducing plasma lipid levels as were those who received diet counselling from a dietician. Tate *et al* (2001) compared the use of a weight-loss Internet education and behaviour therapy programme, consisting of emailed information, support and bulletin board, with one consisting of a web-based information source only, and found that the additional online communication facility led to greater weight loss amongst participants. Goldsmith and Safran (1999) conducted a randomised controlled study of ambulatory patients who had undergone surgery, in which patients were given access to a website offering post-operative care information. An intervention group had access to further password-protected pain management information. Those in the intervention group reported significantly less post-operative pain. Strom *et al* (2000) evaluated the effects of an Internet-mediated applied relaxation and problem-solving training course. A control group were put on a waiting list to receive the educational materials, whilst the intervention group enjoyed a six-week programme delivered in instalments onto a password-only accessible web-site. Results showed a statistically significant reduction in (self-report occasions of) headaches.

Even from the small amount of research undertaken with specific regard to independent use by the public of Internet mediated information there were encouraging signs. The Pew Internet and American Life Project, regularly surveys Internet users with regard to a number of topics, including health and they found (Fox and Rainie 2000) from their survey of over 12,000 users, that 52 million American adults, or 55% of those with Internet access, had used the web to get health or medical information. Forty eight percent of these said the advice they found on the web had improved the way they took care of themselves, and 55% said access to the Internet had improved the way they obtained medical and health information. Nearly half (47%) of those who sought health information for themselves during their last online search said the material affected their decisions about treatments and care. Similarly, 36% of those who sought health information for someone else during their last online search said the material affected their decisions on behalf of that loved one. A recent survey by NoHF (2005) showed that as patients gained easy access to more and increasingly complex medical information, they were seeking to become more involved in decisions about their health.

A Cyber Dialogue (2000) survey came up with similar findings. For example, as a result of using the Internet, approximately half of all health information seekers surveyed advised a family member or friend to see a doctor (something important that will be taken up later), changed their exercise or eating habits or made a 'positive' decision related to their health treatment. Many others joined an illness support group after visiting a disease-specific website. Pastore (2001) reports a study by The Boston Consulting Group (BCG) which found that those who use the Internet frequently were two to three times more likely than infrequent users to take action that affected their diagnosis and treatment. For example, the data that patients found online resulted in their asking their physicians more questions and in greater detail.

However, about 36% made their own suggestions as to the specific illnesses from which they are suffering, and 45% requested specific treatments. For comparison, among those who hardly ever ventured online to find health information, only 16% and 19% of patients, respectively, exhibited the same active involvement. In short, patients who used the Internet to explore health issues reported that the information they found online had a real impact on how they managed their overall care and complied with prescribed treatments.

Impact of digitally informed consumers on medical professionals

Research on how the rise of health information and its delivery electronically has impacted on the work of medical professionals appears to have focused, almost exclusively, on the Internet, probably because of its wide availability and relative comprehensiveness. Much research in this area considers the impact in terms of the doctor-patient relationship. Cox (2002), for example, surveyed a random selection of GPs in the UK to assess their perception of the effect of the Internet on doctor-patient relations. She found that 76% of 560 medical practitioners responding to her questionnaire indicated that patient use of the Internet had affected the doctor/patient relationship (although she did not ask what percentage of patients had actually used this medium as an information source, unlike other studies outlined below). The majority (86%) felt that the phenomenon of patients consulting the web for medical and health information led to a 'challenge to their knowledge' and empowered patients (83%). Most respondents characterised their feelings when meeting a patient who had gathered information from the Internet as 'interested' (78%), or an 'opportunity to learn' (75%). However, a minority felt 'frustrated (15%) or 'indifferent' (8%).

Despite these apparently positive impacts, 87% of respondents felt that the Internet might increase the number of 'worried-well' patients and almost as many, 85%, expressed concern that the information gleaned from the Internet might lead to unrealistic expectations. Finally, 65% felt that the Internet-informed patient is a challenge to the doctor's authority. The authors suggest that this means that, as 'the balance in ownership of clinical information changes, the decision-making role of doctors may come under increasing scrutiny'.

In a similar study, Potts and Wyatt (2002) examined 'Internet-literate' doctors' experience of their patients' use of the Internet and resulting benefits and problems. The study showed that over two thirds of the doctors considered Internet health information to be usually or sometimes reliable; this was higher in those recently qualified. Twice as many reported patients experiencing benefits than problems from the Internet. Patients gaining actual physical benefits from Internet use were reported by 40% of respondents, while 8% reported physical harm. Another study showed that thirty-eight percent of physicians believed that the patient bringing in information made the visit less time efficient, particularly if the patient wanted something inappropriate or the physician felt challenged. The study revealed that the quality of information on the Internet was an important paramount: accurate relevant information was beneficial, while inaccurate information was harmful.

Clearly, both the problems and the benefits may impinge to a considerable extent on professional role and practice. That there is little evidence that patient use of the

Internet has actually affected practice to any great extent is probably to do with the apparently low numbers of patients discussing the Internet with their GPs. In the Potts and Wyatt (2002) study respondents estimated that only 1-2% of their patients had used the Internet for health information within the previous month, a tiny proportion, but probably growing as a study by Brotherton *et al* (2002) indicates. The researchers surveyed oncology patients from two teaching hospitals in Sydney to explore their experience of Internet use and its effect on doctor-patient relationships. The survey was carried out twice, in 1999 and again in 2001. By 2001, 46% of respondents had accessed the Internet for information related specifically to their illness, up from 33% in 1999. Results suggested that accessing the Internet for information had had a positive effect on patients' relationship with their doctors (in the 1999 and 2001 studies, respectively, 26% and 34% felt that this had improved, with 0% and 3% feeling it had deteriorated). Unfortunately, the short paper does not give further details of the ways in which the improvement or deterioration manifested itself. However, with little evidence of poorer relations brought about by the Internet, the authors suggest that Internet use by patients and their families should not be viewed as a problem, but 'as an opportunity for patients and their treatment teams to work together, ensuring that patients have up-to-date information about their illness and its treatment'.

Chen and Siu (2001) surveyed 191 ambulatory patients and 410 Canadian oncologists in order to evaluate the use of the news media and the Internet as sources of medical information by patients and oncologists, and to investigate the impact on patients' treatment decisions and, of particular interest to this section, the patient-doctor relationship. Seventy-one percent of patients actively searched for information, and 50% said they used the Internet to do this. English as the first language, access to the Internet, and use of alternative treatments predicted a higher rate of information seeking. The researchers concluded that Information searching is common among cancer patients in Canada, but that this does not affect the patient-doctor relationship.

Hjortdahl *et al* (1999) looked at the extent to which doctors felt that their clinical work was influenced by 'well-informed patients' who used the Internet for health information. A sample of 1,276 Norwegian doctors responded to a questionnaire survey. Seventy percent of them had experience with patients bringing Internet information to the consultation setting. Most of these doctors found this 'natural and unobtrusive'; a few felt it influenced the doctor-patient relationship in a negative way, while 25% found meeting 'the informed patient' a 'positive challenge'. One out of seven doctors with email access receives electronic mail from their patients. The authors conclude from their results that doctors felt that new information technology has not introduced major changes or created unexpected difficulties in the doctor-patient relationships. A recent study (Xie, Dilts and Shor 2006) investigated the impact of patient-obtained medical information on the physician-patient relationship when patients, as a group, were heterogeneously informed and a physician's interests did not coincide with those of her patients. Introducing additional well-informed patients to the population discontinuously affected the physician's strategy, Alternately, when a sufficient number of well-informed patients existed, increasing the precision of their information allowed all patients to free-ride by receiving more appropriate treatment recommendations. A qualitative study (Hart *et al* 2004) suggested that use of the Internet is contributing to subtle changes in the relationship between health-care practitioners and their patients, rather than effecting the dramatic transformation some people envisage for it.

Wilson (1999) surveyed Primary Care Staff's use of the Internet, their views on the reliability of healthcare information available via the Internet, and their interaction with patients who had presented them with information downloaded from the Internet. Sixty-nine percent of GPs and 70% of practice nurses had looked at the Internet for healthcare information. Fifty-eight per-cent of GPs and 34% of nurses had been approached by patients with information about their condition obtained from the Internet. At first sight, this, and Hjortdahl *et al*'s (1999) findings that 70% of doctors had experience of patients using the Internet, may appear to contradict Potts and Wyatt's finding that an estimated 1-2% of patients had used the Internet (albeit within the previous month). However, neither Wilson's nor Hjortdahl's studies asked about frequency or patient numbers. Considering that only one patient discussing Internet-found information with their medical professionals requires respondents to answer in the affirmative, the finding of both Wilson's and Hjortdahl's studies that only around two thirds of doctors (58% and 70% respectively), and only one third of nurse patients (Wilson 1999), have mentioned patients citing Internet-sourced information would appear to be consistent with the view that there has, as yet, been very little impact on doctor-patient relationships. Although there do not seem to be more current figures, the fieldwork reported for the present study does support these findings. Very few medical professionals interviewed indicated that patients had brought Internet printouts with them to their consultations or, indeed, mentioned the system.

With regard specifically to how the Internet has impacted upon the relationship between medical professionals and patients, both groups reported that the consultation time was 'significantly' increased. However, 39% of practice nurses felt that they were able to use the consultation time more effectively (whereas only 19% of doctors thought this). Respondents were asked to rate how they felt about patients obtaining health information from the Internet. Significantly 53% of GPs were indifferent to patients practising this, and another 12% 'uncomfortable. Nearly a third (33%) of practice nurses felt unsure about this issue, with 20% indifferent and 16% uncomfortable. Thirty nine percent of doctors and 31% of nurses were positive – indicating a certain polarisation of opinion, albeit with over twice as many respondents in the 'positive' camp.

A number of commentators have also looked at developments in information technology – particularly the Internet – and recommended how these might impact on the medical professional and on doctor-patient relationships in the future. Pergament *et al* (1999), for example, recommended three steps that clinical oncologists and other health care professionals can take to direct and control the potential of the Internet so as to optimise patient care. All of these imply a considerable impact on the role and work practices of the health professionals, principally requiring them to be more proactive and to include information provision as an important focus of their work. The recommendations were to:

- find out what type of cancer information is being disseminated on the web;
- use Internet-derived material that patients bring to the clinic as a stepping-stone for patient education;
- become an active participant on the web.

Friedewald (2000) also urged medical practitioners to adopt the new technology in their dealings with patients. He felt that there has been a shift from the paternalistic to the informative model of the relationship between doctors and patients in recent years, occasioned in part by advances in information technology, although, as reported in this review, the evidence for this is sketchy at best. An 'informative' relationship is 'delicately dependent on the assumption that patients could obtain credible information'. He considered that increasing use of the Internet and of email could help doctors steer their patients towards 'credible' information on the Internet. In this regard doctors should become 'URL-proactive.' Including the cultivation of their own professional websites, linking to organisations dedicated to providing current, authoritative information.

Friedewald cited a survey by Medem and the American Medical Association, to prove this is already happening. This showed a 200 percent annual increase in physicians' use of email to communicate with patients, greater physician interest in building practice-related websites and stronger belief in website potential to educate patients. All these phenomena indicated that physicians might be exploiting the Internet to an ever-greater extent.

Finally, Poensgen and Larsson (2001) looked at the future impacts of the Internet on healthcare in Germany and Sweden. Their study 'finds no reason to believe the Internet will empower patients to such a degree that the patient-physician relationship is overturned'. They pointed out that, for example, patients diagnosed with serious diseases will want the comfort and understanding that only a health professional can provide. Their findings also highlighted that the Internet is used as 'an additional source of information, not a replacement for the doctor'. However, the authors opined that the Internet would alter the internal balance and, ultimately, the quality of the patient-physician relationship, by opening new channels of dialogue, remote health monitoring and joint access to medical records.

Summing up the research findings, it appears that use of the electronic information by patients is not being translated into useful interaction with medical professionals. Approximately one third of medical professionals have never been in a consultation with a patient has discussed Internet-sourced information, and in one study (Potts and Wyatt 2002) doctors estimated that even in the early years of the twenty first century, only 1-2% of their patients had used the Internet for health information in the month prior to consultation. Even allowing for the fact that some patients may use such information without disclosing its source, this figure suggests that electronic consumer information is not having a marked impact on the work of the doctor or nurse. However, this situation seems to be changing. In a survey conducted in 2005, 88% of patient-respondents agreed that seeking health information on the Internet improves the quality of consultation with their physician. In the same survey a majority of medical professionals (77%) agreed that patient health information seeking on the Internet improves the quality of patient consultation (HoNF 2005).

In terms of health outcomes with regard to the use of online support groups, Klemm *et al* (2003) noted that there is little known about the short – and long – term benefits. However, Zrebiec and Jacobson (2001) monitored user visits to an online support group discussion for patients of diabetes and reported that '79% of participants rated participation in the chat room as having a positive effect on coping with diabetes'. Further, Ferguson (1997) noted (though) 'There are little hard data on the economic, physical, psychological benefits of online support groups, but some initial surveys have suggested that such benefits may be substantial. In an informal survey of volunteer users by the Better Health and Medical Forum on America Online, 6% said they had avoided one or more emergency room visits because of information they got on this forum. Twenty – six percent said they had avoided one or more doctor visits, and 65% reported an increased ability to cope with a troublesome medical problem'.

Email advice from an online Doctor This can take two forms. Firstly, there is the email enquiry service, where an information seeker sends off an email to seek advice form an online doctor to obtain an answer to a health problem. Secondly, there is the kind of the service where the information seeker corresponds via email with their doctor as part of an ongoing face to face consultation. Mann and Stewart (2000) discussed the nature of email as a hybrid form of communication, which has aspects of conversation, writing, telephoning and note taking, with user-control of its pace and editing. They also mention important issues such as variation in gender-related expression and literacy, and the loss of context. Without context, the provider has few clues to guess the user's level of knowledge and information appetite.

A significant problem for an email health advice service is unsolicited requests for personal medical advice, which need face-to-face examination and awareness of the patient's medical background. Eysenbach (2000) discussed the need for response guidelines. At the new NHS Online email enquiry service, 25% of incoming emails were unsuitable for this reason (Gann 2003). The corresponding figure found by a study of dermatological emails was 27% (Eysenbach and Diepgen 1999). Other problems found in the NHS Direct Online email pilot evaluation was that requests were either too general, or showed unscientific health beliefs (Nicholas *et al* 2001c).

Email is still a relatively new medium for obtaining access to consumer health information. Its use poses a variety of interesting research challenges, involving new ways of using traditional methodologies. There have also been concerns about its limitations. Shepperd and Charnock (2002) commented that digital health information is not exceptional: 'health information and other media has not received the same degree of attention, even though the public is exposed to inaccurate and misleading information from a variety of sources'. But perhaps what is attractive about email is the sheer ease of dashing off a message to obtain an answer your health problems.

Katzen and Dicker (2001) investigated prostate cancer patients' attitudes to follow up patient doctor email contact in a postal survey of 43 users of an oncology clinic. Due to the nature of their condition, all users were over 53 years old (median age 68) and the majority were white. Medical history was accessible to the recipients of their emails. In general, the oncology patients were interested in using email for non-urgent communication with their physician, for repeat prescriptions and non-urgent health questions. Usage increased with the user's level of education. Proportions of patients reporting the following benefits of email were: increased timeliness of message (81%), to ask doctor a health-related question (79%), arranging appointments (73%), eliminating phone calls (70%), for repeat prescriptions (64%). Half the sample (50%) indicated concerns about confidentiality.

Email has taken time to get off the ground. Thus Baker *et al* (2003) in a US study found that only 6% of respondents used email to communicate with their doctor. Conhaim (2003) reporting on a US Deloitte Touche study found that only 23% of doctors used email to communicate with patients, 4% more than the previous year. However, Car and Sheikh (2004) maintained that according to UK national surveys, patients increasingly wanted to be able to communicate with healthcare professionals by email. A more recent large survey of physicians (Brooks and Menachemi 2006) showed only modest advances in the adoption of email communication, and little adherence to recognized guidelines for email correspondence.

To gain insight into doctors' views on patient communication by email, Patt *et al* (2003) interviewed 45 USA physicians who were currently using email with their patients. Many of these found that chronic disease management was improved and that email was convenient for non-urgent replies. However, there were concerns about confidentiality and how to manage emails efficiently. The researchers also gained the impression that physicians identified particular patients as being suitable for this mode of communication. The doctors selected probably represent 'early adopters' of the technology, as they were recruited online. However, the study does give pointers to likely benefits and problems as clinical use of email with patients increases.

Non-use of health information and information systems

The non-use of information resources is, perhaps not surprisingly, an under-researched area. However, it has been recognised both in information science and medical literature, that the acquisition of information may not have solely beneficial effects, and that, as Dervin (1983) suggests, information may actually represent a 'barrier'. The contradictory findings of previous studies indicate the somewhat ambiguous status of information in the treatment cycle. While some studies such as the ones by Leydon *et al* (2000) and McIntosh (1977) on cancer patients showed that many would rather not know more than routine information about treatment, some other studies found the opposite. James *et al* (1999) found that 74% of cancer patients said they wanted 'as much information as possible'.

Studies that have not necessarily been specifically about information need per se have also, nevertheless, highlighted an aversion to information. Pinder (1990), for example, looked at the wider issue of how patients and their GPs managed Parkinson's disease. A major focus of her study concerned communication between doctors, carers and patients. Her qualitative study of 15 patients elicited three patient 'types' based on information seeking. One of these was 'avoiders' who deliberately chose not to find information. For this group the anxiety of not knowing about the disease was preferable to the risk of having their fears confirmed or their hopes dashed. Many doctors she interviewed also felt patients often preferred ignorance in this situation and eschewed the approach they described as, 'We need to discuss this'. However, it seems that patients with cancer increasingly wish to be more fully informed about their disease, treatment and prognosis, and to participate in decision making (Craft *et al* 2005).

There is also literature on non-compliance. For our purposes this can be classed as the conscious decision not to act on, or to act contrarily to, information received. Dervin *et al* (1999) claimed that the worldviews of experts and of laypersons are 'incomparable' and that what medical professionals regard as 'presumed facts' are far removed from the 'complex struggles and understandings ... of lay people'.

In addition to the chosen non-use or take-up of information, there are also the barriers that prevent people who might avail themselves of information from doing so. This may be particularly true with regard to electronically mediated information. There are, for example, many possible reasons why the elderly may have difficulty with IT systems. Ironically, many of the reasons for this could actually be connected with health. Marwick (1999) pointed out that cognitive ability, response time and attention span can all be adversely affected with age, making it difficult to navigate around websites and retrieve appropriate information. It is also common, for example, for people to lose their manual dexterity with age (Hoot and Hayslip 1983; Williamson *et al* 1997) making it difficult to use keyboards or mice. Similarly, the elderly suffer declining vision, which makes computer use difficult. Despite these problems, research has shown that older people can take to information technology, particularly if it is relevant to their own personal needs (Blake 1998). Another group of concern here is people with all kinds of disabilities. There seems to be a lack or research into the usability of the various applications developed for disabled people, and even less concerning those with learning difficulties (Williams, Jamali and Nicholas 2006).

Another barrier to health information is that of poverty. Despite government initiatives to reach the most deprived people with IT services – by planning supermarket, library and other public Internet or touchscreen terminals – there are many reasons why disadvantaged groups might not use services. One such group is ethnic communities. Ethnic minorities are more likely to be unemployed and, consequently, be poor and live in undesirable conditions such as overcrowding. It is likely, therefore, that such groups will have less experience with information technology. Under these conditions it is to be expected that they may not avail themselves of opportunities for access to health information from electronic sources.

Another problem confronting ethnic minorities is, of course, that of language. This has been mentioned earlier, with regard to usability. Jones and Gill (1998a) point out that the NHS was established before the period of greatest migration to the UK, and 'it is far from clear that (it) has changed rapidly enough to meet the challenges posed by patients whose English may not be good enough to communicate adequately with health professionals'. They are particularly concerned with the plight of refugees and itemise a number of problems faced by this group in obtaining health information (Jones and Gill 1998b). Of course, studies have been undertaken looking into the effectiveness of interpreters – including telephone interpretation, (Pointon 1996) and link workers (Gillam and Levenson 1999) etc.

Interestingly, poor command of the English language may be a problem even for native speakers. The NHS Direct telephone service has already had to confront the problem of public misunderstanding of medical terminology. A study by Harrison and Cooke (2000) found that 70% of lay subjects were unable to correctly identify the meaning of the word 'unconscious' in behavioural terms, with many believing that an individual in that condition is able to walk about. Other studies (cited in the 'Readability' section of this chapter) also point to difficulties in information provision due to the inadequate reading ability levels of some information consumers.

Conclusion

This chapter has highlighted a number of important issues pertaining to the provision of electronic health information, ranging from information needs studies to usability and accessibility issues; authority and trust; and impacts and outcomes. The information needs literature suggests a huge variation, both in needs and propensity to seek information. Such disparate findings suggest that electronically mediated health information may play an important role here – the capacity is available not only to produce extremely comprehensive and in-depth information, but, if suitably organised in hierarchies of level and type, also to enable users to control the amount and depth of information to their own needs, far easier than might be possible in a hardcopy environment.

Despite these advantages, a number of potential problems inherent in the digital supply of information have been highlighted. These included, in particular, problems with usability, where studies have shown difficulties with menu lists, site structure, search facility and browser windows. Clearly, much research is still required in the area of organising and presenting electronic information to people yet to become familiar with this new medium. Other problems found were in terms of the quality of information and its readability. The issue of the perceived (and real!) authority of information may present a barrier to usage. Surprisingly, the published literature appears to have ignored this issue. Encouragingly for the National Health Service, studies on public opinion about the authority of the NHS seem to point to continuing high regard for it.

Another positive finding from the literature was the amount of evidence found that suggested that the acquisition and use of information could result in both behavioural and clinical improvements. This is true even from the small amount of research undertaken with specific regard to public use of electronic information. Research into electronic communication by various patient groups also indicated positive outcomes. Networked digital information services are excellent facilitators of communication, and have been shown to meet the needs identified in the literature for people to obtain information, advice and support from others in similar situations.

Despite the apparent benefits of information, the few studies that have looked at the overall impact of the Internet on the work of health professionals, with regard to consumer information and interaction with patients, show that the system has only had a negligible effect on both the work of the health professionals themselves and on their relationships with their patients. The impact of a system physically planted in medical locations – a health information touchscreen – may be greater than that of the use by patients and the general public than that of the diffuse and sprawlingly huge resource that is the Internet. This is one of the questions the present research seeks to answer.

Many questions suggest themselves from the literature. In addition to that of the effect of a strategically placed electronic information system on the relationship between patients and health professionals, as mentioned in the previous paragraph, the impact in terms of behaviour or health outcomes, for example, is one that has not been explored comprehensively in the literature. Issues of usability – the difficulties people face when using digital systems, and how they can be alleviated, are also important. Finally, the important area of 'authority' is clearly a much-neglected one.

Chapter 3

Health Kiosks

Introduction

Touchscreen kiosks have become almost as ubiquitous as Internet terminals, and you will find them at underground stations, banks (cash dispensers) and supermarket checkouts. In fact, a study by the College of Health in London (Boudioni 2003) found touchscreen technology also being used at museums and galleries (e.g. Science Museum) and self-service catalogue systems (i.e. Waterstone's in-Store Online Directory).

The health applications of kiosks have long been recognised, so much so in fact that during the period under investigation the Government issued them 'free' to health centres, libraries and other organisations. The private health sector was also alive to their possibilities and there was some competition between providers, with the following types available during the early part of the new millennium:

- InTouch with Health kiosks
- NHS Direct kiosks
- Wellpoint Health Centres
- The Patient Information for Consent Systems

An evaluation of the InTouch kiosk, possibly, the most successful of them all, takes up the major part of this chapter. A briefer comparative evaluation of NHS Direct kiosks is also made.

We have chosen kiosks as the first platform to evaluate because it was possible to find out much more about their users than was the case with Internet and television users. This was largely because we could paint a much richer picture of the digital health consumer because we knew about the location of use, down to a postcode in many instances, and for many kiosks age and gender information was routinely supplied. We also managed to study them over a considerable period of time, so obtaining data about change and we could monitor them more accurately than we could the other platforms. The kiosk study is therefore not so much an evaluation of a platform but also a deep and robust insight into the digital information consumer in general.

InTouch with Health kiosks

The InTouch with Health's kiosk[1] was a PC based touch sensitive screen health information service designed for public use in doctor's surgeries, hospitals, other medical sites and the workplace. Many kiosks were installed in non-medical locations. The first kiosk was launched on 1st August 1997. The later versions of the kiosk were web-enabled, which allowed for more flexibility and currency. They combined a simple 'touch button' method for viewing a selection of information and printing out fact sheets and a selection of websites were available, which can be chosen by the client and accessed using the kiosk's in-built keyboard and roller ball. The first of these web versions became available July 2001. During the period of our study both forms of kiosks were in circulation.

The drive for the placement of kiosks largely came from Primary Care Trusts (PCTs), which had the mandate for proving general health information to the public. Health matters were also very important to local councils. Councils worked closely with the Health Authority, which had overall responsibility for providing health information to consumers under the government's e-government programme. The councils and Health Authority viewed the health information kiosks as an effective means of divulging information across diverse communities. As such the ultimate decision lay not in making a purchase but in the number to invest in and the strategic distribution of the systems within the community so they could be accessed by everyone.

For illustration, a few kiosks and the activities associated with them are listed below:

- West Pennine Health Authority installed a network of kiosks across primary and secondary care as part of a Local Implementation Strategy project to involve patients in their treatment and help them to manage their conditions better.
- Oldham NHS Trust installed a number of kiosks throughout the hospital in order to provide public access to quality health information which also included sections in Gujarati, Bengali, Urdu and Chinese.
- Edinburgh Royal Infirmary: Two kiosks were placed in the information centre and the A&E department.

The subjects covered by the kiosk included national and local health services, Medical Conditions, Surgical Operations, Support Groups, Healthy Travel and Healthy Living topics. Thousands of individual topics were covered and fact sheets could be printed for each one. The main menu page, shown in Figure 3.1, provides an idea of the range of content.

---

1   http://www.intouchwithhealth.co.uk/delivery_kiosks.htm.

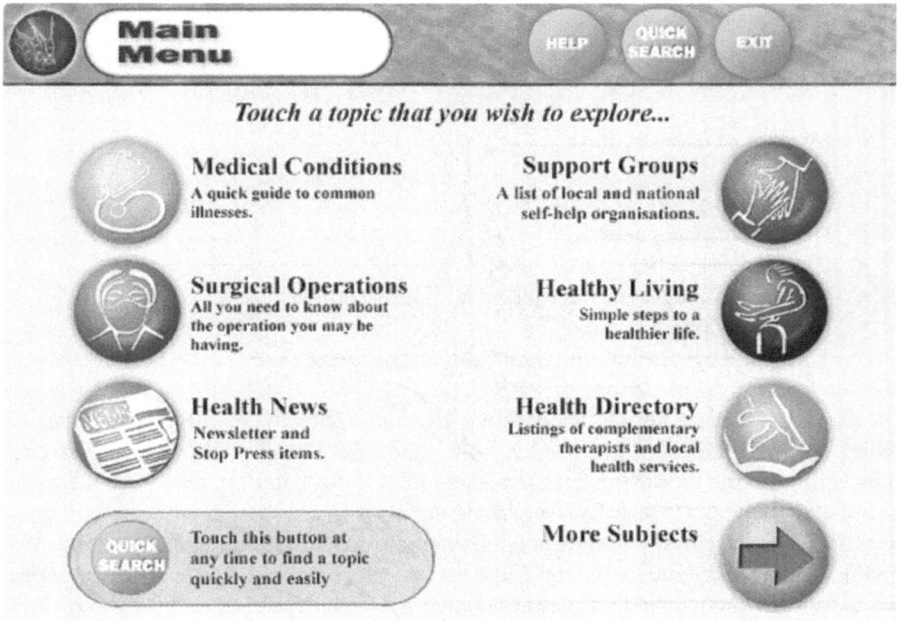

Figure 3.1 InTouch with Health Kiosk – Menu Page

As can be seen, this screen shows six options:

- Medical Conditions
- Surgical Operations
- Health News
- Support Groups
- Healthy Living
- Health Directory

A tab, indicating 'more subjects', was situated at the bottom of the screen. This lead to two more entries:

- A-Z of the NHS
- Travel Clinic

Use and users

Clearly, whether anyone used the kiosks or not was the major concern, and especially whether groups (like the elderly, ethnic minorities or the poor) for whom they were specially (and initially) targeted availed themselves of the kiosks. Logs were largely used to establish this, although they were supported by questionnaire data. The logs provided a range of metrics by which use could be measured, and, sometimes, satisfaction imputed. The following analyses were employed in the evaluation of InTouch kiosks:

- Number of user sessions
- Reach
- Return users
- Number of pages viewed
- Changes over time in use
- Numbers of pages viewed during a visit/session
- Number of pages printed
- Time indices: session time and page view time

Kiosk users were largely anonymous, the only telltale signs they left behind in their logs were their age and gender, which they were prompted to provide before they could use the kiosk (this was requested in order to tailor the health information to the specific type of user). Thus we had to equate a search session with an individual user, hence the use of the term user session employed throughout the evaluation. We had no notion of whether a person came back to search or not, as far as the statistics were concerned each session was conducted by a new and unique user. As plainly people did return, then user number estimates provided in the book overestimate the number of different people searching the kiosks.

It was estimated that on average about 15 user sessions were conducted per day per kiosk (Table 3.1, column 2) and that about 110 pages were viewed. On average just five pages (about 5% of those available) were printed off. Sessions lasted on average a little over a minute and individual page view time was about eleven seconds. The general conclusion obtained from this comprehensive and unique approach to determining use then was that kiosks were used, but lightly and quickly. Kiosks in surgeries (column 2), perhaps surprisingly, were more poorly used in all respects – something we shall return to later.

Table 3.1 InTouch kiosks – summary kiosk metrics

Metric	All kiosks – various time periods covered	Surgery kiosks over 12 month
Average daily number of user sessions per day	14.6	8.7
Average daily number of pages viewed per day	110.2	62.7
Average daily number of pages printed per day	5.0	2.1
Average session length (seconds)	72.9	52.9
Average page view time (seconds)	10.7	9.0

Users

Although on an average day nearly 15 people used a kiosk, there were big differences between kiosk locations and the explanation for this is the subject of this section.

The two best performing kiosks, by some margin, proved to be the kiosks located at Frimley Park Hospital and at a Safeway (supermarket) Pharmacy. These kiosks recorded, respectively, 45 and 38 user sessions and more than 200 page views per day. The Elgin Health Promotion shop and Tawhill Medical Centre performed particularly poorly and recorded fewer than five sessions or less than 50 page views per day. Let us examine what variables if, any, might explain overall differences in the number of user sessions conducted 'between' these kiosks. The particular investigation from which we obtained the data linked kiosk transaction log files of 56 kiosks to a kiosk questionnaire data and postcode data. Variables included in the study included the likelihood of the kiosk's geographical neighbourhood being populated with residents who owned shares and, whether, for example, the receptionist told the patient about the kiosk. The following variables together accounted for about 70% of the variation in the number of user sessions between kiosks.

The size of the host organisation in terms of number of visitors received. The larger the host organisation, the greater the kiosk use in terms of the number of sessions conducted. We call this the 'flow past' rate.

Located in neighbourhoods with children aged between 0-14 years. Again, there was a positive effect, the greater the incidence of under 14 year olds in the geographical area the greater the number of sessions conducted – this we can call the 'kids' effect.

Health professional showing patients how to use kiosk. If a health professional (not a doctor) was available to show how to use the kiosk then this acted as a positive impact on the number of sessions conducted.

Located in neighbourhoods likely to have mortgage homeowners. The incidence of mortgages in the area was a negative coefficient and argued that where the neighbourhood has a high incidence of mortgages generally it would have a lower numbers of kiosk users. This could be because home ownership was related to computer use and use of alternative health information sources and, perhaps, mortgage owners were more likely to have access to a computer and hence may use the Internet instead of a kiosk. Alternatively, mortgage holders may be healthier and hence less likely to visit the doctor.

The availability of a leaflet describing the kiosk and whether health staff verbally referred to the kiosk were. This was also significant, but surprisingly in a negative way. The explanation for this may be that those sites, which provided leaflets, might have considered that this was sufficient and as a result did not really attempt to integrate the kiosk into the workings of the host organisation. The full list of variables included in the study is given in Table 3.2.

Table 3.2 InTouch kiosks – independent variable included in kiosk studied

Geo-demographic Data	Kiosk Variables	Kiosk Variables
House price	Poster at locations telling patients about kiosks	Location type
Acorn Category (6 categories of residential types)	Leaflets at locations telling patients about kiosks	Geographical location
Likelihood to have children aged between 0-4 years	Patient told verbally about kiosk by medical staff	
Likelihood to have mortgage homeowners	Patient told verbally about kiosk by receptionist	
Likelihood to have two car households	Kiosk demonstration sessions	
Likelihood to have unemployed people	Word of mouth information about kiosk from other patients	
Likelihood of share ownership	Doctor will use kiosk together with patient	
Likelihood of ITV viewing	Health professional shows patient how to use kiosk	
Likelihood of households having earnings of £20,000+	Receptionist shows patient how to use kiosk	
Likelihood of microwave ownership	Leaflets are also provided	
	Printouts from patient information system such as INIS	
	Size of location, in terms of number of patients on surgery books	

Four variables were also identified as significant determinates of the number of kiosk pages viewed at a surgery. The four variables accounted for only (a small) 20% of the variation in pages viewed between kiosks.

Gender – females under the age of 55 were more likely to view more pages than other gender/age groups. These users were thought to have a greater health information need.

Ease of kiosk use – those finding the kiosk very easy to use were more likely to view more pages. This suggests a skills factor at work here.

Socio-economic status – those users in skilled employment viewed more pages than skilled unemployed or unskilled (employed or unemployed) users. Again this reflects a skills factor.

Ethnicity – UK born users viewed fewer pages than those users who would not divulge their ethnicity or who said that they were non-UK born users.

The relationship between use and location can further be investigated by calculating how far into the system the user penetrates. This is an important factor that establishes serious use. In many menu-based kiosk information systems the user has to navigate through a number of menu screens to arrive at what can be termed an information page. Clearly what constitutes positive use is that the information seeker navigates beyond the collection of initial menu screens to information pages. For the NHS Direct kiosks it was necessary to navigate through three or four screens to arrive at an information page. People viewing only one to three pages were therefore unlikely to have accessed an information page. By contrast, users viewing over 11 pages were heavy (or interested) users with a good understanding of how to jump between pages and to use the technology to find the information they sought.

There were a quarter to a third more people using kiosks situated in pharmacist, supermarkets and docks who limited themselves to three pages or fewer, as compared those searching from kiosks located in hospitals and walk-in centres. Forty-four percent of these users had viewed one to three pages only, compared to 34% of hospital and walk in centre users. Users at walk-in centres were most likely to view 11 or more pages in a session, while users at kiosks located in pharmacies were least likely to do so: the respective figures being 31% and 15%. Users of kiosks located in a pharmacy were less likely reach an information page and were less likely to interrogate the kiosk system beyond the menu pages. As mentioned earlier, low page penetration is thought to be a result of the greater time constraints that users in pharmacies were under, and the fact that they users may well have been embarrassed to use the kiosk as people queuing at the pharmacist's counter may observe them using the kiosk.

Reach refers to the percentage of users in the exposed population who had availed themselves of the service. However, because kiosk logs did not identify individuals, we cannot estimate the reach figure from the transaction log files alone. However, reach was estimated by questionnaire, for three studies. The data show that reach varied from 5% to 19%, and that a consensus formed around the 17% mark.

It was estimated that kiosks situated in surgeries had a reach figure of about 17%, that is approximately 17% of registered patients would have used the kiosk at one time or another. The figure is obviously lower if one includes non-patients who also visited the surgery – parents accompanying their children or, in some cases, visiting the premises simply to pick up prescriptions. The figure for hospitals was more difficult to interpret. Here the potential audience may be either short or long stay or day patients. Furthermore, family and friends could have visited patients, though this is equally true of kiosks located in surgeries. As we shall see with both the Internet and DiTV, reach can rarely be defined to an individual but usually to a household. However, the weekly reach figure for hospitals can be estimated to be about 5 to 10%.

Overall then, no more than one in six people, or about 17%, who could use a kiosk, chose to do so.

InTouch with Health kiosks did not provide for the identification of individual users – users did not have to furnish a log-in name and they were used in public locations, meaning a whole variety of people could use them. However, return visits were estimated from questionnaire returns. The findings did not point to a high level of repeat use. Nearly 40% of users had not used the kiosk in the past six months. Clearly users were not coming back regularly to use the kiosk, but this might be because surgeries were not locations that users returned to on a regular basis. Sixty % of respondents made three or fewer visits to the surgery in a year and this meant that it was difficult to build a pattern of repeat behaviour.

Use

Kiosks were a novel way for most people to retrieve information/find help and therefore it is very important to review trends in use. In particular, we wished to determine whether usage was spreading as people came into contact with the kiosk or, alternatively, whether the novelty wore off. Figure 3.2 gives the overall picture of kiosk use for 36 kiosks. Combined use as at April 2000 ran at just under 25,000 page views a week. Use fluctuated over the period, however. Increases in use can be put down to the introduction of new kiosks. There was a sharp increase in use in the first half of 2000 by about 74%. From a visual inspection of weekly usage there were three main growth phases of kiosk use: the first, an increase of 174% from February to August 1997, the second a 90% increase from May to December 1998, and the third, a 74% increase, from January to September 2000. Either a falling off or a relative stable use pattern followed each growth period.

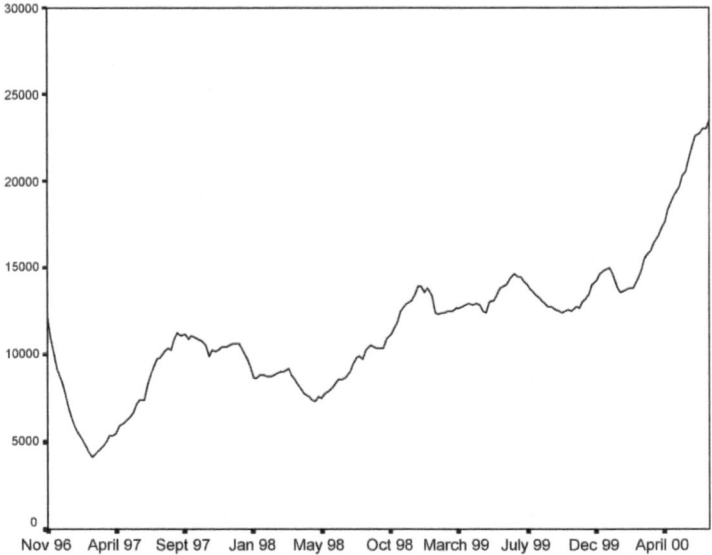

Figure 3.2 InTouch kiosks – weekly use (page views) of 36 kiosks (November 1996 to April 2000)

The swings in use were higher at the beginning of a kiosk's life, and this was true for all the kiosks. The underlying pattern for individual kiosks was one of strong initial interest followed by a waning, and followed in turn by a steady to upward trend. However, there were differences in the patterns of use for different kiosks. Four main distinct patterns of use over time were identified:

- Declining after apex: increase after installation followed by a slow long term decline.
- Steady after apex: increase after installation followed by a decline to a relatively stable use pattern.
- Increasing after apex: increase after installation followed by a decline then an increase.
- No apex: location does not have an apex, relatively stable to no trend pattern.

All kiosks experienced an initial spurt in use, although this was not generally sustained. Follow-up interviews with users indicated that viewing resulted from a combination of factors: patients' (real or perceived) information needs, their natural propensity to actively seek information, and the active promotion of the kiosk by medical staff. Some interviewees were honest enough to mention a fourth factor – curiosity and novelty use.

For many locations use was lower by the end of the survey period. This meant that the increases enjoyed during the first 4 to 6 months of a kiosk's life were not sustained and further there was a net decline in use compared to the volume of use at installation.

A number of possible factors might explain the subsequent long-term decay:

- People were not returning to use the kiosk – often one session was sufficient to obtain all the kiosk had on a subject (this was one of the reasons why web-enabled kiosks were introduced, to provide greater choice and a bigger turnover of information).
- Kiosks merged into their surroundings and largely went unnoticed. Many people interviewed said they simply had not noticed it. This was made worse by poor general care and promotion.
- There was a poor culture of use. Users failed to notice or use it because they do not see others using it – non-use begets non-use.
- System fatigue – health professionals ignored (or forgot about) it after a while.

Another way of examining the number of pages viewed is to group user sessions by the number of pages viewed. In part this was necessary to get a better grip on a metric that was highly skewed. Figure 3.3 shows the distribution of the number of pages viewed in a session at a surgery. The chart is highly skewed. Eight percent of users just viewed one page, 15% viewed just two pages and 15% just viewed three pages.

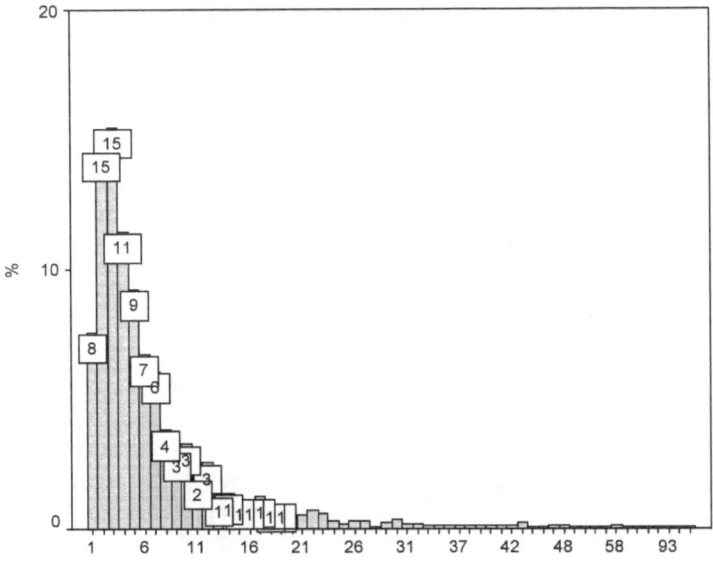

Figure 3.3 InTouch kiosks – distribution of the number of pages viewed in session at a surgery kiosk

Well over a third of users undertook sessions where three pages or fewer were viewed. As these users had to navigate at least that number of pages to view a content page they were not really getting to information content. Clearly positive use comes with the information seeker navigating beyond the collection of initial menu screens to the actual information pages.

Sixty three percent of kiosk users viewed four or more pages and probably reached an information page, whilst 19% of users viewed 11 or more pages. People viewing over 11 pages could be described as heavy (or interested) users with a good understanding of how to jump between pages and to use the technology to find the information they sought. Hence this metric not only provides an idea of page use but also says something about the quality of that use.

We sought to determine whether any variables explained whether a user reached a content page rather than a menu page. The variables found significant in explaining whether the users at one kiosk location arrived at a content page were:

Employment status. Skilled workers were twice as likely to access a content page as non-skilled workers. This is thought to have something to do with educational background and technological skills, which is further discussed below.

Gender and age. Females under the age of 55 were three times more likely to find an information page compared to both men and women over the age of 55. Males between 56 and 75 were seven times more likely to find an information page.

These users made up a small proportion of respondents, about 2%; however, their perseverance in finding an information page was clear.

Ease of use. Those people finding the system very easy to use were about twice as likely to find an information page compared to those who found the system not easy to use. Ease of use is further discussed below.

Pages printed are a very useful metric because if someone is bothered to print out a page this provides a strong indication that they found something of particular interest. This section looks at the estimates of the number of pages printed and attempts to account for the number of pages printed at a kiosk. It was decided to examine what variables, if any, explained the printing of a page at a kiosk location. The following variables were significant:

- Skilled employed workers were one and a half times more likely to print material off from the kiosk. This probably reflects a skill in using the technology.
- Females under 55 were also one and a half times more likely to print off a page compared to other users. These users were thought to have a greater information need and searched on behalf of others.
- Males aged between 56 and 75 were about three times more likely to print off a page, while users aged over 75 were about three to four times less likely to do so. Again this user group were thought to have a greater health information need.
- Those who were told to use the kiosk by health professionals were three times more likely to print a page and those with a specific inquiry just over twice as likely to print a page off compared to curious users. This was a very significant finding, and emphasises the importance of health professionals being pro-active with their patients regarding the use of information systems.

Time indices Session time is the time it takes to conduct a search. Session time varied, not only between kiosk sites but also between users. The high rate of failed search sessions viewing three or fewer pages meant that many users did not find anything and explains in part the low search session times. Little could be accomplished in a search lasting 30 seconds and suggests aborted or truncated use. Just under half of all users recorded sessions lasting one minute or more. Just over a quarter of users could be expected to have spent sufficient time on the system to get something from it – those spending more than two minutes on a session.

We examined what variables, if any, explained session view time differences between kiosks. The model explaining 'session time' identified two variables that together explained about 47% of the variation of page time between kiosks. These variables were:

- Incidence of the 'age 0-14' children in the neighbourhood. This has a negative impact on page view time. This indicates that young people (accompanied

by parents) might touch it out of play and then leave the kiosk without really using it.
- Likelihood of households having earnings of £20,000+. Areas more likely to have a population earning £20,000+ were likely to have a longer session time. This might indicate a previous IT experience and hence users might spend more time online because they know how to use the technology.

This study was repeated for some other kiosks and four variables were identified as significant determinates of session view time between users. The four variables accounted for a small, 23%, of the variation in pages viewed within a kiosk.

- Gender. Females under the age of 55 were more likely search for longer. These users may have had a greater health information need.
- Gender. Males aged 56 to 75 were more likely to search for longer. These users may have had a greater information need.
- Ease of kiosk use. Those finding the kiosk very easy to use were more likely to conduct longer searches. This may reflect skills attainment.
- Socio-economic status. Those users in skilled employment recorded longer session times than skilled unemployed or unskilled (employed or unemployed) users. This may reflect skills attainment.

It is possible to determine the duration of time the user spends viewing a page or screen. On average the view time was 11 seconds. This is low. However, it should be remembered, that about 37% of users undertook sessions where only three pages or fewer were viewed. These users did not generally view pages for any length of time and this had a disproportionate effect on the average figure.

We looked to see what variables, if any, explained differences in page view time between kiosks. The model explaining 'page time' identified three variables that together explained only about 25% of the variation of page time between kiosks. These variables were:

- *Incidence of 'age 0-14' children in the neighbourhood.* This had a negative impact on page view time and suggests that young people might touch it out of play, and then leave the kiosk without actually using it (and observation confirmed this).
- *'ITV viewing'.* Those people in areas where ITV was watched a lot recorded low page view times. This might indicate an educational constraint and suggested that pages may have been too technical (medical) to read.
- *Health professional shows the user how to use the kiosk* had a positive impact. The presence of a health professional may have a positive impact on the user's attitude towards the kiosk and they may spend longer reading the information as a consequence.

What variables – if any – explained page view time differences between user sessions at the same kiosk location? By linking questionnaire responses to kiosk transaction log files four variables were identified as significant determinates of session view time at a particular kiosk location. The four variables accounted for a small 19% of the variation in pages viewed within a kiosk.

- *Gender*. Females under the age of 55 were more likely to spend more time viewing a page.
- *Gender*. Males aged 56 to 75 were more likely to spend more time viewing a page.
- *Gender/Status*. Male unskilled users spent less time viewing a page.
- *Ease of kiosk use*. Those people finding the kiosk very easy to use were more likely to spend more time viewing a page, while those finding the kiosk difficult to use recorded shorter viewing times.

Categorising users

Users can be defined by a wide range of characteristics. As mentioned earlier, InTouch with Health kiosks required the user to enter their age and gender and via a questionnaire it was also possible to obtain data on ethnicity for some people. The type of organisation in which kiosks were housed was also known and it was also possible to place the kiosks geographically by postcode.

Differences in use between kiosks could be clearly ascribed to where they were housed and this was examined by grouping kiosks into location types and comparing metrics. For this purpose twenty-one kiosks were grouped into four location types: Information centres, Pharmacies, Hospitals and Surgeries.

Kiosks located in pharmacies performed relatively poorly and scored particularly badly on session time (50 seconds) and number of pages viewed in a session (6). Pharmacies recorded the lowest number of pages viewed in a session, below 6 page views as compared to about 7 at other locations. Furthermore, they recorded the lowest session time of less than 50 seconds. Kiosks located in hospitals (10) and information centres (10) recorded the longest page view time, saw a greater number of pages viewed in a session (7 seconds in both cases) and the longest session time compared to kiosks located in either pharmacies or surgeries. Sessions at hospitals and information centres lasted approximately 80 seconds, about twice as long as sessions in pharmacies.

Use differences between surgeries and pharmacies and hospitals and information centre locations can be ascribed to search disclosure (something we shall return to later), integration of the kiosk at the location, information authority, time anxiety/ uncertainties, flow past rates and the problems associated with an information stagnant kiosk.

To obtain an overall measure of how well used a kiosk was shall turn to the number of sessions per hour metric as this is not sensitive to the number of hours a kiosks is open (Table 3.3). The frequency distribution over hour of day was not normally distributed and the mean, median, 5% trimmed mean and Huber's m-estimator are reported.[2] Here we will compare kiosk use employing the robust 5% trimmed mean estimator.

Table 3.3 InTouch kiosks – average number of sessions per hour by type of kiosk organisation

	Information centre	Pharmacy	Hospital	Surgery
Mean	1.17	0.72	0.98	0.59
Median	1.23	0.60	0.37	0.37
5% Trimmed	1.15	0.69	0.85	0.52
Huber's M	1.14	0.62	0.42	0.38

Kiosks located in information centres performed best according to this metric and recorded just over one user session per hour. The next best were kiosks located in hospitals, just under one session per hour. Surgery kiosks were the most under deployed and recorded on average just over one session every two hours. It is of interest that kiosks in surgeries did not perform so well, because they might have been expected to (and certainly so by health policy makers). One explanation for this is that some users may have been too intimidated to use the kiosk in a public environment. This factor, called 'search disclosure', is further examined below.

Hospitals – a special case   Interestingly, hospitals scored well in terms of user numbers, with a session approximately every hour. Hospitals (and information centres) also scored well in terms of session times. This may be for several reasons for this, including:

- More pro-active interaction by nurses as compared to doctors, either using the kiosk with patients or endorsing its use, as described in the section on impacts.
- Greater throughput of people, which might affect sessions per hour, although not time online (unless people ended their sessions because others were waiting to use the kiosk, which observation had shown was unlikely).
- Greater anonymity in hospitals. Hospitals obviously take in-patients from a wider catchment area than doctors' surgeries, reducing the possibility, mentioned by one interviewee, of being seen by a friend while looking, perhaps, for personal information. Also, it may be that the kiosks were located in more open spaces. Certainly those in the main reception areas of hospitals visited were in very open-plan areas.

---

2   Huber's M-estimator is a weighted mean estimate where extreme values are given less weight.

- Fewer time constraints. Hospital visitors maybe on the premises without an appointment (e.g. outpatients, Accident and Emergency), or be visiting someone.
- More incentive to use: Hospital patients were likely to have more serious conditions, which might be longer term and require more managing. It is logical, therefore, that there may be a greater use of the kiosk in hospitals than in surgeries.

Because of its novelty and future potential, it is worth comparing the supermarket (Safeway) kiosk with the other kiosks. The kiosk located at Safeway had a higher percentage of men users – 55% compared to 48% for all the other kiosks (which is, perhaps, not what would be expected – possibly, men using the time when there partners shopped?). It also recorded a higher percentage of use by those under 15 and those over 75 – 36% and 9% respectively as compared to 26% and 6% at other locations. Those aged 36 to 55 made less use; this group accounted for 15% of users compared to 25% at other locations. Table 3.4 provides the key use metrics. In nearly all cases the figures are quite different, suggesting that supermarket kiosks attracted quite a different audience.

Table 3.4 In Touch kiosks – use of Safeway supermarket kiosk

	Page view time (Seconds)	Number of pages viewed in a session	Session view time (Seconds)	Sessions per hour	Prints per hour	% of users viewing 0-3 pages
Safeway	6.9	5.3	39.2	1.33	0.46	40.7
Other locations	9.4	6.7	68.5	0.54	0.23	32.8

Session view time and page view time were substantially lower at the Safeway supermarket. This is partly explained by the higher percentage of use by the under 15s. As mentioned above, a higher proportion of children's use will be associated with short sessions and a short page view times (the 'Kids' effect). However, the evidence suggests that users tended to give up on their session soon after beginning viewing. In part this may be due to reluctance on the part of the user to engage in what maybe a new navigational system. Alternatively, users may have taken a look at the opening menu and were willing to try to locate a page; however, finding this not to be particularly easy decided to give up – in a menu heavy structure users might just not bother.

Males were more likely to conduct shorter searches and view fewer pages. Although both males and females found the afternoons most attractive to conduct their searches, men appeared to prefer 10–11am, 2pm–3pm and 5pm–6pm and women 4pm–5pm, possibly as a consequence of taking children to the surgery after school.

Of course, touchscreen kiosks were introduced into health environments because they were thought to be easy to use by groups who typically frequent these environments and who might not have access to alternative sources of information, like the Internet. We are talking here about the elderly, single parents, the infirm and the poor. InTouch health kiosks required users to enter their age and this data provides us with the basis for the following analyses.

Unsurprisingly, perhaps, those aged over 75 made the least use of their kiosk session, they viewed a smaller number of pages, recorded the shortest session length and the lowest page view time. The reasons for this are explored below. Fifty-seven percent conducted sessions of less than half a minute and 51 percent had sessions where they viewed only three pages or fewer. That is, about half were unlikely to have found an information page: a high failure rate, but one that might have been expected, especially with so little help being afforded in the kiosk locations. The over 75 year old users were more likely to terminate their kiosk session soon after starting.

36 to 55 year olds viewed the most pages (6) and conducted the longest sessions (96 seconds), suggesting that when this group used the kiosk they used it well. The 36 to 55 years old were the most likely to conduct long sessions: 21% of this group recorded sessions of over four minutes. This group of users showed the greatest appetite for health information, probably, because they experienced greater health problems than younger users and, in addition, were more likely to be carers for younger and older people.

Users aged 16 to 35 and those aged 56 to 75 years old viewed, respectively, between 5.4 and 5.8 pages in a session and conducted sessions of about 81 seconds long.

The under 15's recorded the second shortest time viewing pages (9 seconds) and the second shortest session length (5.3 pages). Telephone interviews with a number of kiosk host organisations established that the under 15 year olds played games on the kiosks. In fact some kiosk sites had rules to limit the use by the under 15s. The under 15 age group were responsible for just under half of all use for these kiosks and were clearly an important user group. The relative short page view time and session length suggests a less motivated user (they were unlikely to have anything seriously wrong with them or come into the category of the health worried consumer). An analysis of pages viewed by youngsters showed that 32% of content pages were made up of Travel pages a section that featured cartoon like animated graphics. Interestingly though, the under 15s were the heaviest users of Healthy Living pages, making up 17% of pages viewed by this group. We need, therefore, to be careful when interpreting the data.

There is much to concern (interest) us about kiosk use by children. Log statistics indicated that, at 31% of users, the under 15's were by far the biggest user group. They were not, however, a group at which the kiosks were originally targeted (but initially neither were mobile phones – they were originally designed for farmers and sales people). This raises several questions about motivation for use, the kinds of information accessed and the use to which the information was put. Children's use of the kiosk could not be examined directly, because of the difficulties in obtaining ethical approval. Nevertheless, a wealth of data were obtained from interviews with health professionals and medical location reception staff, having direct experience of children, interviews with adult patients (some parents) at kiosk site locations, and non-participant observation. Of course, the log data themselves also spoke volumes about children's use.

Several respondents suggested that age statistics might be unreliable because many users entered details for others – specifically those for whom they were making enquiries. Thus, it may be that parents entered the age of their children when using the system. It is reasonable to suppose that these might include predominantly young children or, as mentioned later, the elderly. More than one interviewee suggested that the requirement to enter age and gender details may cause some users to assume that information provision was then tailored to the needs of the particular group entered. It is worth noting that other research by the authors (Nicholas *et al* 2001b) has shown that there was a considerable amount of searching on behalf of other people (or, 'intermediary searching') in the health field. According to questionnaire data, almost one in two (48%) searches conducted was undertaken on behalf of someone else. There appears to be some evidence, albeit slight, in the topics accessed by those giving their ages as under 15, to support this possibility. Arguably, one could say that children would not be worried about cancer prevention.

According to health staff interviewed, Travel pages, 'simply for the animation', and pages sexual in content were liked by children. But the logs do not support this, which raises all kinds of questions about adult perceptions of children's behaviour. The 'top ten' pages chosen by children were in fact:

- Good eating
- Exercise
- Alcohol
- Brazil
- Asthma in childhood
- Weight
- Cape Verde
- Cancer prevention
- Enuresis
- Egypt

Health professionals were positive overall about children's kiosk use. Various interviewees said they had been involved with or had seen at close hand children undertaking all of the following activities:

- Researching homework tasks ('I quite often have children come in when I am here, and ask if they can use the machine to look up something for school. They are not even here to see us [i.e. for a consultation']).
- Showing parents or grandparents how to use the kiosk ('Often their parents will let them play, and then the youngster will call them over and show them something of relevance').

- Searching the kiosk as intermediaries, on behalf of family members ('they have asked me to spell something – like varicose veins – because their parents have been complaining about them').
- Looking up information for their own conditions ('I often tell youngsters to look on the kiosk for information related to their problems – as they are more receptive to doing this than adults').

The majority of parents felt that their children simply had a natural curiosity in 'all things electronic', and that the relative tediousness of 'being dragged round with me' was somewhat alleviated by the possibility of 'playing' on the kiosk. However, gentle probing revealed several reasons for their children's use. These were:

- School work of all descriptions (including project work, homework, 'something to do with school' etc.), as also mentioned by health professionals.
- Sports information (apparently unsuccessfully sought, although much 'Healthy Living' pages, in fact, were relevant).
- General 'Healthy Living' (those mentioned were diet and exercise).
- Specific conditions with regard to the children themselves (asthma; sprained wrist; 'Osgood's disease').
- Specific conditions with regard to other family members, as also noted by health professionals (diabetes; glaucoma; blood pressure). This appeared in each case to be personal volition on the part of the children, rather than as a result of a request from adults.
- Alternative medicine (for their own information).

Observational studies provided valuable insights into children's kiosk use. Interesting use amongst teenagers was observed, much of it corroborating parents' and health professionals' accounts of children's behaviour. A number of fairly lengthy sessions (i.e. longer than 10 minutes) carried out by members of this group were viewed when, clearly, genuine information tasks were being carried out. Most of these were by children either apparently alone – 14 or 15 year olds – or accompanied by an adult. On one occasion two girls of about 13 were seen consulting the terminal in concert. Confirming what the nurses said, there were instances also of children calling to their parents or other accompanying adults and apparently showing them things and using the kiosk with them.

Plainly then, children used the kiosks for a number of reasons – for projects, for (and with) parents, and also for recreational purposes. Even in the latter case it could be argued that such use should be encouraged, providing it did not prevent others in need using the kiosks. This is because, as a result of their play, these children were learning to become digital information consumers, a skill they certainly would not acquire purely from school. And for those people who would ban their use, there should be consideration of children's undoubted role as carers. Those against children's use of kiosks also ignore what has happened in the case of mobile phones, where children profitably use the technology in huge numbers. The lesson appears to be that when you come across an information or communication system that proves attractive to children you should take advantage of it, not put it off limits. Information and communication leads to knowledge and education and this will hold children in good stead for the world of digital health information that will surely confront them in their old age.

Kiosk use by ethnic groups was investigated through an online questionnaire of users of a kiosk in a Nottingham surgery. Forty two percent described themselves as white British, and 31% as Pakistani – which corresponds quite well with the distribution of patients across the practice. In other words, ethnicity was not a kiosk use determinant or barrier at this level. Seventy two percent reported that they were UK born, 15% as being born outside the UK and 13% did not say (Figure 3.4).

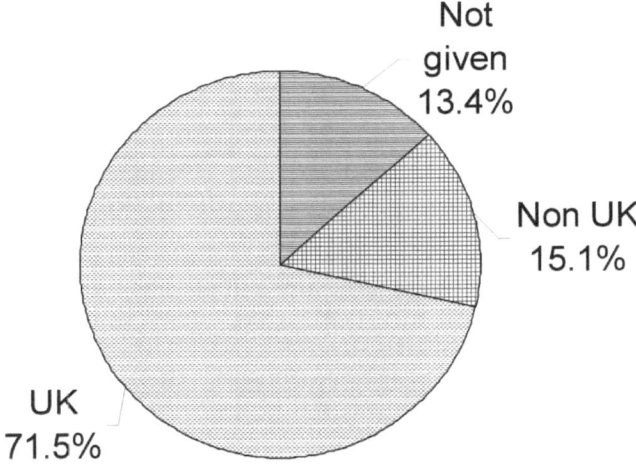

Figure 3.4 InTouch kiosks – distribution of users by place of birth

While females constituted the majority of UK born users for this kiosk (63%), almost the exact opposite was true for non-UK born users (Figure 3.5). Sixty one percent of non-UK born users were male. Perhaps, reflecting cultural patterns, in that men may well be responsible for family health for some ethnic groups. The age distribution between UK and non-UK born users was much the same (Figure 3.6). However, rather more over 75s and fewer under 15 year olds did not give their place of birth and may reflect a confused cultural identity.

Health topics sought

This is probably the most interesting analysis of them all as it tells us something about the health concerns and interests of the digital consumer, and sometimes on a very large scale indeed. We have been able to examine content use by gender, age, and ethnicity. This information is, of course, of critical importance to health authorities. Why people looked at the topics they did is just as important, and that data were largely obtained via interview and questionnaire.

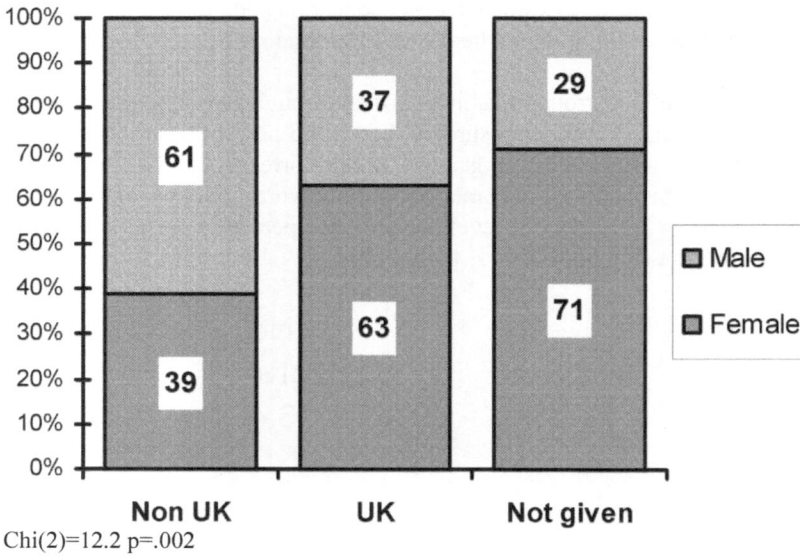

Chi(2)=12.2 p=.002

Figure 3.5 InTouch kiosks – users by gender and place of birth

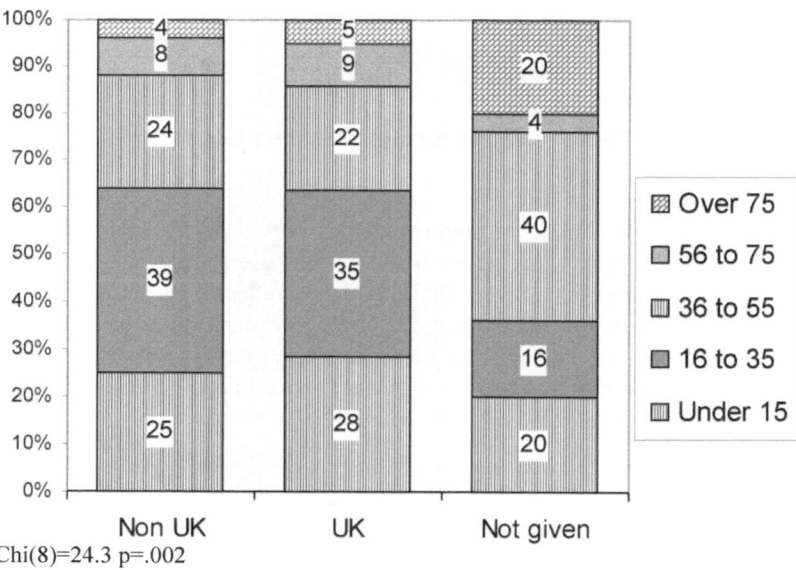

Chi(8)=24.3 p=.002

Figure 3.6 InTouch kiosks – users by age and place of birth

Plainly, people can only view what is available, so we need to remind ourselves of what the InTouch with Health kiosks covered and how the content was presented and sectioned. The following example illustrates the set up within the main contents entries:

- Main menu entry: Surgical Operations
- Second level index: List of operations and body parts that may require operations (Blood vessel system, for example)
- Third level index: List of types of operation (Amputation etc.)
- Fourth level: List of details user might require about operation chosen (Body parts involved, the operation etc.)
- Fifth level: information provision.

More information on the content and structure of the kiosks can be found in the section on usability, below.

General picture of health information topics required   Figure 3.7 shows the percentage use of each health section across 21 kiosks located throughout the UK The most popular section viewed was Medical Conditions, suggesting that people were interested in helping themselves or a relative/friend to information in respect to a particular illness. Most (50%) views to this section were made at the Peak Pharmacy. This is interesting as it might constitute evidence of people using the pharmacy as a substitute for going to the doctor, a course of action some NHS advertisements have encouraged. However, there is considerable variation between kiosks and, significantly in this regard, the lowest use of this health section was in a surgery, that of Dr Merali – just 27% of views concerned the medical section. Overall the next most important section was the Healthy Living section. Most views to this section were made at the Associated Chemist, where 20% of section views being accounted for by this Healthy Living. The Travel Clinic section was also well used though the variation in use of this section was considerable, from under 10% to 22%, probably reflecting the times when people go on holiday. Most use of this section was made at the kiosk located in Dr. Merali's surgery and 22% of section views here were to this section. It is thought that the explanation lies in the large number of children that searched the kiosk at this particular location.

Table 3.5 compares the use of four health sections in regard to a range of use/ users variables. The variables included in the analysis were age, socio-economic status, reason for use, users' birthplace and gender. Age was found to be highly associated with socio-economic status and this resulted in estimation problems and it was decided to drop age from the analysis. This should not imply that age was not significant, but that age and socio economic status compete to explain the same area of variance. Fourteen percent of those aged 16 to 35 fell into the other category. This was true of 6% of 36 to 55 year olds and 11% of those aged 56 to 75, arguing that this category included people who had not entered full time employment or had left the labour market.

Users were classified into broad economic grouping: skilled or unskilled, employed and unemployed. It was decided to add to these groupings those under the age of 15 and those aged over 75. Both these age groups should not appear in the socio economic groups, the first age group being too young to work, the second too old. The 'Other' category of Socio-economic grouping is likely to include those in retirement or early retirement and those who have not yet entered the labour market. The use between men and women was fairly even (7.8% compared to 6.2%).

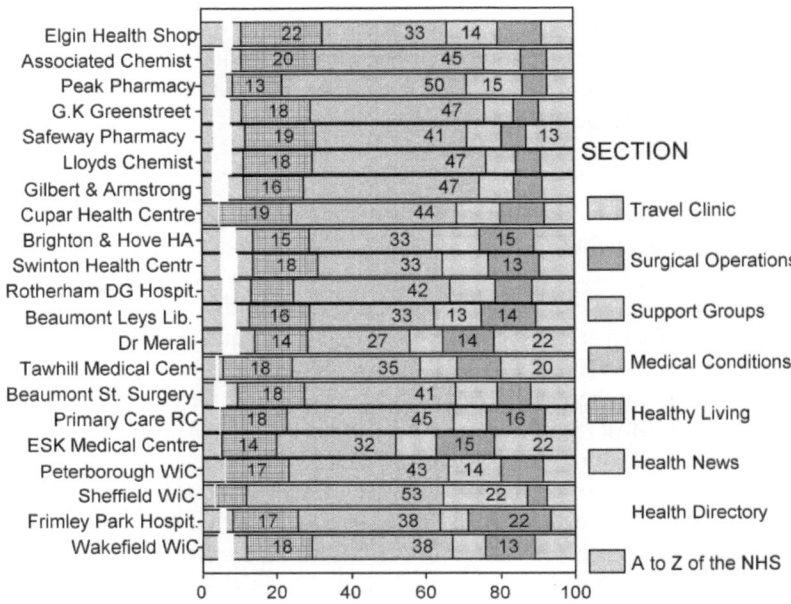

Figure 3.7 InTouch kiosks – percentage use of each health section across 21 kiosks

Socio-economic status. Those in skilled employment were far more likely to view Healthy Living section pages and less likely to view the Surgical Operation pages. The skilled employed were at least twice as likely to look at Healthy Living pages compared to the unskilled, the unemployed, those over 75 and those under 15 years old. However, the skilled employed were found to be least likely to view Surgical Operations. The over 75s' were about four times more likely to view a Travel section page (4.2) or a Surgical Operations pages (4.3) and were less than half as likely to be interested in Medical Conditions (.44) and Healthy Living (.50) as compared to those skilled employed. The unskilled and employed used Surgical Operations (4.3) and the Travel section (2.6) but were less likely to use Healthy Living pages (.30) compared to skilled employed. Those unskilled and unemployed were about twice as interested in medical condition pages (1.84) but half as interested in Healthy Living pages (.44) compared to skilled employed. For this analysis, those aged under 15 were nearly seven times more interested in the Travel section and over 3 times more interested in Surgical Operations (3.5) but were half as likely to be interested in Medical Conditions (.43) and Healthy Living pages (.46) compared to skilled workers.

Table 3.5 InTouch kiosks, modelling health section use

		N	Medical conditions	Healthy Living	Surgical Operations	Travel Section
Socio-economic/ age status	Skilled employ	865	-	-	-	-
	Skilled unemployed	225	.69* (.16)	.25*** (.27)	6.01*** (.24)	1.38(.32)
	Unskilled employed	133	1.03 (.19)	.30*** (.31)	4.32*** (.29)	2.61*** (.26)
	Unskilled unemployed	119	1.84** (.22)	.44* (.34)	.16t (1.0)1	.93 (.75)
	Other	151	1.24 (.19)	.18*** (.38)	10.6*** (.24)	.13* (1.0)1
	Over 75 years old	106	.44** (.27)	.50* (.32)	4.25*** (.31)	4.15*** (.33)
	Under 15 years old	576	.43*** (.13)	.46*** (.16)	3.45*** (.21)	6.68*** (.19)
Reason for use	Curious	1095	-	-	-	-
	Specific enquiry	393	1.48** (.13)	.23*** (.23)	1.29 (.22)	.14*** (.43)
	Told to	283	1.02 (.16)	.54** (.24)	1.85** (.21)	.1*** (.40)
	Other	404	.67** (.14)	1.24 (.17)	1.30 (.18)	1.04 (.19)
Birthplace	UK	1518		-	-	-
	Not given	370	.85 (.14)	-	.70 (.24)	.64t (.28)
	Non UK	287	.56*** (.14)	-	1.41* (.18)	3.23*** (.18)
Gender	Female	1386		-	-	-
	Male	789	1.8*** (.10)	-	.78t (.15)	.40*** (.18)

Reason for use. Not unsurprisingly, those with a specific inquiry were about one and half times more likely to look at a Medical Conditions page compared to either curious users or those told to use the service. However, those with a specific enquiry were four times less likely to use a Healthy Living page and about eight times less likely to use the Travel section compared to curious users. Those with a specific enquiry may have viewed Healthy Living pages as not as medically important as Medical Condition pages.

Those told to use the service were just under twice as likely to view a Surgical Operations section page, half as likely to view a Healthy Living page and 10 times less likely to view a Travel section page, as compared to curious users. Again, a surprisingly poor use of Healthy Living pages by this group. Further, unexpectedly, this group was just as likely to view a Medical Conditions page compared to curious users. The question is raised as to why these users, who appear to have a clear information need, were not making use of the Medical Conditions section – one would imagine that this section was the most important, in terms of content, on the kiosk, for this group.

Birth place. Those born outside the UK were three times more likely to view the Travel section (confirming what we would have expected), were half as likely to view Medical Condition pages and just under one and half times more likely to view Surgical Operation pages compared to UK born users.

Gender. Men were just under two times as likely to have viewed a Medical Conditions page compared to women, but were about a quarter less likely to view a Surgical Operations page and half as likely to have viewed a Travel section page.

Individual health topics viewed

We can get much closer to what needs people have with regard to health information (Table 3.6). The table furnishes the top 15 pages and the bottom 15 pages viewed for 21 kiosks located throughout the UK, with each topic being generally represented by a single page. In all 864 health topics were viewed. Some topics were much more popular than others. Thus the top 15 pages, about 2% of the 864 pages available, accounted for about 30% of all pages viewed. Health policy makers will be glad to note that Good Eating even accounted for 6% of all page use. Some of the worst performing pages proved surprising. For example, although Cancer Prevention made up about 2% of all pages viewed, cervical screening made up less than half a percent of pages viewed. This may be due to the visibility and prominence given to each subject. Clearly how easy a page is to find (which we term 'digital visibility') will impact significantly on page use. In this specific case, Cancer Prevention was available two menus down from the home page while that for Cervical Screening was further down the hierarchy.

It is worth noting here that there is a wide variation in the number of levels a user was required to traverse in order to arrive at a desired page. This was because it was impractical to include a large number of menu items on the kiosk screen, as each entry in the various contents lists needed to be large enough and far enough from its neighbours to be activated by the touch of a finger. For this reason the kiosk had a large number of menu layers, and thus, users may only arrive at an information page after traversing several screens of options. In some cases, 'Medical Conditions' for instance, a shortcut can be created by various methods. One way was to touch the relevant part of a body diagram to limit the list to entries related to that part of the anatomy. An alphabetical index also helped overcome the directory hierarchy.

Table 3.6 InTouch kiosks – most popular and unpopular individual health topics viewed

Top 15 pages viewed		Bottom 15 pages viewed	
Good Eating	5.8	Appointment	.0
Alcohol	4.8	Artificial Limb	.0
Exercise	4.8	Artificial Limb Service	.0
Weight	1.9	Bed Wetting	.0
Cancer Prevention	1.8	Cancer	.0
Back pain - Strain	1.7	Cervical Screening	.0
Abnormal Heart Rhythms -	1.2	Child Protection	.0
Smoking	1.1	Chiropractic	.0
Stress	1.0	Choice	.0
Asthma In Childhood	.9	Citizens Advice Bureau	.0
Mastitis - Mastalgia	.9	Commissioning	.0
Brazil	.9	Community Health Council	.0
Enuresis	.8	Contract	.0
Asthma	.6	Council Tax	.0
Iron Deficiency Anaemia	.6	Curvature Of The Spine	.0
As a % of all page views	29%		

Several variables appeared to have affected the individual health topics viewed. Key ones were:

Time of the day. There was a lot of variation here and some of it particularly interesting. Thus, for example pages on Smoking and Contraceptives were viewed more in the evening (7pm) and Stress and Antidepressants pages viewed more in the morning (12am).

Kiosk host organisation. The top 20 list relating to hospitals tended, unsurprisingly, to have more topics related to operations and topics such as 'Hip Replacement' were not repeated on the lists of other kiosk locations. There was a greater use of pages under the category Travel Clinic in surgeries, which might be because more children used kiosks in surgeries.

Geographical location. Although there was a lot of variation here, too, the effect of geographical location on the health information needs and seeking requires further research. It could have something to do with the age profile, socio-economic class, or the occupational profile of the area, or possibly the result of a particular health campaign.

Reason for use. While more than half of the participants in one survey said that they used the kiosk out of curiosity (perhaps, while waiting for the doctor), 17% of patients had a specific inquiry and 12% were instructed to use it, presumably by their

GP or nurse. Plainly, curious users were much more likely to look at Healthy Living issues, while those with a specific inquiry or who were told to use the kiosk were more likely to visit more specific medically related pages. The data indicated that the users' information need and circumstance was important in understanding how they interacted with the kiosk.

Gender. In one study it was revealed that the total number of unique pages viewed for all users was about 30% more than the total unique pages viewed separately by gender, implying a substantial difference in the unique pages viewed between men and women. This in part can be seen by the differences in the ranked top 15 pages between women and men. Women were more likely to view pages on cancer prevention, breast biopsy and lumps, and smoking, while men tended to view pages on back pain, the bladder, brain tumours, hair thinning and fractures.

Age. The popularity of Good Eating, Exercise and Alcohol pages declined as age increased. Alcohol dropped out of the top 15 ranking for the 36 to 55 year olds, while exercise and good eating dropped out of the ranking for those aged 56 to 75. This apparent lack of interest is surprising, given that these topics should become more important, purely on health grounds, for these age groups (so, maybe, it is an example of information avoidance?). The under 15 year olds, and users over 75 were more likely to view Travel Clinic pages.

Usability and accessibility issues

Kiosks, of course, were specifically designed to be easy to use by a whole range of people who might have difficulties in using computers. In other words their great strength was supposed to be their usability and accessibility. We researched whether this was really the case or not. The section on non-use, of course, should be read in this context.

The following issues were identified as important factors in the usability of the kiosks:

- Readability/terminology, and the general ease with which information could be read and understood.
- Navigation and use of search facilities.
- Deficiencies in the functioning of the kiosk.

Although the construction and layout of each of the sections of the kiosk mentioned at the beginning of this chapter, is not quite the same, activating any of the main menu items leads to a further list of contents. In some cases, 'Medical Conditions' for instance, the list – often considerable – can be shortened by one of two methods. These were:

- an alphabetical listing. This facility is offered by, for example, the Support Group entry, and allows users to key in the first letter of the topic/organisation they seek.

- a body diagram, whereby users are instructed to touch the relevant part of the body which interests them (Figure 3.9).

Often an activated menu entry results in further content selections being displayed. Indeed, in some cases, five screens were required to arrive at the required information.

The following example illustrates the set up:

- Main menu entry: Surgical Operations
- Second level index: List of operations and body parts that may require operations (Blood vessel system, for example)
- Third level index: List of types of operation (Amputation etc.)
- Fourth level: List of details user might require about operation chosen (Body parts involved, the operation etc.)
- Fifth level: information provision.

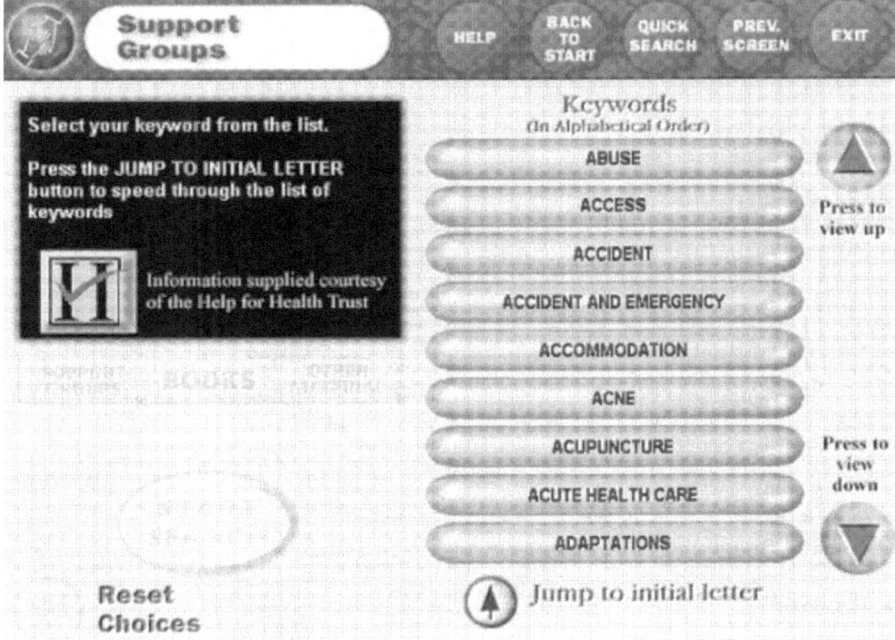

Figure 3.8 InTouch kiosk – alphabetical menu, showing scroll arrows

Navigation and orientation facilities within a digital system are, of course, vital for effective and efficient use. Users were asked how easy the system was to navigate; how they found the menus, and whether the site was easy to read and understand. Only just over a third of users thought that the kiosk had easy menus 'all the time' and just under a third (30%) thought the kiosk was easy to navigate 'all of the time'.

Furthermore, 40% said that the touchscreen area was easy to use 'all of the time'. The significant difference between the use of menus, navigation and touchscreen is best understood by comparing how easy they were perceived to be either 'at times' and 'not really'. Nearly one in three (30%) of respondents thought that the menus were 'not really' easy or 'only sometimes' easy compared to 20% of respondents finding navigation and touchscreen areas easy only 'most of the time'. This indicates that menus were a problem and more so compared to navigation and the use of the touchscreen areas. Kiosks are a menu heavy information system and this may result in users terminating their session early and, maybe, one reason why so many users were giving up on their session after just viewing thee pages. Clearly menus, and topic visibility, are features that can be improved on.

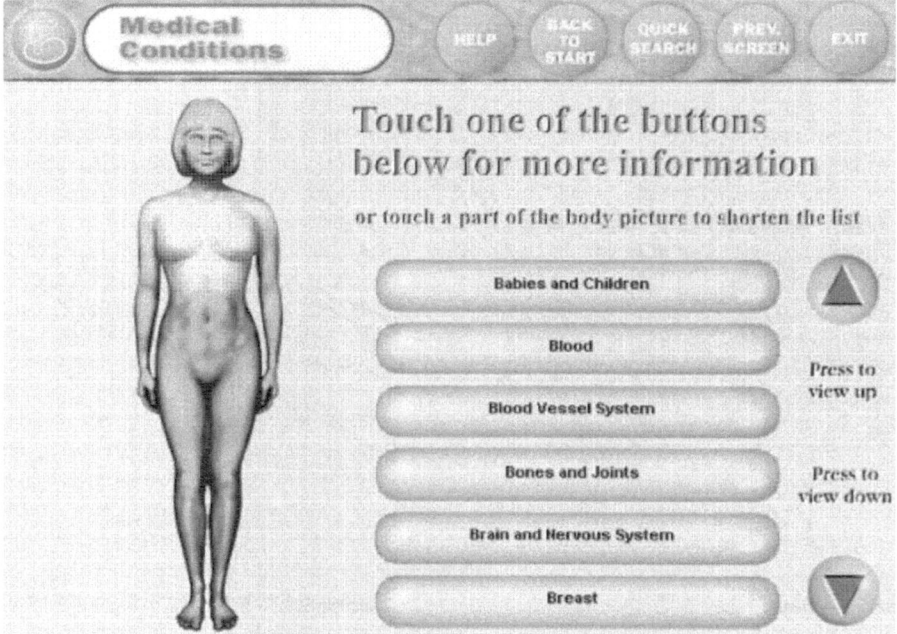

Figure 3.9 InTouch kiosk – body part navigation (showing instruction to 'touch a part of the body picture')

With regard to navigation, the health professions interviewed raised some possible problems with navigation. One person said that those not used to the Internet would not understand the meaning of the 'Back' button. This was in fact borne out in the DiTV study where, in usability sessions, some participants did not equate a 'Home' button with a link to the main or title page. Guesses as to the meaning, included 'Health in the home' or 'Home-based product advertising'.

Important factors in determining whether a system is easy to use is the type of information content offered, language employed and how easy the content is to understand. Our studies showed that 30% of respondents found the kiosk easy to understand 'all the time', 50% understood it 'most of the time', 15% understood it 'at times' and 5% did 'not really' understand it at all.

Interviewees indicated that they found no problem with the terminology, either in terms of headings/signposting or medical language used in information pages. Indeed, at one kiosk site, four of the six interviewees thought the language patronising ('...in some instances, the language seems almost condescending ... persons might feel offended', '...it's a bit insulting to intellectuals, I think.'). A majority seemed to be pleased with the fact that medical jargon was simplified, so that complex medical terms could be easily understood. Use of diagrams was also thought to be adequate, with only one person of the opinion that more diagrams and illustrations could be used to simplify some issues. However, some medical professionals complained that often medical expressions were used in the system. Thus users typically searched under a common name – the example of 'piles' was given by one interviewee, for information which could only be successfully retrieved by using the term 'haemorrhoids'. Staff at a pharmacy in Sheffield found the problem so common that they made sure there was always a medical dictionary handy to help them search the kiosk with and on behalf of their customers.

Many health professional indicated that they would not recommend the kiosk to, or retrieve information on behalf of, all patients. Some patients were described as 'clearly unable to read even basic leaflets'. Jones and Gill (1998b) pointed out that the NHS was established before the period of greatest migration to the UK, and 'it is far from clear that (it) has changed rapidly enough to meet the challenges posed by patients whose English may not be good enough to communicate adequately with health professionals'. InTouch with Health were aware of this problem, and produced an innovative kiosk containing content in various ethnic languages. This highlights a problem that was being addressed by researchers in Sheffield working on an ethnic health initiative[3] – that of illiteracy amongst speakers of foreign languages. The head of the project explained: 'We had to find a way to break down the communication barrier faced by ethnic minorities. Some languages only have a verbal tradition; so many people are unable to read their mother tongue.' To overcome this, a handset was included on the kiosk to enable users to listen to oral versions of the information pages. A short video loop also played on-screen, showing someone approaching the terminal and lifting the receiver.

Even many native English speakers had difficulty with written leaflets, kiosk printouts etc. This has long been recognised as a problem, with various commentators suggesting that documents should be written for a reading age calculated as 12 (Albert and Chadwick 1992) and 9 (Griffin and Griffin 1996). Of course, it has also been recognised that this practice itself brings with it the problem of patients finding such literature patronising, uninteresting and lacking in authority (Kenny *et al* 1998). Health professionals could only offer the solution of speaking very clearly to patients suspected of having a low reading level, and writing down the bare minimum for them, such as bullet lists of recommended actions ('rest', 'take one tablet every four hours', 'no alcohol' etc.)

---

3   http://www.intouchwithhealth.co.uk/ethnic_health.htm.

Two problems were noted by health staff at various kiosk locations, which would affect the usability of the system. These concerned calibrating the screen and using the printer. In addition, some interviewees complained of the machine simply being 'broken'.

Usefulness, benefits, outcomes and trust

It was, of course, important to look beyond the usage logs and ask questions to determine the usefulness, benefits and outcomes of using the kiosk. This is also the place to look at the related issue of trust and authority. This chapter is structured as follows:

- Relative usefulness of kiosks compared to other health information sources
- Usefulness in meeting information needs
- Range and quality of content
- General benefits of the kiosk
- Trust and authority of the kiosk
- Outcomes: information and dealing with medical professionals

Of course, the non-use section (following) says volumes on usefulness, and it should be read in that context.

Questionnaire respondents using a surgery in Scotland were asked to rate a number of health information sources on the scale 4 = very important, 1 = not important. The two most important sources of information proved to be their own doctor (3.6) and the practice nurse (2.8). The kiosk scored a relatively lowly 1.8, but this was in fact a little better than the web (1.6), and only just below the well established NHS Direct telephone line (1.9), which must be a big surprise given the personal and diagnostic nature of the latter. Nevertheless, the message to be taken away from this analysis is loud and clear: personal, face-to-face health consultation with a health professional, especially a doctor, is what consumers wanted.

The highest correlation between topic of interest and importance of the kiosk as a source of information was recorded for alternative medicine. Medical research and medical news were also relatively high correlated. Information on drugs, diet and a particular condition scored poorly and argues that these subjects were not so well covered. The score for a particular condition is surprising and, possibly, argues that the section covering Medical Conditions was not meeting the information needs of users or that users were not using this section in the surgery environment. Perhaps users received better information on this topic from their doctor and kiosk pages were not sufficiently detailed.

Interviews and questionnaire data suggested that, whilst people did access information on specific conditions, they used this in concert with the information they obtained from their doctors. It may be that those who obtained information as an alternative to contacting or visiting a medical professional may value kiosks more highly. This could be particularly true of information seen as being unobtainable from (traditional) doctors. Thus it may come as no surprise that the kiosk was highly regarded by those with an interest in alternative medicine. The kiosk hosted several pages on this topic, which contained information a doctor might not agree with or even have time to explore.

We can draw on a number of studies for evidence, which show how kiosks met health information needs – studies of kiosks in Cornwall, Nottingham, and Edinburgh. Thus Cornish users were asked whether the information found on the kiosk answered their question and whether the user had more questions as a consequence. Just over two-thirds thought the information had answered their question, which has to be regarded as a satisfactory result; although 16% chose not to answer. It is, of course, possible that some of these users might not have had a specific question in mind when using the kiosk – being the kiosk equivalent of web surfers. Excluding non-respondents, 8% said that the kiosk did not answer their question and 16% said that they were not sure, which suggests that the kiosk answered some, but not necessarily all, of their query.

A logistic regression was fitted to the outcome variable 'did it answer your question'. The best model fitting the outcome variable included the four variables – gender, seeking information on a medical condition, ease of finding the topic and readability. Women were found to be three times more likely than men to say that the information found answered their question. This may reflect the women's important role as carer in the household and that, as a consequence, were more open to seeking a wider range of health information. Furthermore, and backing up findings described already, the analysis indicates that if the person was searching for information on a medical condition then they would be about three times less likely to say the information they found answered their question.

Regarding ease of use, unsurprisingly, those people who could not find their topic easily and who found the topic difficult to read were less likely to say they had their question answered. People who did not say yes to finding the topic easily were four times less likely to have their question answered and users who did not respond yes to finding the information easy to read were about 13 times less likely. The results reinforce the belief that the ease with which the kiosk was used and the readability of the information found had a profound impact on whether the person found what they were looking for.

People searching for a medical condition were three times less likely to have their question answered. This finding seems to indicate that the InTouch with Health kiosks performed less well in this area, and confirmed the result that information on a particular condition was insufficiently covered by the kiosk.

The Cornwall hospital patients were asked if they had more questions to ask as a consequence of using the kiosk. Respondents could either answer yes, no, not sure or could decline to answer. Fifty seven percent of respondents said that they did not have more questions to ask after using the kiosk, while 28% said that they still had a question to ask, 6% of users declined to answer and 8% said that they were not sure. Of course, it is possible that the receipt of information – especially in the health field – triggers off another information need, by disclosing an information gap. The survey therefore included a follow up question in which respondents were asked where they would go if they had more questions. The survey offered five alternatives: a health professional, telephone helpline, a manned information centre, re-use the kiosk or other, and adds to our understanding of source selection. Sixty-four respondents, or 16% of the total sample, ticked at least one of the options. Of the 64, 22% said that they would visit at least two sources to get an answer to their query.

Half of those seeking more information said that they would use the kiosk again to search for an answer to their query and this suggests that the kiosk was a possible launching pad for their query.

A final analysis modelled those saying they would go to another information source, other than the kiosk, to answer their question. Three variables were found to have an impact on whether the user said that they would seek an alternative information source. These were whether the user found it easy to find, whether the information was understandable and whether the information being looked for was to do with a medical condition.

If the person did not answer yes to finding the topic easily they were about 4 times as likely to seek an alternative to the kiosk information source as compared to those who found the kiosk easy to use. In addition, those who did not understand the information found on the kiosk were about three and half times as likely to seek out another information source compared to those who did understand the information. These findings argue that those people either finding it difficult to use the kiosk or understand the information will look elsewhere. People were plainly evaluating and making comparisons. Again the numbers involved were small and this analysis must be regarded as only indicative of likely relationships that need to be further researched.

The analysis also shows that those viewing a medical condition kiosk page were about three times more likely to go on to another information source compared to those not viewing such a page. This is a further indication of the inadequacy of the kiosk in supplying medical condition health information, possibly this is an impossible task for a stand-alone, general public machine. However, it does show that users in general do critically assess kiosk content and where the content is lacking that they will go on to seek information elsewhere.

The absence of the variable of those users finding the kiosk 'difficult to read' argues that these users did not go elsewhere for information. That is, there was no evidence that those users who found the kiosk 'difficult to read' went on to look for information elsewhere. It is as if these respondents blamed themselves and their perceived inadequate reading skills, rather than the kiosk, for not understanding the information and did not then go on to seek information elsewhere. Perhaps kiosks should state that if users do not understand the terminology then they should telephone NHS Direct. However, those finding the kiosk difficult to read, made up only a small proportion of kiosk users, less than 10%, though they were 12 times less likely to have their questions answered. The kiosk may in this circumstance reaffirm their ineffectiveness in seeking and finding health information, though this group may traditionally be poor users of health information sources generally. A further study is needed to look at the specific health information needs and sources used of those with poor reading skills.

Bivariate analysis indicated a relationship with age and whether the information found answered a user's question. Older people were less likely to say their question was answered. This study, additionally, found that those users born in the UK and who were employed as skilled workers were just over half as likely to find the kiosk very easy to use as compared to non-UK born users, and UK born unskilled users. This suggests that educational level might impact on how easy people find the kiosks and, following on from this, whether people find what they are seeking.

The Safeway kiosk evaluation previously described sought to discover whether the information found on the kiosk met the consumer's needs. Results were extremely positive. One user who had a life-long (unspecified) illness said that he was now in better control of his health condition. Many interviewees stated they had recommended the system to others, because they found the information so useful. Others, who said that they had not referred the system to other people, stated they would do so when necessary because they thought it was 'a useful resource'. A majority of users did indicate, however, that the kiosk had answered their questions. For some it appeared that it was not one piece of information, or one fact etc. that was required. There was an element of either checking the information to see what gaps existed in one's own knowledge. Other respondents thought of the kiosk as providing background information or an overview: 'It helped. It's a good basis for understanding my body and how it works or doesn't.' However, not everyone was satisfied.

At the Nottingham kiosk people were asked about the general usefulness of the kiosk but only 58% of users answered this question. This implies that a little under half of the users either did not understand the question or did not feel that their feelings regarding the information provided would fit comfortably into any of the three options – useless, useful or very useful. Of those who did answer, 39% said the information found was 'useless' – which is quite a strong condemnation of the kiosk, 30% said it was 'useful' and 31% found it 'very useful'. Users who found the information 'useless' were compared with those who found it useful or very useful. Again a logistic regression was used to fit the outcome.

The three variables found to be significant determinants of whether the user found the information of any value were: 1) whether the system proved easy to use; 2) reason for use and; 3) age of user. Users who either found the touchscreen easy or very easy to use were about 10 times less likely to find the information 'useless' compared to users who found the system not easy to use. This reaffirms the importance of kiosks being easy to use. Fifty-five percent of those finding the system very easy said the information found was very useful, this compares to 30% of those finding the kiosk easy and 8% of those finding it not easy to use. Seventy five percent of people who found the system not easy reported that the information found was 'useless' to them, a figure which says it all.

Only 10% of kiosk users had been advised to use the kiosk. Surprisingly, these people were just under four times less likely to find the kiosk useful. They may have perceived the kiosk to be an inferior information source compared to their doctor. There was evidence that this dissatisfaction may well be linked to health section use. There was no difference between the curious and those told to use the service in terms of viewing a Medical Conditions section page, although those who were told to use the service were twice as likely to view a Surgical Operations page. Users here may be cutting short their session when they realise that the medical condition page is not giving them any new information.

Age was also a significant factor. Ninety four percent of people aged over 75 reported that the information found was 'useless'. They were 10 times more likely to report that the information found was 'useless' compared to those aged under 15. Users aged between 36 and 55 were most likely to find the information either useful or very useful. Eighty percent of these users found this to be so. Forty percent of age group 56-75 and the under 15s found the information 'useless'. Interestingly those users who had been told to use the kiosk were just under four times as likely to say that the information was useless.

There were substantial differences in the responses of doctors and nurses regarding the benefits of the kiosk. The former tended to concentrate more on practical issues – space/time saving, easier access to information etc., whilst the latter pointed to the medical benefits patients might accrue. Benefits cited can be broken down into three types:

- Educative/informative
- Intrinsic
- Practical

The kiosk was seen, particularly by nurses, as an educational service to complement other available materials. Thus, patients were encouraged to both use the service independently, and as a complement to the instructions or advice offered by the health professionals. One nurse pointed out that it was not possible to go through all the details of treatment, recovery etc. in a consultation, and that kiosk information emphasised the major points. This was described as particularly important when patients needed an operation. Also, printouts from the kiosks served, as with information leaflets, as a patient aide memoir. This was considered as being of great importance. As the nurses stated from their own practical experience, retention of orally transmitted information was generally poor. Medical research confirms this anecdotal view. Kitching's (1990) studies show that patients generally forget half the information provided to them within five minutes of leaving a consultation. Having a written document to take away clearly should go some way to remedying this situation, although, of course, a formal examination of the advantages of kiosk printouts would, of course, require a study of its own.

Interestingly, the benefits in terms of educating users were all re-active, referring to managing an existing condition, rather than preventing one (as 'Healthy Living' pages on both SurgeryDoor and NHS Direct were designed to do). The information was said to give patients control over what was a pre-existing condition, which in turn helped them manage it better; facilitating more self reliance. Some hoped that this would lead to a reduction in re-consultations, relieving the overloaded system – although no such effect had been noted. Surprisingly, no one mentioned any possible benefits of the kiosk in terms of disease prevention or the use of it to provide information promoting a healthy lifestyle.

Edinburgh kiosk users were asked whether they felt better informed about their condition. Reflecting the findings of earlier studies (Cyber Dialogue 2000; Nicholas *et al* 2001b) most people (94%) said they felt better informed about a condition after having used the service.

The intrinsic benefit of the kiosk was that it fulfilled the same function as leaflets in being a 'gift' for the patient, this role being a phenomenon noted as long ago as 1970 (Balint *et al* 1970). Not only were the patients happy to accept this token, but referral to the kiosk, or a kiosk search on behalf of the patient, served as a signal that the consultation was terminated. Doctors were quick to point out the advantages of this – being ever conscious of the time element, although an astute practice manager also mentioned this. Of course, there were intrinsic benefits also in that the kiosk represented a symbol of both the high regard for patient information (and, as a logical extension, of care) and information content in maintaining a healthy lifestyle.

Doctors highlighted the practical and administrative advantages of the kiosk more than the advantages relating to an improved service for the patient, which nurses tended to highlight. Chief amongst comments was the view that easier retrieval of information was possible. Also, the high number of leaflets that would be required to provide the same level and coverage of information afforded by the kiosk would be prohibitively expensive and administratively difficult to maintain. Several doctors mentioned time and space-saving advantages. Doctors at one practice said the kiosk was helping them create the 'paperless surgery'.

It was not considered appropriate to ask members of the public what they felt about the range of content. This was because each person would have particular information and health needs and would be unlikely, therefore, to judge the kiosk on its broad range of topics, about which they would probably be ignorant. This was not the case with medical professionals however. It was much more likely that they would use the kiosk to answer a wide range of queries stemming from patient consultations.

Views, collected from a series of in-depth interviews, on the range of contents centred on four main areas:

- Specificity of information
- Variability of information
- Gaps in information provision
- Currency of information

Many felt that the depth and breadth of information provided was far more than leaflets could offer. This range meant that access was available to documents with a higher level of specificity, meeting the individual needs of patients far better than previously (i.e. when only leaflets were available). However, there was some feeling that the information content was 'too variable'. Several respondents indicated that for some conditions (such as dyslexia) information consisted 'merely of an address from where a leaflet could be obtained'. Others, by contrast, 'provided very detailed information written at a level that may not be accessible to many people'.

Nearly all of the kiosks were networked, so there was a facility to add, remove and update information centrally (i.e. from the offices of InTouch with Health). Indeed, one of the selling points was the possible inclusion of a health alert service, whereby current health issues could be highlighted and explained. Information was updated every three months, unless an urgent modification of information is required.

The majority of professionals appeared to be very happy with this frequency of updating.

People's views on the authority of the information provided by the kiosk and the trust they exhibited in it are possibly related to whether they find the information useful or of value. The particular position of kiosks located in non-medical locations such as supermarkets, where the information might take on another persona, is of particular interest.

Interestingly, not one interviewee in any location or context (i.e. medical/non-medical) raised the issue (trust). When the topic was mentioned by interviewers, users did, indeed, tend to say that they had 'every trust in the information'. This was true even in non-medical locations. Here the host organisation was generally vested with the degree of responsibility necessary to only permit quality information to be disseminated on their premises 'Well, they wouldn't let any cowboy stick a kiosk here, would they?'

Non users might be expected to mention trust or authority in their explanation for not using the kiosk. In fact, this issue was not raised, despite a large number of non-users having been interviewed. Those who were vague or not forthcoming about their reasons for not using the kiosk were asked specifically about the issue of authority. It seems that there had never been any doubt in anyone's mind that the information would be trustworthy and authoritative. Again, there was an assumption that 'they would not allow incorrect information on the kiosk'.

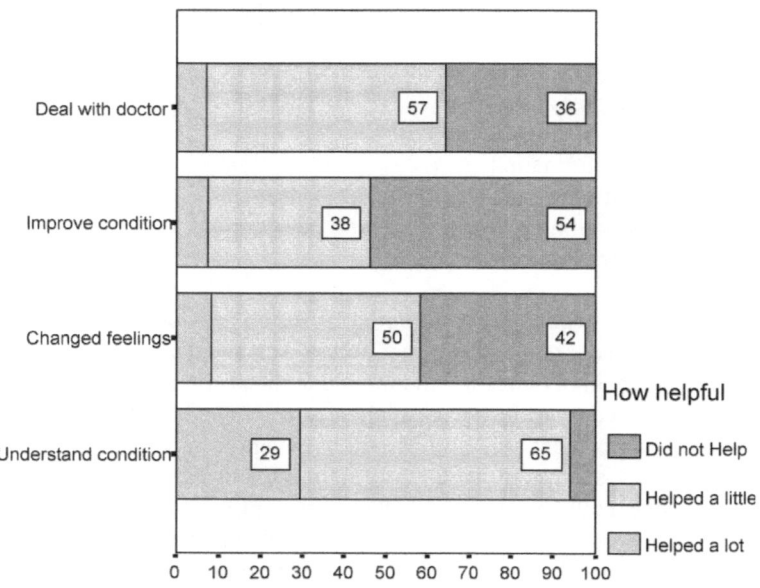

Figure 3.10 InTouch kiosks – how helpful has the information found on the service been in relation to the following

It is one thing to know that people were satisfied with the information they obtained from a kiosk, it is quite another – and more important – thing to determine what they did with it or how they benefited from it. Figure 3.10 shows what people told us. Plainly most people felt that it helped them understand their condition – 29% thought it helped a lot and 65% felt it offered some help. Two-thirds felt that the information they found had helped a little or helped a lot in their dealings with the doctor and nearly one in ten said it had helped a lot. Indeed, nearly one in ten actually felt it improved their condition.

Some of the users interviewed considered that the kiosk could give them the supporting information they required in order to make an informed decision regarding their own health. Such information was said to supplement that obtained from medical professionals. For example, one respondent was put on anti-depressants and she wanted to know whether unpleasant side effects she was experiencing only happened to her. She thought the information she found from the kiosk helped her in making decisions with regard to her own medical treatment, rather than just letting the doctors tell her what was good or not good for her instead.

Thirty percent of the Edinburgh surgery patients said that they had used health information that they had found (from whatever source) as a substitute for visiting the doctor. A statistical model was used to explore which information source was likely to have an impact on whether the person substitutes the information for a visit to the doctor. In terms of information sources used, only medical books were found to have a significant impact on the outcome. Surgery kiosk users who were fairly or very interested in medical books were just under four and half times more likely to use information found as a substitute to a visit to the doctor, compared to those not at all interested. The kiosk was not found to be a significant information source and had no impact on the person in terms of its use as a substitute for a visit to the doctor. We might expect this, clearly the kiosk is located at the surgery and users were unlikely to cancel their appointment.

In terms of personal characteristics age was a significant factor. Those aged 56 and over were about half as likely to use information from sources found as an alternative to a visit to the doctor compared to users aged 35 and under. Younger people seem more receptive to information from a variety of sources, and less worried about authority issues.

All of the kiosk users in medical and non-medical locations, however, thought that the information obtained definitely played a part in helping them to deal with health professionals (rather than substituting for them). A common theme (as we found also in the studies of DiTV health information users was that doctors did not have enough time to explain everything or even if the doctor were able to verbally impart sufficient information, they probably would not understand or remember it all. Another patient said that the few times she made an appointment to see her GP, they were usually booked up at least two to three weeks in advance. In the meantime, she could get some rough idea from the kiosk as to the seriousness of her problem, or get some self-care advice, so that it might ease her worries.

The issue of whether the health professionals actually wanted their patients to 'know everything' or 'know too much' came up with interviewees as well. One patient said she needed to know more details of the medication she was prescribed than the doctor appeared to want to tell her, and how it would affect her life. She therefore used the kiosk to arm herself with the information she needed to discuss things with the doctor so they would not be 'condescending' towards her.

Two other users thought getting the information for the kiosk helped them in asking the right questions during consultation and having a meaningful discussion with the doctor.

Role and impact of kiosks on health profession and services

Now we turn our attention to the medical professionals, and the impact consumer health information had on their work and practices. The role of the kiosk and its potential impact on this group might be expected to be extensive amongst the men and women in the front-line: the doctors, nurses and other medical professionals. The research looked at the impact at an individual level, interviewing those whom the kiosk was expected to effect. Several issues related to the role of medical professionals in the provision of information in general, and that from kiosk terminals in particular, were explored. These included:

Reasons for kiosk purchase,
- The extent to which expectations have actually been met.
- The use of kiosks by health professionals.
- To meet their own information needs, and any consequent displacement of other sources for health professionals to refer patients.
- The displacement of other sources for patients, and the degree to which this has been encouraged or necessitated (by the diminution of leaflet provision, for example).
- The degree of internal monitoring and evaluation of kiosk use occurring or already undertaken, by whom, and the impact this has had on their professional work practices.
- Impact on professional practice, in terms of relationship with patients, with particular regard to:
  - The quality of consultations – are patients more knowledgeable? Is that a good thing, or does it undermine the consultant?
  - Work load – has wider information provision for the public meant more background reading and current awareness by doctors? Are there more visits to doctors as a result of information acquisition by patients (as mentioned earlier)?
- Practical issues such as delegation of responsibility, technical/mechanical problems, dealing with misuse etc.

Differences in responses between doctors and nurses, and between health professionals and practice managers, were of interest, and are discussed in the text. Finally, in addition to exploring how the kiosk impacts upon the work and role of the health and other staff, we look at the reasons for kiosk purchase.

Those directly responsible for kiosk purchase tended to be senior practitioners, although towards the end of the study it appeared that health authorities themselves were taking the decisions and were the force behind the expansion, particularly of web-enabled kiosks. In the case of our study however, 8 out of the 16 doctors interviewed had some say in kiosk purchase or were privy to knowledge of how the purchase came about, and all nine of the practice managers claimed some involvement. Interestingly, the reasons stated were not as numerous – and often not as fundamental or detailed – as the benefits generally proclaimed for kiosk purchase. The main reason for this is that often it was nurses, not doctors, who trumpeted the system, despite the former being responsible for purchase. Also, some benefits were not anticipated, and only manifested themselves as the kiosk began functioning. Indeed, few reasons were given for actual kiosk acquisition. Considering the high cost of purchase, outlined above, during the time of the study, there was a very surprising lack of deep and well thought out deliberations of the issues entailed.

Reasons given were:

- A general belief in the importance of patient information.
- The enthusiasm of a single individual committed to greater patient information provision.
- Practical and/or administrative benefits.
- External offers of financial contribution.

As mentioned earlier, the kiosks were principally for use by the general public – the lay user. However, assessing the impact of the kiosk upon the work of the professionals meant examining how they used it themselves, for their own information needs, and also, whether – and to what degree – they did so in an intermediary capacity, on behalf of their patients. We were also interested in the extent to which they referred patients to it.

Use of the kiosk for the benefit of the health workers themselves or for their jobs was higher than may have been expected considering the system is primarily targeted at the lay consumer. There was a discrepancy between nurses and doctors, with the former being by far the bigger users. Nurses described a number of information needs, the principal enquiry being for holiday vaccine details. The kiosk provided more current information than leaflets, and this type of information was always in demand.

By contrast only one doctor we came across indicated any personal use of the kiosk – and he was the person instrumental in its purchase and was therefore already committed. He said he had cause to consult it on various occasions. As an example he described a lady who wanted to donate her body to medical science. He (perhaps surprisingly) found out how to do this on the kiosk.

Referral takes two forms. Firstly, the health professional can indicate orally that the patient may find appropriate information on their condition on the system and direct them to it. Secondly, the patient can be given a written 'information prescription', described later, for use in retrieving information from the kiosk.

There was a marked difference generally regarding the referral (be it oral or using written chits) of the patient to the kiosk, as with other issues, between opinions and practice between doctors and nurses. The latter were far more likely to refer patients to the kiosk than their doctor colleagues, although doctors at one site, felt 'obliged' to refer patients to it, as they were trying to create a 'paperless surgery' and were reducing the number of leaflets stored. Only one other doctor indicated that he specifically referred patients to the system, whilst the others generally felt that patients 'knew it was available and made their own choices'. One doctor claimed he used to talk to patients about their information needs and how the kiosk might help them, but that he found it far too time consuming. Another said that as there was no guarantee patients would 'rush out and look at the kiosk as advised' there was 'little point in referring patients to it'. By contrast, nine of 11 nurses mentioned this practice. Ironically, one of the reasons given was that 'left to their own devises' many patients would not use the system.

For those who did refer patients to the kiosk or use it with them, the reasons cited were:

- To encourage use (both to become better informed and because: the system is there, costing money – the patients should use it);
- To encourage a greater involvement by the patient in their own condition and treatment;
- To save nurses' time in not having to hunt for leaflets.

Interestingly, InTouch with Health regard the referral of patients to the system by doctors as very important in maximising use and, thus, helping to better inform patients generally. To encourage this, the company has produced what 'Patient Information Prescription' (PIP) pads, alluded to above. These are chits of paper on which doctors write key words relative to a patient's condition, which they can use to retrieve information from the kiosk. These were, unhappily for the company, almost universally ignored. Of all the interviewees, only one doctor used them.

The reasons for non-use of PIPs amongst doctors were almost exclusively practical. They were time constrain and the fact there was no guarantee that patients would use the information.

Apart from the impact of the kiosk with regard to professional practice, there were other ways in which the kiosk impinged upon the work of staff. Practice managers and administrative staff, however, almost exclusively felt the impacts here. Two major themes emerged – dealing with children, and managing the upkeep of the kiosk. With regard to the first of these, practice managers were almost universally negative, with a common comment that children often 'play', but rarely used the kiosk correctly.

Kiosk maintenance was a big issue with the practice managers, who were de facto, charged with the day to day running of the kiosk. The workload caused some resentment. Clearly, having a more formal allocation of responsibility for the upkeep of the kiosk, and a more engaged approach by the medical professionals, would help enhance its usage and benefits.

Our enquiries into the role and impact of the kiosk on medical and other professionals elicited a number of important findings. Of particular interest were the differences in outlook and practices between the three 'players' on the staff at kiosk locations: doctors, nurses and practice managers. The differing views between doctors and nurses is of much importance, as the degree of pro-activity regarding kiosk use appears to be a strong factor in its take up by the general public. An editorial in the British Medical Journal (Smith 2000) described the divisions between doctors and nurses as including sex, background, philosophy, training, regulation, money, status, and intelligence. Perhaps, therefore, it is not surprising that their views and experiences of the electronic information system may be so different. It may also be expected that nurses appear to engage more with patients. Research shows that when nurses do the work of doctors, it is often to the greater satisfaction of patients (Shum *et al* 2000). Similarly, nurse consultation over the telephone can safely reduce hospital admissions for both adults and children (Lattimer *et al* 2000) and that there is evidence of high levels of satisfaction with nurse-manned NHS Direct telephone service (O'Cathain *et al* 2000). All of this research seems to point to very high public regard for nurses, and indicates a certain receptivity for any suggestions by them with regard to information seeking – from the kiosk or otherwise. By contrast, whilst nurses appear to be gaining in public esteem, doctors are, apparently, losing theirs. A report from the BMA (2001) claimed that 'family doctors are demoralised. They are angry that despite ever increasing hours of work and coping with an agenda of constant government-imposed change, they are often not able to give their patients the service they deserve'. Similarly, studies have reported poor records of doctors in perceiving patients' underlying worries (Stewart *et al* 1979) and have trouble in recognising those seeking support (Salman *et al* 1994).

Time constraints, an issue connected with the comparative work of doctors and nurses, was a major factor determining employment of and attitudes towards the kiosk. Whilst research (e.g. Shum *et al* 2000), indicates that patients express greater satisfaction with professionals, be they nurses or doctors, who spend longer over their consultations and give them more information, doctors just do not have that time to give – hence their lack of knowledge of kiosk information content, non-use of Patient Information Prescriptions or other referral of patients to the system.

The difference between health professionals' and practice managers' views was also important. There was a clear problem for the latter at many locations – exacerbated by printer and other malfunctions – regarding staff responsibility and delegation, and some resentment that the kiosk had resulted in extra work for them. It is possible that this led some practice managers to talk negatively when describing use by children. This is in contrast to the way the kiosk was seen by health professionals, none of whom mentioned any of these issues.

Non-use

Clearly as important as why people choose to use a health kiosk is why they do not. And as we know, the majority of people chose not to use the kiosks for a whole variety of reasons. The following issues emerged as factors in contributing to the non-use of kiosks:

People-specific factors:

- Experience and confidence in using Information Technology
- Cultural and social issues
- Health

System-specific factors:

- Usability issues
- Preference for other delivery systems
- Deficiencies in the functioning of the kiosk

Environmental factors:

- Location
- Promotion

Questionnaires sent to patients in surgeries with an InTouch kiosk addressed the issue of the use of Information Technology generally, as a lack of experience or confidence in using electronic systems was considered to be a likely barrier to use. Patients were asked how they described their feelings towards computer-generated information. Just over one third, 36%, said that they had used and felt comfortable with this. However 58% – just under two thirds – of respondents said that they had used IT but 10% of this IT 'literate' group said that they did not like it and 28% said they did not have the time to use it. In all 42% of the potential user group said that they avoided computers. Those who used and felt comfortable with IT were more likely to have used the kiosk: 21% of these computer literate users had done so compared to 6% of users who avoided computers. Half of the users who avoided computers and two-thirds of users who used computers, but did not have the time, reported that they knew about the kiosk but had not used it. IT experience seemed to be an important factor as to whether a patient used the kiosk. However, it should be emphasised that approaching a half (42%) of those who used and felt comfortable with information technology did not actually like using computers. Open-ended questions also suggested that a lack of understanding of or confidence with information technology is a significant barrier to use. Eighteen percent of those who had visited a surgery with a kiosk said they did not use it because they did not know how.

Clearly the kiosk, though touchscreen activated, was still viewed as a technology that is difficult to use. The barrier to use here, however, may be more attitudinal rather than practical. In-depth interviews with users and potential users showed that the 'computer literate' interviewees found the system extremely easy to negotiate. Research reported above indicated that kiosks were more likely to be used in areas where the local population had a high incidence of microwave ownership. This indicates that even previous use of touchscreen technology has an impact on kiosk use.

By 'cultural and social factors' we mean:

- Reluctance of some people to seek health information from any source
- The need for human interaction
- Privacy and anonymity concerns

With regard to the reluctance to seek health information from any source, there is much evidence to show that certain kinds of people in certain situations are reluctant to seek health information – from whatever source.

Medical professionals interviewed spoke particularly of the elderly, in regard to the attitudes many of them have about their GPs and other health professionals, which may inhibit them seeking health information. Elderly people were described as coming from a generation where professionals such as teachers and doctors were exulted figures whose word was never questioned or even confirmed. A consequence of this is that this group would not regard it as appropriate to inform themselves of medical matters. One could argue, of course, that with fewer educational opportunities when they were younger, and a higher proportion working in manual jobs that did not entail handling information, there was no culture of information research in any sphere. Patient interviewees did, indeed, appear to reinforce this view.

Running through all our studies of the use of information technology is the issue of first hand human information sources ('real people') versus second hand pre-prepared information (be it text, audio etc.) Whilst we have shown that information from electronic sources was used as a substitute for visiting a doctor, nevertheless, there is much evidence to show that information imparted by someone on a one-to-one basis was valued more highly. There is a great need, in other words, for human interaction. Thus in one survey three quarters of non-users said that their doctor or nurse told them all they needed to know so that had no need for the kiosk. Clearly in these circumstances the authority of the kiosk is undermined by the close proximity of a more highly considered source of information. The need for the active involvement of a human was manifest also in non-users stated preference for written or printed information from the doctor.

When users were asked to rank the importance of health information sources (out of 5) the two most important sources of information proved to be their own doctor (average rating 3.6) and the practice nurse (2.8). Friends and family and leaflets were also considered important and, respectively, scored 2.4 and 2.3. Health books and newspapers scored 2.0. Electronic sources scored poorly. The kiosk scored 1.8, two decimal points above the web (1.6) and one decimal point below the NHS Direct telephone line (1.9). DiTV was the least important source of information and scored just 1.3. Clearly, personal contacts – be they medical professionals or the lay public – count far more than mediated information.

Interviews showed that even for kiosk users, information imparted face to face, principally by a health professional, but also from other valued figures, were far more valuable than that obtained from personal research. 'You can't beat the doctor telling it to you face to face'.

There are several reasons for considering that, ironically, health may itself be a factor in the non-use or underemployment of the kiosks. The reasons emerged from interviews with health professional, although log data did support these findings. Firstly, many elderly people, of course, suffer declining vision with age (Marwick 1999). If those with poor vision used a finger to guide their eye when reading, this would inadvertently activate the system to retrieve an unsolicited page. One can imagine a user stopping after two or three unexpected and unwanted page retrievals have occurred. This may be why the average number of pages viewed by the over 75s is so low – a point which has serious implications for their take up of services.

Interestingly, and perhaps worryingly, only a tiny minority of health professionals mentioned particular problems either physically or mentally disabled people might face in accessing digital information. A nurse spoke of problems a wheelchair-bound person would have in using the terminal. As it can only be accessed from a standing position, this immediately precludes unaided use by the wheelchair bound and those who find standing for any length of time difficult.

Even a cursory glance at the kiosk indicates other potential problems that those with a disability might face. Firstly, despite the larger font size on the kiosk than on the corresponding website, the screen may be too small for those with a visual impairment. The choice of white lettering on a beige/sandy background for the main orientation buttons on the top of the screen white on a pale green for many pages does not help here. The attitude of some doctors at one site was not helpful, either, who joked about 'the blind' using the kiosk. Secondly, a problem no-one mentioned was that the touchscreen access system precluded use by some people with physical disabilities. Unlike computer 'mice', which could be adapted for disabled use, the mechanism does not appear to readily lend itself to suitable modification. Indeed, no-one at any of the locations visited even considered this possibility.

Besides usability issues and technical problems (paper jams etc.) there was some evidence that people who were confident in information technology and who were happy to seek health information from digital sources nevertheless did not use the kiosk. Thus nearly a quarter of non-users said that they preferred to use the Internet to search for medical information and younger respondents were more likely to say this.

Several issues arose regarding the location of the kiosk. One concerned the appropriateness of the location of the kiosk in a medical location. Many interviewee patients suggested that as they were already about to see a doctor there was little point in researching for information from inside the building, be it from the kiosk or from any other source: 'my doctor is there to give me the answers'. It had been speculated that patients might indulge in casual use of the kiosk, in the way they might flick through a magazine, but in fact there was no evidence of any 'electronic browsing' or pre-consultation information seeking of any kind.

Factors pertaining to the peculiar circumstances prevailing in doctors' waiting rooms may also inhibit kiosk use in surgeries. First, people are usually on edge and uncomfortable in the relatively intimate company of strangers, and they are disinclined to do anything that sets them apart from the others. Secondly, they are also very conscious of the time dimension – they are, after all, waiting for the doctor. Interviewees at non-medical locations said they would feel least comfortable using the system at a GP surgery. Furthermore, the searching for information may be perceived to be something that is not really legitimate behaviour. This also came out in interviewees with patients, and has already been discussed. Finally, people might not want to use the kiosk for the very reason that they are unwell and, as such, lacking in both mental and physical energy.

Taking all these circumstances into account, counter intuitively; a GP's waiting room may actually be a pretty poor place in which to put a kiosk. A more appropriate location might be somewhere more private, or at least more anonymous, where people could feel that they can spend as long as they need in order to find the information they require. The government seems to be right to consider locations such as supermarkets and libraries, where members of the public can access health information both anonymously and without the need to seek a medical appointment. This raises the issue, of course, of the purpose of kiosks, and whether they should be considered different depending on the location. In a medical setting they might be regarded as an adjunct to a doctor consultation, in which case they might be utilised, as suggested, by staff in tandem with patients. In non-medical locations, the role would be more that of an alternative to or substitute for an appointment with a medic. There are clear implications for the type of information each plays host to that requires further research in these alternative locations.

Log statistics also inform the debate on the suitability of kiosks in doctors' surgeries. In an examination of the performance of kiosks in various types of locations: information centres (i.e. libraries, community centres), pharmacies, GP surgeries and hospitals, results supported the view that these locations might not be ideal.

Another factor proving to be a barrier to use was that of the promotion of the kiosk. Several kiosk users at the Safeway supermarket pharmacy pointed out it would be helpful if the system was signposted, stating what the system was used for and how to use it. This they felt could be beneficial in attracting potential users, especially those who might not be computer literate. The kiosk was not, in fact, signposted at all, apart from a notice placed by the researcher recruiting interviewees. Also, the kiosk was not located in a particularly appropriate place. It was placed sideways on to a wall, and it was hard to see, as it blended into the decor of the location. One could not readily tell what it was or whether it was working or not. Props/display racks were even placed in front of it, blocking its view from customers.

This lack of signage led to two major problems: lack of awareness of the existence of the kiosk, and misconceptions regarding the purpose of the kiosk and for whom it had been provided.

As shown below, however, even where kiosks were publicised by posters and people encouraged to use them, this problem still manifested itself. Thus in the case of patients asked why kiosk use was declining at their surgery no fewer than 41 out of 150 non-users who had visited the surgery (i.e. 27%) stated that they had not noticed it. This was surprising, as it was not possible to enter the reception area and waiting room without passing the kiosk, which has a poster above it explaining its function and inviting people to use it.

Many people who did notice the kiosk declined to use it because of misconceptions about its function and/or the information it held. Further questioning showed that 13 of the 150 patients (9%) who did not use the kiosk did not realise it was for patients to use.

InTouch with Health Web-enabled Health Kiosks

During our investigation, InTouch with Health introduced a web-enabled kiosk, which attracted much interest amongst health trusts and surgeries. This form of kiosk has proved very popular and now constitutes InTouch's main kiosk product.

A pilot investigation of these kiosks was conducted to see whether they performed differently to the original, stand-alone kiosk.

Web and non web-enabled InTouch kiosks shared the same 'kiosk' content. However, the web-enabled kiosks also allowed users to access other health websites. This way the main weakness of the stand-alone kiosk, its (relatively) limited content, could be overcome. Web-enabled kiosks also allowed content to be updated remotely and more frequently. Both types of kiosks studied were PC based touch sensitive screen health information systems. For web-enabled kiosks the host organisation for the kiosk chooses the other websites users can visit. InTouch with Health recommended they choose no more than 15. The kiosk was set up to be a 'walled garden' in that it had links to and promotes certain sites, which users were tacitly expected not to stray from. However, with a keyboard available, and a URL location box on screen, it was possible to access other sites be they medical or not (the latter described from here on as 'non-sanctioned' sites).

Web-enabled kiosks dialled up to the Internet via an ISDN dial-up connection and used a dynamic IP address to connect to the server, so each time they connected to the web they were given different IP addresses. The kiosks, however, log the URL (Uniform resource locator) of the sites visited by kiosk users and also the date, day and time of the visit.

The main kiosk screen is divided into three columns. The left hand one consisted of the main traditional kiosk menu items. (Surgical operations; A-Z conditions, support groups etc.). Users were not required to log in with age range and gender information. The centre screen announced 'Health information for speakers of other languages'. Touching this activated a short video showing someone approaching the kiosk and picking up the telephone receiver. This resolved into a list of languages 'Chinese, Gujarati, Bengali and Urdu'. A series of instructions appeared in the language chosen, and a moving arrow pointing to icons of a printer, information page and scroll buttons.

The right hand side consisted of web links. Three were visible without scrolling on the terminal: SurgeryDoor, NHS Direct and the Department of Health. Pressing the scroll button revealed one more link at a time (each link being a rectangle with the name of the site and a logo). On one particular kiosk examined, the other websites accessible were:

- National Childbirth Trust
- British Heart Foundation
- NICE
- The Stroke Association
- Organ Donor Register
- Meningitis Trust
- Contact a Family

Activating the link opens the website of the organisation. Internal links can be activated by touch or mouse-ball and clicker button.

Web-enabled kiosks were compared, firstly, by location – within a hospital and between hospitals, and, secondly, they were compared with non web-enabled kiosks.

Each kiosk recorded user transactions in a log file. Web-enabled kiosks produce a transaction log file listing the websites visited and a file recording use of the InTouch database. The non-web-enabled kiosk recorded a single log file of use made of the InTouch database. The database was the same on both types of kiosk. In all, nine InTouch kiosks were selected for the study, six of them web-enabled, distributed over three hospitals.

Web-enabled kiosks provided access to two databases, the accessible websites and the standard InTouch database. For the InTouch database there were on average 4.6 user sessions per day per kiosk (Table 3.7). For the web part it was estimated that about one and half user sessions were conducted. It is difficult to determine whether users crossed between the two databases, hence they may not have been more than about 5 daily sessions, two of which might have included some web content. This was lower than might have been expected given the extra choice offered; traditional kiosks recorded an average of about 15 user sessions. The Table also provides key use metrics too. The average number of pages viewed in a day per kiosk was about 63 pages. This was again lower than expected for the traditional kiosk (110). The low figures recorded here may well reflect the specialist locations of the kiosks, 3 of the kiosks were located away from the main reception at one organisation and another kiosk was located at a specialist hospital. Users may of course have been dissuaded to use what seemed like a complicated home page menu structure – more complicated than the traditional kiosk. However, and this shows how important it is to employ a range of metrics, sessions lasted on average just about seven to eight minutes, considerably longer than the one to two minutes recorded for traditional kiosks. This argues that some users did start a traditional kiosk session then went over to the web based area. Individual page view time was about 12 seconds and was much the same, though a little higher, to that recorded for traditional kiosks.

Table 3.7 InTouch web-enabled kiosks – summary kiosk metrics

Metric	6 Hospital based Kiosks	
	InTouch Database	Websites
Average daily number of user sessions per day	4.6	1.6
Average daily number of pages viewed per day	62.8	N/A
Average daily number of pages printed per day	N/A	N/A
Average session length (seconds)	465.6	N/A
Average page view time (seconds)	12.2	N/A

As mentioned earlier, use of websites was prescribed by the host organisation; however, it was still possible for a determined and skilled user to search other, non-sanctioned sites. In all, 10% of all users' web accesses were to non-sanctioned sites and 57 non-sanctioned sites were accessed. Seventeen percent related to ad.doubleclick.

net, an organisation that counts accesses to certain pages. This suggests that users were clicking on online adverts. Significantly, four of the sites appearing in the list were medical – not surprising, given that they were links from sanctioned medical sites. Of the sanctioned or promoted sites, the most accessed were SurgeryDoor, the Internet arm of the InTouch with Health kiosk, and NHS Direct Online: accounted for, respectively, 42% and 25% of accesses.

Health topics sought

Kiosk pages were grouped into six broad menu sections: Medical Conditions, Surgical Operations, Travel Clinic, Support Groups, Healthy Living and A to Z of the NHS. Medical conditions followed by Surgical Operations were the most popular sections visited and made up between 60 to 70% of kiosk use. Given that we were talking about hospitals, the health topics sought were those that we might have expected. The least used sections were the A-Z of the NHS and Support Groups; however, these two sections had far fewer pages available to users. There tended to be a greater difference in the use between sections within a hospital location rather than between the two kiosk types (web-enabled and traditional). Hence, there were more than expected views to Surgical Operations pages in the kiosk located in Day Surgery clinic (Conquest) compared to other kiosks located at other locations in the hospital. Approximately 34% of views were made to Surgical Operations compared to about 17% made to this section at other kiosks.

The variation in InTouch pages viewed related more to kiosk location differences than to differences in the kiosk type (Table 3.8). The kiosk at the mental hospital Lynfield Mount had more views to Schizophrenia and Brain Tumour pages than at any other hospital reported here. Users of this kiosk however viewed few pages. Only 97 unique pages of InTouch were viewed compared to about 300 recorded at the Airedale Hospital (main reception) and St Lukes. This is thought to reflect the poor kiosk content on mental health issues. This argues that there is a link between kiosk location and type of information consulted, and that the menu structure should reflect easy access to content likely to be viewed at the location.

In terms of unique pages viewed and the percentage share accounted for by the top 15 pages there was little difference between use of the web-enabled kiosks and non-enabled. About 300 unique pages were viewed and the top 15 pages accounted for about one third of all page views – about the same between kiosk types. Table 3.9 gives the ranked topic pages at the Conquest Hospital. The non-web kiosk at the main reception at Conquest did record just fewer than 500 unique page views. However, the kiosks located in the outpatients (Conquest) and Day Surgery (Conquest) had much the same number of unique pages viewed as the web-enabled kiosk in A&E reception (Airedale) and Children's Outpatients (Airedale) – about 300. Day surgery (Conquest) did have more pages linked to Surgical Operations that did not appear in the top 15 page view rank compared to the Main Reception and outpatients (Table 3.9).

Table 3.8 InTouch web-enabled kiosks – ranked top 15 pages viewed

Main Reception Airedale Hospital	%	Lynfield Mount	%	St. Lukes	%
Exercise	4.4	Good eating	5.4	Good eating	6.6
Good eating	4.3	Alcohol	4.4	Exercise	5.5
Alcohol	4.2	Schizophrenia	3.1	Alcohol	4.3
Cancer prevention	2.7	Breast biopsy	2.7	Weight	2.1
Cataract lens repl.	1.8	Abdomino-perineal r	2.3	Backpain - strain	2.0
Cor. heart disease	1.7	Alcoh. liver disease	2.3	Cancer prevention	1.8
Retained tooth -root	1.7	Brain tumours	2.3	Enuresis	1.7
Breast lumps	1.7	Knee replacement	2.3	Stress	1.5
Backpain - strain	1.6	Renal failure - chronic	2.3	Mastectomy	1.4
Iron def. anaemia	1.4	Slapped cheek synd	2.1	Renal failure - acute	1.3
Duodenal ulcer	1.3	Wisdom teeth remov	2.1	Croup	1.3
Urinary tract Inf.child	1.3	Adenoidectomy	1.9	Iron deficie. anaemia	1.2
Leukemia - acute	1.2	Angola	1.9	Hip replacement	1.1
heart rhythms - atrial	1.2	Hallux valgus	1.9	Abn. heart rhs - atrial	1.1
Weight	1.1	Belize	1.7	Knee arthroscopy	1.0
% of top 15	32	% of top 15	39	% of top 15	34
Total no. of unique pages viewed	**300**	**Total no. of unique pages viewed**	**97**	**Total no. of unique pages viewed**	**308**

At the time this study represented the first study made of web-enabled kiosks, a form of kiosk that has captured the interest of Health Trusts, who have held back from employing kiosks in their attempt to provide patients with improved information provision. The added content and greater versatility of the new kiosk was plainly the great attraction, but the cache of being able to say you are providing web-access must be an important factor too. The main conclusions were:

- This finding confirms previous research that higher patient throughput levels were linked with the higher kiosk use.
- There was no significant evidence that web-enabled kiosks attracted more kiosk users compared to non-web-enabled kiosks. It might be that people are still to wake up to the fact that kiosks have changed and now offer much more choice in terms of content.
- There was strong evidence linking kiosk location to the type of website consulted. The kiosks were used to lookup information relevant to the user needs as generally defined by location within the hospital or by type of the hospital. Web-enabled kiosks support a limited number of links and kiosk administrators need to think carefully about the links provided that best suit potential users; matching site selection to information needs, in other words.
- Users at Lynfield Mount, a specialist mental hospital, were more likely to use the web facility rather than the kiosk. This was linked to the specialist nature of the user needs. These needs were not adequately met by the InTouch kiosk

content and hence users were more willing to use the web services. Users were clearly content sensitive.

- Less use was made, as estimated by the number of pages viewed, for the same static InTouch with Health database when it was offered along side a web based information service. It argues that less use will be made of an information service when it is offered alongside competing information sources.
- The variation of InTouch pages viewed was related more to kiosk location differences than to differences in the kiosk type (traditional or web-enabled). This links kiosk location to type of information consulted.
- Despite efforts to make the kiosk as 'user-friendly' as possible, there were nevertheless issues related both to navigation and to kiosk functionality. This is almost inevitable, given the complexities of providing information stored on a local directory, using a particular structure and menu system, whilst also offering access to a number of disparate and independent websites.

Table 3.9 InTouch web-enabled – ranked top 15 pages viewed at Conquest Hospital (traditional kiosks)

Main Reception	%	Outpatients	%	Day surgery	%
Good eating	5.3	Exercise	4.9	Alcohol	5.3
Alcohol	4	Alcohol	4.4	Exercise	4
Exercise	3.3	Good eating	4.4	Good eating	2.6
Cancer prevention	1.9	Abn. heart rhy'ms - atrial	3.5	Cancer prevention	1.7
Subarach haemorrh	1.7	Abn. heart rhys ventricula	2.2	Cancer of the colon	1.6
Hip replacement	1.7	Weight	2.1	Knee replacement	1.6
Weight	1.5	Smoking	1.5	Abn heart rhy ventricula	1.6
Backpain - strain	1.3	Raynauds syndrome	1.4	Cataract lens replac	1.6
Mastitis - mastalgia	1	Ankle sprain	1.3	Cholecystectomy	1.6
Breast lumps	0.9	Warts	1.3	Knee arthroscopy	1.5
Abn. heart rhms - atrial	0.9	Balanitis	1.1	Discectomy slip disc	1.4
Cerebrovas' diseas	0.9	Cancer prevention	1.1	Abdomino-perineal re	1.3
Caesarean section	0.8	Breast lumps	1	Wisdom teeth removal	1.3
Knee replacement	0.8	Cape verde	1	Haemorrhoidectomy	1.2
Urinary tract child	0.8	Coronary heart disease	1	Nasal polyp removal	1.2
% of top 15	27	% of top 15	32	% of top 15	29
Total no. of unique pages viewed	**486**	**Total no. of unique pages viewed**	**310**	**Total no. of unique pages viewed**	**271**

NHS Direct kiosks

The evaluation of NHS Direct kiosks was a small part of the overall kiosk evaluation. The intention was simply to cross-check some data that what was being found in regard to InTouch kiosks.

One hundred and eighty six touchscreen NHS Direct kiosks were made available in various locations in England at the time of the study. This service formed part of the Government's NHS Plan, aiming to provide a convenient out-of-hours health service. The NHS Direct information points had twin aims: to give the public greater information about how they can look after their own health and also to give information about health services. The health information on the kiosks was provided by NHS Direct and was similar to that found on the NHS Direct Online website. The kiosks were situated in key public locations such as pharmacies, supermarkets, libraries, shopping malls, universities, sixth form colleges and more traditional NHS locations such as hospitals and NHS Walk-in centres. The decision on where to locate kiosks was the responsibility of each of the 22 local NHS Direct Centres.

The Department of Health commissioned independent consultants to help develop the specifications for the kiosks, including disability and access options. The first NHS Direct kiosk was installed in September 2000. Eighty-one kiosks were installed by February 2001, 136 by October 2001, and 180 by January 2003. A number of the NHS Direct Information Points featured telephone handsets enabling the public to contact their local NHS Direct Call Centre free of charge, for additional support and healthcare advice (Boudini 2003).

A description of the menus and content of the kiosks follow:

Menus and content
Hot Topics
Take care of yourself this winter
      How should you treat a cold
      What to do if you get flu
      How to treat coughs and sore throats
      Antibiotics
Healthy Living
Eating for health –
      Eating for health
      The balance of good health
      Glossary of nutrients
      How to eat more starchy food and fibre
      How to eat less fat
      How to eat less sugar
      …, …
      …, …
Maintaining a healthy weight
      …,
Getting active
      …,
Thinking about drink
      …,

Quitting smoking

…,

Managing stress

…,

Keeping your teeth healthy

…,

Staying healthy at work

…,

Childhood immunisation

…,

Self Help Guide (uses same algorithm as NHS Direct telephone service)
How to use the guide
About the self help guide
Body key –
        Head & chest –
Breast Changes – (user needs to answer a series of Qs by choosing Yes or No, before getting advice info)
                Breathing difficulty in children
                Chest pain in adults

                …,

                …,

        Skin
        Limbs
        Abdomen
Symptom or a condition –
Index
        ABCDEFGHIJKLMNOPQRSTUVWXYZ
                Tablets
                Tapeworms
                        Worms
                Teenage pregnancies
                        Teenage pregnancies
                Temperature, high
                        Baby rashes
                        Backache in adults
                        Breathing difficulty in adults
                        Colds & flu

                        …,

                Tendons, damaged

                        …,

                        …,

                T…,

Glossary of conditions
        Acne
        Allergies
        B…,
        C…,

        …,
Reference section

Accidents to children
A...,
Bereavement
B...,
C...,
Dietary supplements, vitamins and minerals
Female puberty
How do I know my baby is ill?
...,
About NHS Direct
About home page
NHS Direct telephone service
NHS Direct Online
NHS Direct self help guide
NHS Direct self help points

The extent of kiosk use was of chief interest and especially whether groups (like the elderly, ethnic minorities or the poor, for instance) at which they were specially (and initially) targeted availed themselves of the kiosks. Logs were the principal source of data, although these were supported by a questionnaire survey.

The 123 kiosks investigated were NHS produced kiosks for which logs were supplied for the month of July 2001.

On average the NHS Direct kiosks recorded 12 user sessions per day per kiosk (Table 3.10). This was slightly fewer than that recorded for InTouch with Health (14.6). The average number of pages viewed in a day per kiosk was 70 pages, down on the: InTouch figure of 110.2. Sessions lasted on average just about two minutes, half a minute more than for InTouch users, and individual page view time was about 16 seconds, again some five seconds more than for InTouch users. The general picture then was that NHS kiosks were used, but lightly.

Table 3.10 NHS Direct kiosks – summary kiosk metrics

Metric	123 Kiosks – July
Average daily number of user sessions per day	12
Average daily number of pages viewed per day	70
Average daily number of pages printed per day	N/A
Average session length (seconds)	122
Average page view time (seconds)	16.2

Across all 123 kiosks 46,394 user sessions were recorded and 306,302 pages were viewed in the survey month. On average, users at NHS Direct kiosks viewed between five to six pages in a search session. Kiosks located in areas with a high incidence of microwave ownership recorded 20% longer session, measured by the number of pages viewed, compared to kiosks located in areas which have only a 'low or medium incidence of microwave ownership'. There is evidence to support that prior use of technology, such as microwaves, will impact on kiosk use. Pearson *et al* (1999), in a study of kiosk use by cancer patients, found that those with a previous experience using a video, microwave and cash card were more likely to find a kiosk easier to use and would have a longer session time.

Table 3.11 NHS Direct kiosks – ranked top 20 pages viewed
(hospitals, walk-in centres and supermarkets)

Hospitals		Walk-in Centres		Kwik save	
Topic	*%*	*Topic*	*%*	*Topic*	*%*
Is it ok to drink while pregnant	5	Is it ok to drink while pregnant	4.5	Is it ok to drink while pregnant	8
Eating for health	5	Eating for health	4.3	Eating for health	6.3
Rashes	4.1	Rashes	3.9	Rashes	5.6
Maintain healthy weight	3	Maintain healthy weight	3.1	Maintain healthy weight	2.8
Hands and feet	2.8	Managing stress	2.7	Joint pains	2.6
Accidents	2.5	Losing weight	2.4	Hands and feet	2.5
Quitting smoking	2.4	Quitting smoking	2.4	Getting active	2.5
Losing weight	2.3	Hands and feet	2.3	Managing stress	2.5
Managing stress	2.3	Accidents	2.1	Quitting smoking	2.3
Getting active	2	Thinking about drink	1.9	Thinking about drink	2.1
Thinking about drink	1.9	Getting active	1.8	Losing weight	1.9
Joint pains	1.8	Joint pains	1.8	Accidents	1.8
Burns and scalds	1.2	Burns and scalds	1.6	Burns and scalds	1.7
Itchy rashes	1.2	Itchy rashes	1.4	Child breathing difficulty	1.3
Child breathing difficulty	1	Child breathing difficulty	1	Baby rashes	1.2
Adult chest pain	1	Rashes with fever	1	Rashes with fever	1.2
Smoking and stress	0.9	Baby rashes	1	Smoking stress	1.1
Baby rashes	0.9	Smoking and stress	0.9	Itchy rashes	0.9
Rashes with fever	0.9	The risk of obesity	0.9	The risk of obesity	0.9
Reducing risk	0.9	Adult chest pain	0.8	I would exercise but	0.9
Pages account for	43	Pages account for	42	Pages account for	50

In terms of pages viewed kiosk location was also plainly a significant factor. The top four locations by this metric were kiosks located in docks (173 pages), hospitals (157), walk-in centres (135) and Kwik save supermarkets (104). The most used kiosk, however, was situated at a dock and recorded approximately 173 page views a day. The findings are surprising, especially with regard to docks. However, high volumes of use are in part attributed to the number people passing through each location locations with a large throughput of people, like docks, hospitals and supermarkets, will logically record higher levels of use.

Walk-in centres recorded the highest number of pages viewed in a session (six pages in a session), followed by hospitals (five) and information centres (five). This is, perhaps, not surprising, as one might expect kiosks in a medical location to be more fully consulted than those in other environments.

Hospitals and walk-in centres, both of which performed well in terms of the number of pages viewed in a session and session time, are almost by definition places to research health information. Furthermore, they are places where users might well have the time to search what may well be a new information system. This may not be the case for kiosk users in supermarkets or pharmacies, where there is pressure to perform shopping tasks; locations that did not perform above average by the number of pages viewed in a session and session time.

The most popular page viewed was that detailing the safety issues of drinking while pregnant. Healthy eating, rashes and maintaining a healthy weight were also popular pages. In terms of view time the page on losing weight was viewed the longest (42 seconds) followed by itchy rashes (33 seconds) and adult chest pain (30 seconds). Getting active and maintaining a healthy weight obtained only cursory looks by comparison (both much less than 10 seconds).

Table 3.11 shows the top ranked 20 medical pages viewed for kiosks located in hospitals, walk-in centres and supermarkets (Kwik save). The top 20 pages in each case accounted for approximately 40% of all medical pages viewed.

The ranked top 20 pages viewed by users was very much the same for all three locations, which is perhaps surprising given the very different locations and the different reasons why people would be at these locations. The explanation perhaps lies is the limited content available on the kiosk. In all there were only 500 pages available on NHS Direct kiosks, about half that compared to InTouch with Health kiosks that have about 1,100 pages available though only about 850 pages were generally used.

With 46,394 user sessions being conducted in a month and 306,302 pages viewed, by any standards this has to constitute a significant consumption of health information by the general public. An upward trend in both the number of pages viewed and the number of user sessions was identified, which suggests that the kiosks were possibly becoming increasingly popular, although the date range was of course rather limited to be certain.

Postscript

The Government's direct interest in kiosks came to an end in 2005 and NHS kiosks are no longer a feature of the digital health consumer environment created by the Government, which is somewhat puzzling given their success in other walks of life.

Chapter 4

Health Websites

It has been long established that health information is one of the most frequently sought topics on the Internet. The consumer uptake of electronic health information has been truly phenomenal, especially in the United States. In order to evaluate its impact in the UK we choose to study three leading UK based consumer health websites – SurgeryDoor,[1] NHS Direct Online[2] and Medicdirect.[3] As the first is a commercial site, the second a government funded one and the third run by a consortia of doctors this provided a representative selection of sites. The SurgeryDoor investigation was the lead evaluation and obtains greater coverage, especially in regard to some of the methodological issues that have to be dealt with when evaluating web use. The Medicdirect evaluation provides largely comparative data.

SurgeryDoor

When surgerydoor.co.uk launched on 27th January, 2000, it became one of the UK's first Internet health portals, offering electronic versions of official NHS information, and the country's biggest online health multi-store UK-specific health website (M2 Presswire 2000). The company had formed partnerships with a number of other interactive service providers including well known Internet portals and retail and lifestyle sites.

The site used health advice and information supplied by leading health bodies including the NHS, the Health Education Authority and the Red Cross.[4] It comprised over 5000 pages of content with access to an additional 40,000 pages of local health service maps and listings. The site sold products and services ranging from pharmacy items to healthy foods and health related insurance through the multi-store. Content is closely tailored to a British audience who might find generic or US-influenced health sources off-putting. A home page can be seen in Figure 4.1.

SurgeryDoor provided access to the following content:

* Medical facts covering minor and major conditions and operations.
* First electronic version of NHS Home Healthcare Guide including self-treatment and first aid advice.

---

1   www.surgerydoor.co.uk/
2   www.nhsdirect.nhs.uk/
3   www.medicdirect.co.uk/
4   The editorial team responsible for content was led by the television doctor, Dr Mark Porter, during much of the survey period.

- Maps showing all UK hospitals, general practices, dentists, opticians – searchable by postcode.
- Alternative therapies.
- Full information on all prescription drugs.
- Healthy Living online magazine.
- An online health shopping multi-store.
- Health related weather forecasting and warning service.

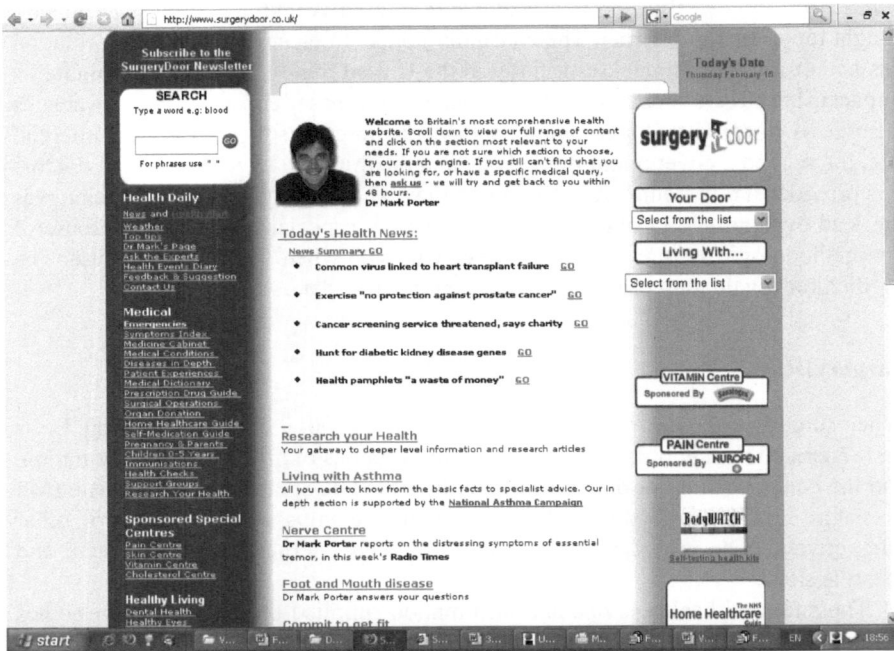

Figure 4.1 SurgeryDoor – homepage

The site featured targeted sections, providing health advice for groups such as teenagers, carers, women, travellers and disabled groups.

Site content was divided into the following sections, each of which appeared as main content entries on a side bar, and contained a series of subheadings:

- Health daily (news and health alert, weather, tips etc.);
- Medical (emergencies, medical dictionary, drug guide etc.);
- Healthy living (preventing accidents, dental health, advice on alcohol etc.);
- Sponsored special centres (e.g. Skin Centre sponsored by Balneum);
- NHS and benefits (leads to external pages such as 'Health in your area');
- Complementary medicine (an A to Z of Complementary Medicine);
- Travel health (vaccination, travel health kit etc.);

- Community and fun, and (feedback, suggestions, patients experiences and so on);
- Shopping (to buy online).

The site offered many facilities for user contributions and feedback. These were:

- Patient experiences, which allows patients to post messages describing various aspects of their condition and their experiences of it;
- Message boards; inviting users to 'swap ideas, questions and answers';
- Feedback and suggestions, which is an email link to SurgeryDoor, and
- Health surveys. The current, and first, one of these was about the SurgeryDoor site itself.

Use and users

During the 12-month survey period, October 2001 to September 2002, there were approximately 1,926 users per day. The average number of pages viewed in a day was about 8,369 pages. Sessions lasted on average about five minutes and individual page view time was about 30 seconds. The site was visited by 381,704 separate IP (Internet Protocol) addresses (excluding declared robots) over the survey period. Figure 4.2 provides a breakdown of the pattern of return visits for robot and non-robot users over a 12-month period. Robots or electronic agents were more likely to return to the site, 69% did compared to just 14% of non-robot users. Robots and agents will return to monitor changes in content. Individual users (non-robot users) were less likely to return to the site, nearly nine in 10 users only visited the site once, approximately 11% of users visited between two to five times and 3% visited six or more times. However, this does not give a correct picture of the pattern of return visits. The analysis does not allow for the problems of proxy servers and floating IP addresses; both of which impact on the pattern of return visits and give a distorted picture. The impact of proxy servers overestimates returnees as lots of users share the same IP number while floating IP numbers underestimates returnees, as users may be allocated a different IP number, by their provider, for each Internet session.

Web logs provide an Internet Protocol (IP) number to identify the user. However, as mentioned, the IP number cannot be traced back to an individual, only to a machine. And the use of proxy servers connections mean that the IP address cannot be assumed to relate to use on a specific machine, use in this case relates to a group of users, rather than an individual. Furthermore, access to a site may be via an IP number allocated temporarily to a client's machine. Net providers have a bank of IP numbers that are shared out as requested to users and returned to the bank ready for use by another user. Both the use of proxy servers and the use of floating IP numbers means that the tracking return visits via the IP number is not a reliable procedure.

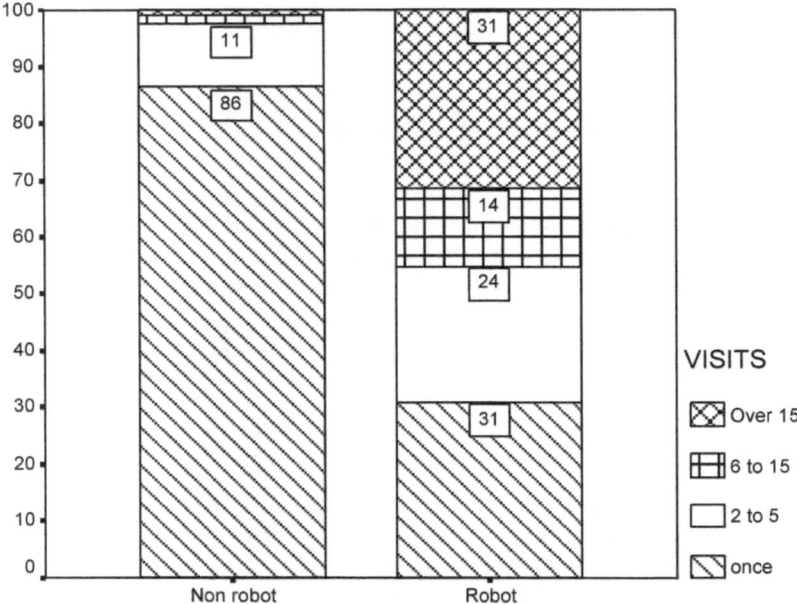

Figure 4.2 SurgeryDoor – number of times users visited by type of user

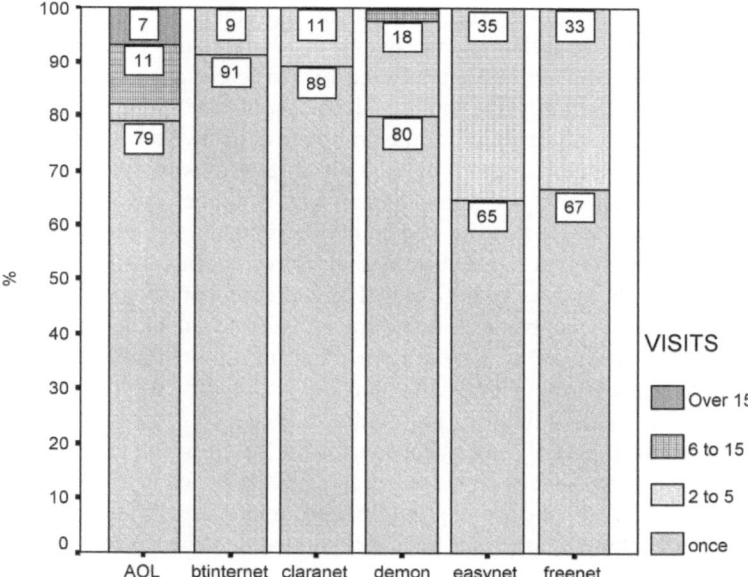

Figure 4.3 SurgeryDoor – number of times users visited by net provider of user

However, not all IP providers use the system of allocating users with a floating IP addresses. Some providers allocate a dedicated IP number to each of their users. In part the IP allocation policy of a Net provider can be guessed by looking at the structure of the IP address or the reverse DNS (Domain Name Server) look up. Easynet, which accounts for less than 1% of users, for example, allocates a separate IP number to each user and also does not operate as a proxy server for users. Figure 4.3 compares the estimated return visits for six IP providers, AOL, BtInternet, Claranet, Demon, Easynet and Freenet. For example if we used Easynet users to estimate returnees, on the basis that these users were not allocated with floating IP addresses and hence, arguably, gives a more robust estimate of returnees, then 35% visited more than once in the 12 month survey period and 65% just visited once. This still produces a high figure for those not returning but it is lower, and more realistic, than the original estimate of 89% given above.

3,680,453 pages were viewed during the survey period (Figure 4.4). Average daily use numbers in the 12-month period remained stable. The average daily figure over the year was 8,369 page views.

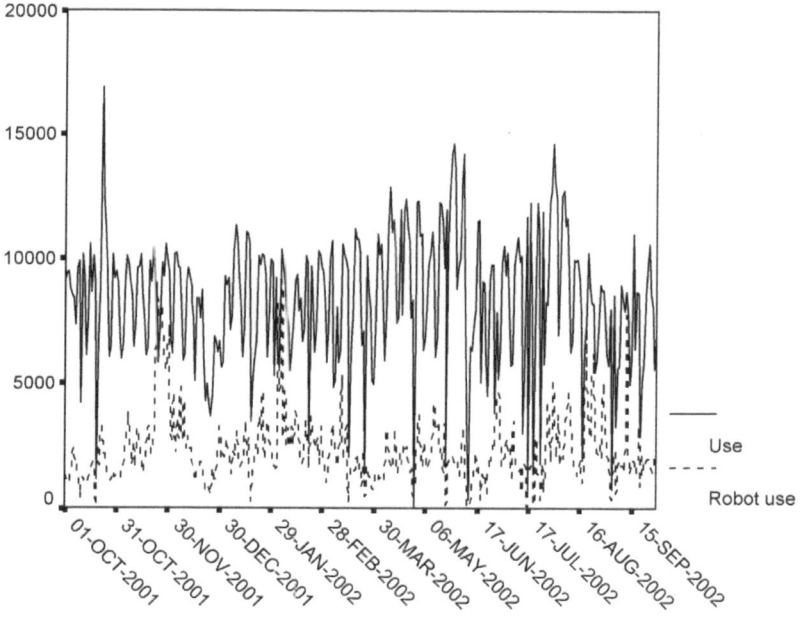

Figure 4.4 Daily use of SurgeryDoor website

A slight rising pattern in the weekly frequency of IP numbers (users) was recorded over the period. The daily average for the year was about 1,926 different IP numbers accessing the site a week. The figures seem to reflect a mature market with both use and users remaining much the same over the period. There was a small rising trend in the number of users over the period. This was not accompanied by increases in use, suggesting that there has been an increase in the number of users looking, but not making significant use of the site.

Estimates of use maybe under-reported as a result of caching. Caching is an Internet browser feature which is switched on at the client's machine and means that pages once viewed are available from the terminal being used. Thus, any pages re-viewed do not have to be downloaded again from the server, obviously saving considerable time. From the point of view of evaluating logs, however, this practice creates a problem. Views of previously seen pages are made from the cache and are therefore not recorded by the server access log file as files used. Caching can significantly result in the under recording of the number of pages viewed, especially where single HTML pages contain information on a number of topics, with a menu structured as internal links at the top of the page. In these cases users would have cached a multiple topic information page and a menu page by downloading just one page. The user could then access the cached information and menu page 'exploring' a number of related topics without requesting further pages from the server. Caching creates a false picture in that it negatively impacts on two key metrics: it under-reports the number of pages viewed and provides incorrect page view times. Caching only concerns web logs and, thankfully, is not an issue with the logs of kiosks and DiTV, which we shall deal with later.

There were, on average about two pages viewed in a session. However, the distribution was heavily skewed and sessions were grouped into how many pages were viewed. This metric gives an idea of how much of the site was penetrated. Approximately 74% of user sessions featured three or fewer views, 20% between four and 10 and 6% had 11 or more.

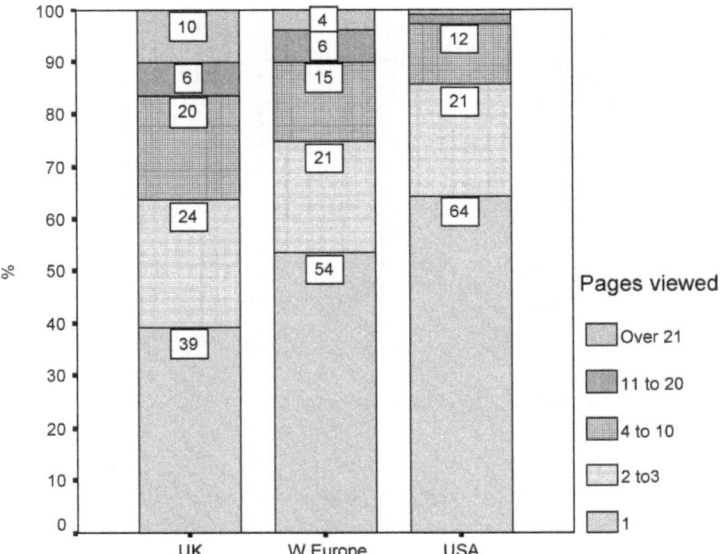

Figure 4.5 SurgeryDoor – pages viewed in a session by country (academic IP addresses only)

Figure 4.5 groups the number of pages viewed in a session by location for academic institutions only. The analysis is limited to academic users as they provide a fairer indication of their true geographical location, as academic institutes are much more likely to register their domain name server in the country where they are located – see below. The Figure shows that UK users were more likely to view a greater number of pages in a session compared to either US or other Western European users. Only 39% of UK users viewed one page only, as compared to 64% of US users and 54% of Western European users. This is thought to reflect a preference among health consumers to view home-based sites.

On average, a user session lasted for about five minutes. Users may have left their browser open on the site while they did something else and this resulted partly in the skewed distribution, however the problems of a skewed distribution were met by using the robust estimator (Huber's M-estimator). Figure 4.6 looks at median session time in seconds by grouped number of pages viewed. As expected, users who viewed more pages conducted longer sessions. Hence, users looking at 11 to 20 pages in a session recorded a viewing time of approximately 20 minutes and users looking at between one to three pages conducted sessions that lasted just under one and half minutes.

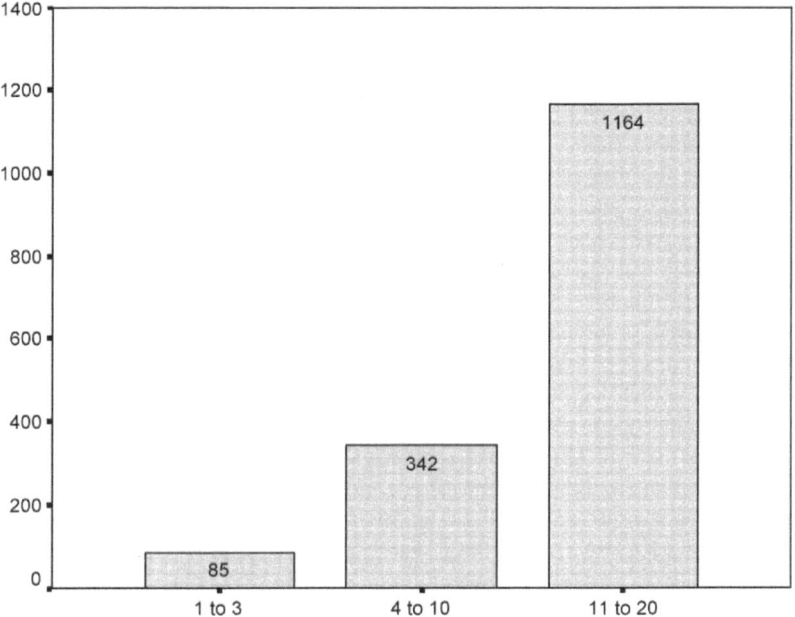

Figure 4.6 SurgeryDoor – session time (median) by number of pages viewed (grouped)

Page or screen view time is determined by calculating the difference between time stamps. Just under half of all page views, 47%, had a view time of 30 seconds and under. Sixteen percent had a page view time of between 30 seconds and a minute, 12% had a view time of between one minute to two minutes and 10% between two to five minutes. About 15% had a view time greater than five minutes, which is a high page view time and suggests that these users have in fact left the page open while they do something else.

In terms of views by day of week Mondays and Tuesdays were slightly more popular than the rest of the week. This may reflect postponed use from the weekend, with people taking advantage of free work place access. Weekends were generally not very popular times to search the service. Afternoons and early evenings were key viewing times, however.

Categorising users

The geographical categorisation of the users was based on their IP addresses. However, as hinted earlier, it should be noted that the IP address is not a wholly reliable indication of either the user's location or organisation affiliation. This is because non-USA users can choose to have a USA registered IP address. Quite a few UK based commercial companies and UK Net providers will have USA registered IP addresses. Use related to these companies will be attributed as USA when in fact the users were located in the UK and this results in an over estimation of users coming from the USA This phenomenon was discussed in detail in Nicholas *et al* (2000). This is less the case with academic institutions because they do not follow this practice and tend to register their IP number in the country in which they are located. Academic IP numbers are therefore a more realistic basis for comparing use by geographical location.

The largest number of users – nearly one in eight – had a USA IP address and only 9% had a UK address. In terms of the use (number of pages viewed), again most use – nearly 71% – came from IP addresses registered in USA and 22% of use originated form UK registered IP addresses. Comparing use and users, it is apparent that USA users left the site without having viewed as many pages as UK users. As we have mentioned earlier this seems to suggest that a good number of users preferred websites that originate in their own country.

Fifty eight percent of users accessed the site via a commercial institution, although these users made up nearly three-quarters (73%) of pages viewed. About 36% of users accessed SurgeryDoor via a net provider (home users probably); however, these users only accounted for 20% of use. A result which indicates that these users were perhaps not penetrating the site and were bouncing out of their session early on (maybe, to go elsewhere in their search for health information?). These users were more likely to have used a search engine, such as Google, employing the links supplied by Google to jump from site to site.

Looking at just academic users and extrapolating the figures to the whole population of users, it can be concluded that 35% of users and 70% of use originated from the UK This is a more realistic country distribution compared to the distribution of 9% and 20% indicated originally.

Well over half (55%) of respondents who used SurgeryDoor were women and this compared to 44% of respondents who used other health Internet sites. The comparative figure for health touchscreen kiosk users varied between 50–55 %. Comparing age distribution for those respondents who had used SurgeryDoor and those that had not, it was found that SurgeryDoor had a slightly older profile and 56% of respondents who had used this site were aged 45 and over as compared to 47% in the same age bracket who used other health sites.

Health topics

Clearly content must be one of the most important reasons for using a health website, but precisely what type of content interested people? Users were asked to score their preference for 12 health topics, such as new treatments, natural health, pregnancy etc. The scores were 1 to 4, from not important to very important. The two most importantly rated topics were general health information (3.3) and diet (3.2). Relatively poorly performing topics included information on medical conditions (1.8), pregnancy (2.2) and support groups (2.3). This may well reflect user interest in coming to this particular site and, possibly, they obtained the latter information topics elsewhere.

A factor analysis identified specific user groups by topic of interest. The four following types of 'topic' user groups could be identified. The combined factors accounted for about 60% of the variance.

- 'alternative remedy' users,
- 'keep fit and healthy' users,
- 'keeping up to date' users, and
- 'ill but want to know more' users.

'Alternative remedy' users rated the two topics, natural health and complementary medicine most highly, while the 'fit and healthy' group rated healthy living, general health and diet topics most highly. The third user type was those people that rated medical news and research highly and suggested that these users 'wanted to keep up to date'. The fourth group rated prescription drugs and new treatments highly, which suggested a type of user who maybe 'ill but wants to know' about what they've been prescribed and about new treatments.

Age, gender and for whom the person was searching were significant characteristics of the alternative remedy group. Thus, 'alternative remedy' users tended to be women under the age of 34 and tended to search on behalf of friends and children. However, these people were also using this information for themselves and for their dependants. The alternative remedy user was young, maybe considered this interest as 'fashionable'; however they were developing an interest in health information from their interest in alternative and complementary medicines.

The fit and healthy information user group was found to relate to the user's current health status, and, not surprisingly, those who were currently healthy, scored highly. These users, it seemed, were accessing content so as to 'stay' fit and healthy and to check health requirements. A low positive correlation (0.27) was also found between 'content' attributes and this type of user, suggesting that these users were interested in the depth and quality of content. This may indicate a wealthy or educated user who understands the value of health information in looking and staying healthy.

The 'ill but wants to know more' type of user, was found, perhaps unsurprisingly, to relate to the person's current health status, with carers, those currently suffering and those who had a long term illness being more likely to feature in this group. These users have been put into the position by reason of their health to seek and understand the importance of health information. This was also true to a certain extent for users identified as wanting to keep up to date. Those people with a long-term illness also sought to keep up to date with health information. Furthermore, those users searching for other people and for children also featured strongly in the 'ill but wants to know more' user group. The two groups, 'ill but wants to know more' and 'keeping up to date', may differ in their illness type, there attitude towards the limitations of the health information on the web.

Health topics viewed (Logs) Logs were also a source of information on what topics were viewed. The top ranked 20 pages for each month accounted for approximately 80% of page use (Table 4.1) – quite a concentration in use. Views to menu pages accounted for about 45% of use and can easily be spotted on the first line of each month's listing. Child Health, Health Lifestyle and Exercise, Pharmacy, Health News and Sexual Health were popular topics and appeared in the top ten topics viewed for each month. Winter illness appeared in the top 20 topics only twice – in December 2001 and February 2002. The separate sections, Women's Health and Men's Health, were also popular, suggesting that users liked the health distinctions made. Alternative Medicine appeared in the top 20 each month for the six-month period October 2001 to March 2002 but dropped out of the ranking for the period June 2002 to September 2002. The topic Communicable Diseases appeared in the top 20 only once for November 2002.

The amount of time spent viewing different health topics varied. The longest viewing time was for Drug miss-use (54 seconds), Research (51 seconds) and Allergies (50 seconds). Interestingly, the NHS obtained the shortest viewing time, just five seconds. Addiction (9 seconds) was another topic to obtain only cursory treatment.

Usability and accessibility issues

Usability was assessed with the aid of a number of volunteer participants and also by including usability issues on an online questionnaire which was part of a UK national study of the use of the Internet for health information. Respondents in the latter study were asked how they accessed the site. Most people had arrived at a health site via a search engine (30%) or had found the site after having read about it (28.5%) – the latter provides a good example of how the various media entwine. We might have expected far more respondents to have found the site using online methods. Only just over half of respondents used online methods to find SurgeryDoor: 30% had found the site via a search engine, 19% via casual browsing and 11% had found it via online or off line advertisements. This might indicate a difficulty, for some users at least, in finding sites online. The Internet is not a plug in and go information platform, users are confronted with significant complications with regard to finding, assessing and navigating between sites. Interestingly – and maybe worryingly in the light of our comments about information source relationships and partnerships, very few people (2.3%) were recommended to the site by their doctor (Figure 4.7).

Table 4.1 SurgeryDoor – ranking of pages viewed grouped by subject category (October to December 2001)

October	%	November	%	December	%
Menus	38	Menus	44	Menus	45
General	6.1	Unclassified	4.9	Unclassified	4.8
Unclassified	5	General	4.3	General	4.2
Child Health	3.8	Search	3.4	Health lifestyle exercise	3.6
Health lifestyle exercise	3.2	Child Health	3.4	Child Health	3.4
Pharmacy	3	Health lifestyle exercise	3.2	Search	3.3
Search	2.8	Pharmacy	2.7	Pharmacy	2.9
Health News	2.8	Sexual Health	2.4	Health News	2.4
Diet	2.3	Diet	2.3	Women's Health	1.9
Sexual Health	2.2	Women's Health	2.1	Dental	1.9
Pregnancy	2.2	Health News	2	Sexual Health	1.8
Accident and Emergency	2	Pregnancy	2	Pregnancy	1.8
Women's Health	2	Dental	1.7	Diet	1.6
Ear Nose and Throat	1.8	Men's Health	1.7	Research	1.6
Alternative medicine	1.6	Ear Nose and Throat	1.6	Men's Health	1.6
Communicable Disease	1.6	Alternative medicine	1.5	Alternative medicine	1.5
Dental	1.6	Accident and Emergency	1.2	Ear Nose and Throat	1.5
Men's Health	1.6	Communicable Disease	1	Winter illness	1.1
NHS	1.1	NHS	1	Accident and Emergency	1
Travel	1	Alcohol	0.9	Migraine and Headaches	1
% of all page views	85	% of all page views	87	% of all page views	87

People were further asked what online methods they used to locate health information sites. Respondents were questioned as to whether they used a search engine, re-visited a site, clicked on a health link or clicked on a banner advertisement. The results are reported in Figure 4.8.

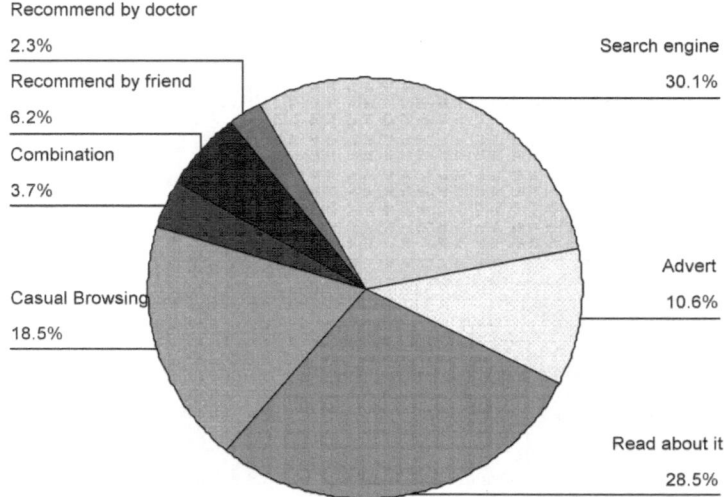

Figure 4.7 SurgeryDoor – how users found the site

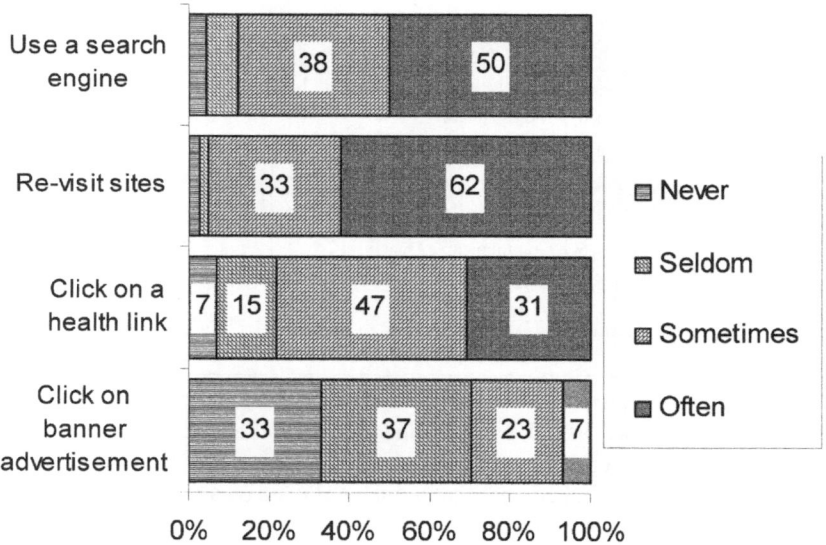

Figure 4.8 SurgeryDoor – in general, when searching for health information on the Internet, did you ... ? (%)

Most SurgeryDoor users located health information by re-visiting sites that they had previously visited: 62% of respondents often did this, 33% said that they sometimes did this (the log studies would show that people might have been exaggerating the extent to which they did this). Using a search engine was also popular and 88% said that they had often (50%) or sometimes done (38%) this. Clearly people were using both methods – returning to favoured sites but also comparing information with additional sources found by using a search engine. A surprisingly high percentage said that they had clicked on health links: 31% said that they had often done this, while 47% said that they sometimes did. Respondents, it seemed, did value and will use health links and references placed on web pages. Clicking on a health banner advert was, unsurprisingly, found to be the least popular way of finding health information. Only 7% said that they had often done this while 23% said that they sometimes had. Most respondents, 37%, said that they seldom clicked on a health banner advert while 33% said that they never did. Banner advertisements may not be a particularly good method for directing people to health sites.

There were differences between the various user groups. Thus women were more likely to have clicked on a health banner advertisement: 31% had either sometimes or often done this, compared to 21% of men.[5] Furthermore, Sun newspaper readers were most likely to do this while Guardian newspaper readers were least likely to: 53% of Sun readers had clicked on a banner advertisement either sometimes or often compared to only 8% of Guardian readers[6] – a significant difference. Additionally, those earning less than £30,000 were more likely to click on such adverts – about 35% did as compared to about 23% of respondents earning £30,000 and over.[7] There appears to be a social divide here, with those earning less and tabloid newspaper readers being more likely to view banner adverts. We believe that this may reflect differences in engaging with digital text menus and that tabloid readers may well respond better to pictorial or icon based menu objects.

Those in full time employment were more likely to use a search engine: 91% did so compared to 82% in other employment groupings.[8] This group were also more likely to have revisited sites, 98% did so compared to 93% for the others.[9] However, it seemed likely that these users were more experienced and more regular web users and may have had access to the Internet at work.

What then were the key barriers to using SurgeryDoor? The focus here was on reading from a screen, navigating around it, or downloading information. We examined usability issues in a controlled environment (see also Williams *et al* 2002b; 2002c). It was carried out with 20 research volunteers, who were first asked to examine the site in their own way, looking at pages of personal choice and navigating through the system as they desired. Secondly, directed use was undertaken, where information retrieval tasks were set.

Four retrieval tasks were set as described below:

Task 1: What is the telephone number of the British Red Cross? This task was included as a simple fact finding one; however, it was not as straightforward as

---

5   6.4 2df p=.04 (chi-square test).
6   24.2 10df p=.007 (chi-square test).
7   17.8 10 df p=.059 (chi-square test).
8   7.3 2df p=.026 (chi-square test).
9   11.8 2df p=.003 (chi-square test).

envisaged. A large majority of users (75%) took the search engine route at some point in the conducting of the task, 12 (60%) of them doing so as a first step in the exercise. Problems arose when the term 'Red Cross' without speech marks, lower or title case, did not yield any page containing the required information. Using the correct procedure, however (i.e. with phrases in parentheses), generated a hit list that did. Other users accessed the required page by browsing.

Task 2: Find the names and addresses of all the GP surgeries in your own area. This proved to be a surprisingly simple task. Eleven (55%) users accessed the information easily, using the map of Britain at the bottom of the home page. The successful completion of this task was attributable to two 'signposts' on the home page. These were the map of Britain and a menu link to 'your home area', both of which obviated the need either for browsing menus and links, or for undertaking a direct search.

Task 3: What are the causes of and treatments for shock? It was hoped that this question would yield a variety of answers and information retrieval methods. There were, indeed, several search avenues explored in carrying out this task, each one leading to the same page and the same information. The most common tactic (undertaken by 30% of users) was to look at the First Aid menu first. Unlike the first task, more people adopted this form of browsing behaviour rather than use the search facility during the search, because there was a main menu item of clear relevance available as a starting point.

Task 4: To what extent does diet play a part in the prevention of cancer? What types of cancer are most affected by diet, and what types have little or no relationship to it? This was more of an investigative question, for which more time was required, and one to which perhaps the site was not best suited. Many participants spent up to the allotted 20 minutes trying to find something relevant. No one found a satisfactory page, although the required information was to be found within the pages devoted to individual types of cancer. Interestingly, although the search facility was used by all but one of the students, not one person included the word 'prevention' as a search term.

By the end of the session, all users had managed to find pages on various different types of cancer, and, given more time, could have researched the topic from these individual pages. No one, however, was able to find a page presenting information about the disease in general terms and including a section on diet. This prompted two users to say that, as cancer was such an important topic, about which a great many SurgeryDoor users probably seek information, it would be a good idea to include the topic as a main menu item in its own right.

Many implications for site creation and development, construction and layout could be drawn from the study. For example, a larger and better-placed logo and other measures were needed to provide a clear identity for a site.

A number of salutary points emerged regarding site navigation. As the present writers found with a study of newspaper sites (Williams and Nicholas 2001b) contents lists and indexes liberally scattered over various pages – in an attempt to provide a sense of organisation – do not always aid the navigation process. Nielsen (1994) too, has found from his usability studies that users ignore navigational aids where these are perceived as being excessive. In the study reported here, users simply became confused as to which list to consult. Some even spent time trying to work out the criteria by which some entries appear on each particular list. Equally problematic was the way the left menu bar changed appearance and content when certain sections of the site were accessed. Users feel comfortable with consistency, and a constant point of reference would have been a positive feature.

Retrieving information by direct searching rather than site navigation proved popular. As mentioned above, many users either did not use the required parentheses or did so inappropriately (i.e. by enclosing individual words of a search term rather than the phrase itself), In consequence information that was on the site was not retrieved. As described, operators were used, but generally after no relevant articles had been retrieved from an initial search.

A clear message emerged that users were by now so familiar with inputting terms without operators, parentheses or any other additional element, that to do otherwise was confusing. It may be that there was an assumption that the site search engine worked in the same way as Yahoo! or AltaVista – by the simple input of a number of words. The concern about retrieving items that contained the search terms but were only marginally relevant implies that if a site is to contain a search facility, a best match term weighting system would be the most appropriate.

What the students did not comment on was also revealing. The lack of attention to issues of authority, attribution and currency has already been discussed. The lack of interest in interactivity is also noteworthy. This aspect of the web is often considered one of its main attractions, although previous work by the present writers (Williams and Nicholas 1998) and others has also shown a surprising lack of take up and interest in this facility. Chapman (1998), for example, notes in his account of use of a regional newspaper online, that take up of the interactive element 'has been noticeably (and interestingly) lacking'. Our participants may have been different from some other users, however, in that they were not looking for emotional support or the reassurance of shared experience, which might be relevant to people concerned about their health, or that of a close relative.

To measure the readability of the SurgeryDoor website, four pages were taken from different sections of the site, and Microsoft Word's readability scores taken of them.

The results showed that SurgeryDoor was written at a level that many people would not understand. The mean score for the Reading Ease measure is 53.4, ten points below that recommended by Word. This is classed as 'fairly difficult', readable only by US High School students or above – roughly equated in England to GCSE level. The researchers also used Flesch scores (from Smith 1998) to test the readability of the site.

The main conclusion from all this is that the site may have contained information that was too difficult for some potential users to understand, requiring, therefore, some thought on the part of the site developers. In an article by the present writers with regard to non-use of information systems (Williams *et al* 2003b) the idea was floated of organising information into different levels of detail. That paper sought to address the problem of a lack of interest on the part of some people for detailed health information. However, the suggestion offered applies equally to readability. Touchscreen and web 'point and click' interfaces both facilitate such hierarchies of information. What may be beneficial would be to provide 'vertical' layers of pages offering information on each topic at different depths or levels of detail and complexity of language. This would complement the more common 'lateral' arrangement of material organised by topic. Those who found it difficult to read to an 'adult' level (e.g. GCSE standard) would be able to obtain information from the top level of the site, whilst other users could drill down to an appropriate level dependent on their interest and reading capacity.

Not all users will respond or relate to the site's attributes in the same way, and it is a valuable exercise to classify them according to the characteristics to which they did relate. Of course, some attributes might be seen to conflict with each other – for example, ease of navigational structure and breadth of content. Thus, as content increases, the navigational structure becomes more complex and might prove to be difficult to understand. There are conflicts between other characteristics as well; thus where advertising is thought to be intrusive there is a reduction in the perceived trustworthiness in the site.

A factor analysis, which identifies un-correlated or independent combinations of variables in the responses of how users rated each attribute, was conducted to see if meaningful groupings could be found, and the following relations were revealed.

- Site visitors who favoured content were interested in breadth, depth and trust. Users most interested in facilities were happy with advertisements, shopping and email facilities, while 'system people' related favourably to the characteristics of speed of delivery and navigational ease.
- The user's rating fell as the number of sites visited increased. This suggests that that there is a group of people who believe they have to visit many sites to find what they want. We can call these people 'site checkers' or 'end-user evaluators'. They largely do this checking on the basis of long-experience of searching the web, a lot of practice in making constant comparisons and a through a process of trial and error. The Web provides a huge opportunity to 'suck it and see' and these people take full advantage of this.
- The older the users, the less happy they were with the system. This might result from a number of factors, including the fact that older people would be less familiar with Internet technology, like chat rooms and emails, have more fears about the security of online shopping and disapprove more of advertisements.
- Women were more likely than men to be happy with facilities. Women also tended to be more satisfied and less critical with regard to speed of delivery and navigation ease.
- Those people who visited the site less frequently scored lower on system attributes (speed and navigation). Logic suggests that these people were irregular users because of these factors (which they didn't like) or, perhaps they were just unhappy with a site with which they were not familiar. Furthermore,

some users may have had a slow Internet connection and consequently blamed the site rather than their own computer set up for this.
- Carers and those users currently suffering from an illness were found to be much more positive in regard to the site's system attributes.

Usefulness, outcomes and trust

This section is concerned with the following:

- Relative usefulness of the Internet compared to other health information sources
- Usefulness in meeting information needs
- Range and quality of content
- General benefits of the Internet
- Trust and authority of the Internet
- Outcomes: information and dealing with medical professionals

Of course, the non-use section says volumes on usefulness, and it should be read in that context.

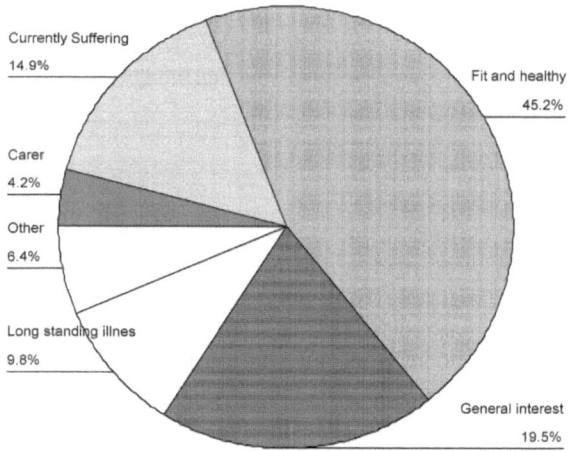

Figure 4.9 SurgeryDoor – user's first health interest

Significantly, although users were accessing the site for information on a particular condition, the largest percentage (45%) of people searched for information connected to being fit and healthy (Figure 4.9). The second biggest group were those who said that they only had a general health interest (19%). It is just as well to remember that up to 40 to 45% of users will be searching on behalf of someone else, and were perhaps not suffering themselves but searching on behalf of people who were suffering; although clearly many users will be searching to stay fit and healthy.

15% of visitors to the site were currently suffering from an illness and 10% as a result of a long-standing illness. Respondents were asked about a second health interest but most people (61%) did not have another although, plainly, general interest and curiosity loomed large.

The majority (66%) said they were searching the site for a specific purpose. Just under a quarter (23%) were at the site simply to browse the general health news. There was a relationship between the reason for using the site and the importance of the topic for the users. For example, those users with a long standing illness were, not surprisingly, more likely to find information on prescription drugs, new treatments, medical news and medical research very important compared to those users who described themselves as having a general interest.

Commercialism has always proved a contentious issue in the health information field, so health consumers were asked how helpful they found health information distributed by commercial companies' websites. In all, over half (53%) of respondents said that they had not returned to a site because it was too commercial. SurgeryDoor respondents were asked as to how helpful they found health company links, health warning links, publicity material and drug company information.

Surprisingly, health-warning links were considered less helpful than the online information put out by drug companies. Most respondents (55%) thought that drug company information sites and links were either very (15%) or fairly (40%) helpful.

Educational background proved to be important regarding the responses to how helpful health company advertisement links were. Those with a post graduate or a degree qualification were least likely to say that health company advertisement links provided fairly or very helpful information: 11% of postgraduates and 16% with a degree qualification said this compared to 33% with a GNVQ or O level qualifications. This seems to indicate that the user's level of education impacted on how critical they were of this link.

A further factor in the reason for use is whom the user searched the site for. Almost one in two (48%) searches conducted on the Internet were undertaken on behalf of someone else (Figure 4.10). Around 17% sought information for a partner, 16% for a child and 14% for a relative. Thus it seems that, while family and relatives were not consulted for health information, they were key information triggers. These users may function as health information gatekeepers or gateways for an inner social circle of family and friends. Further, this is not really so different to how other health (non-digital) information sources are used. However, this whole topic clearly needs further investigation and if it really is the case that there are many people mediating on behalf of others in this field then the NHS and other health organisation will have to take cognisance of this in the design and delivery of their information systems with this in mind.

Users of SurgeryDoor website were asked how they rated the trustworthiness of the site. Perhaps, unsurprisingly, very few respondents rated SurgeryDoor's trustworthiness as poor. Three quarters of respondents either rated the site as either good or excellent. We might have expected this as people were unlikely to use the site if they did not trust the content.

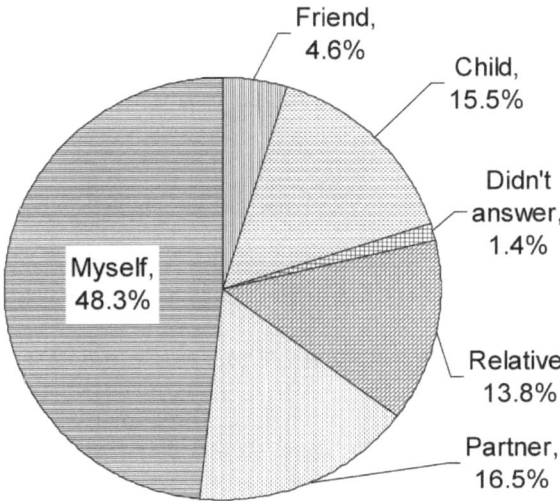

Figure 4.10 SurgeryDoor – on whose behalf people searched

A number of factors seem to have impacted on the way users rated trustworthiness of the site. There was a relationship between how the respondent heard about SurgeryDoor and the site's rating. Those respondents who were recommended the site were least likely to say that site trustworthiness was poor or OK. Users who arrived at the site via an advertisement or a search engine were most likely to rate trustworthiness as either poor or OK. Those who had read about the site were more likely to rate the site as excellent.

Advertisements on the site also impacted on views as to the site's trustworthiness. Those finding the number of advertisements as either poor or OK were more likely to report that the sites trustworthiness was also only poor or OK. One third of users who found the advertising content poor also rated the trustworthiness as poor or OK. The issue of advertising was also raised during a usability study. Some participants were very sensitive to the commercial aspects of the site, and felt a certain distrust of the commercial part of the site. This may be due to the fact that, in Britain anyway, there is a widespread perception that health care (and, by implication, health information) should be free at the point of delivery. A questionnaire study of SurgeryDoor, a site that carries advertisements, found that just 53% of respondents said that they had not returned to a site because it was too commercial.

A person's trust in a site was also found to be a significant factor on health outcome, with those users demonstrating the greatest trust being more likely to claim a positive health outcome. Importantly, it was found that those rating the site's trustworthiness as either good or excellent were more likely to say that they had been helped a lot and were less likely to say that the site was of no help.

Outcomes and impacts

SurgeryDoor visitors were asked the following questions about possible health outcomes and were given three possible answers (helped a lot, helped a little, no help):

- how the Internet information they located had helped them in dealing with their doctor;
- whether they felt better informed as a result of using Internet health sites;
- if the information found on the Internet had changed the way they felt about their condition; and
- whether their condition had improved as a result of finding information on the Internet.

Most (80%) users felt that the information that they found had helped in their dealings with the doctor and nearly half (41%) said it had helped a lot. Supporting the findings of earlier studies, (i.e. Cyber Dialogue, 2000), most people (97%) said they felt better informed about a condition after having used the site and two-thirds felt they were helped 'a lot' in becoming better informed. Again, the vast majority (82%) of SurgeryDoor users felt that the information they found had changed the way they felt about their condition. With the obvious caveats, most important amongst them being that this was a self-selecting online sample, these results seem encouraging for digital health providers, and especially the NHS as it embarks on a costly programme of digital information provision. Even better news was contained in the answer to the question whether the respondent's condition had improved as a result of finding information on the site. Approaching three-fifths (59%) of respondents went on to say that their condition had improved after having visited the site, with 11% saying that information found had helped a lot in improving their condition. This must surely be of great significance – and offer comfort to NHS Direct, whose telephone hotline has been roundly condemned by many health professionals (Marsh 2000) and had not impressed the British Medical Association (Carvel 2000). Indeed, even their fledgling NHS DIRECT website has attracted criticism (BMA 2000).

Some factors affected the answers by the users to the aforementioned questions. Significantly, who they searched for had an impact on their response – specifically in regard to how they felt about the condition and if the information found improved it. Respondents were more likely to say 'No help' if searching on their own behalf. They were more likely to say the information was 'helpful' if they were searching for someone else.

Users were also more likely to report 'No help' in the improvement to their condition if they were currently suffering or had a long-term illness. Of course, it may be that those who were into a cycle of a long term illness may well have gained much of the information they required to manage their condition from alternative sources. It was really people who were seeking fitness and general information who reported the most improvement and this might have been expected.

Users were more likely to say that they had become better informed if they were regular users of the Internet. Those using the web once a day were twice as likely to report that they had been 'helped a lot' in terms of being better informed from information found on the Web as compared to those who surfed the web only once a month.

People were likely to say that they had been 'helped' if they were regular users of the SurgeryDoor site. This was true on all four measures of health outcome. People using the site regularly were more likely to say that they found the information 'helpful' compared to users who use the site infrequently.

A person's trust in a site was also found to be a significant factor on health outcomes, with those users demonstrating the greatest trust being more likely to claim a positive health outcome.

People were also asked if they ever used information found on the Web as an alternative to seeing the doctor. In other words, was the information found sufficient, in their judgement, to meet their health query and substitute for a visit to the doctor? Ninety eight percent of users answered this question of which 27% confirmed that web information had indeed replaced a visit to the doctor. This is plainly very significant data, with self-help being one of the NHS' goals in providing health information. However, this result needs to be put into context. It should be noted that the percentage (27%) is no different from what we might expect regarding the use of most health information sources, that is we expect around 30% of those using health information, from any source, to use it in this way. It has been found that those respondents 'very interested' in the Internet, though, were twice as likely to use information in this way compared to those not interested, not very interested or fairly interested in the Internet. We suspect that the Internet is used as a source of information to substitute for a doctor's visit, but this is particularly true for those respondents who are both technically proficient and confident in using the Web.

Those people who were currently suffering from a health problem were more than two and half times, as likely compared to respondents with a long standing illness, to say that they had used information from the Internet as an alternative to seeing their GP. Those visiting only one health site were less likely to use Internet information as an alternative to a visit to a doctor compared to those visiting more than one site. Trust of the site was a factor, with those rating the site as excellent, more likely by half to use web-based information as an alternative.

Importantly, who the user was searching for was a significant factor. This was particularly so when the searcher wanted information for a child. This group were almost twice as likely to use web information as an alternative to a visit to a doctor compared to users searching only for themselves. Interestingly, age was also a significant factor, with those aged between 55 and 74 being 50% less likely to use web-based information in this way. The respondent's positive rating of the importance of complimentary medicine was also found to be significant and may say something about the information users' belief in traditional medicine and the willingness to try something found on the web. Respondents using the web to look for alternative health advice were an important group. Those respondents who were currently fit and healthy or who were currently suffering were twice as likely to have used health information found on the Internet as a substitute for a visit to the doctor compared to those with a long-standing illness. This may indicate that a site like SurgeryDoor was unlikely to be particularly helpful to those suffering from a long-term condition; perhaps, because these people were already quite knowledgeable about their condition, or because it does not take long to assimilate the limited information found on any particular condition from the SurgeryDoor site itself. In addition, those people that rated the trust of the site as being excellent were about one and a half times more likely to have used information as a substitute compared to those just visiting one site. Preliminary chi-square analysis indicated that recognition of an affinity with Dr. Mark Porter, the television celebrity associated with the site, was also a factor. SurgeryDoor provided a facility by which its users could email Dr Porter for medical advice. Forty three percent, compared to the sample (population) of 27%, said that the 'Dr Mark Porter' section proved an alternative to seeing the doctor. However, the small number answering this question and the way the question was framed prevented inclusion of this in the full analysis.

Use of other health information sources

An online questionnaire hosted on the SurgeryDoor Website for a month asked visitors about the information sources they went to when they needed medical information. Most used a combination of sources, with only 12% of respondents claiming to use only one information source. Sixty percent used up to three sources. Just over 50% said they used their doctor as their first port of call, while 38% said they used health leaflets first (Figure 4.11). It is interesting that leaflets, a grey literature source, still held their own in the light of increased consumer health coverage in the media and the growing presence of the Web. The Internet came a distant third (7%) – but easily beating the once 'trusty' friends (3%), family (1%) and the media (1%). Given that family and friends are so accessible it is perhaps surprising that they were so low down the health source pecking order.

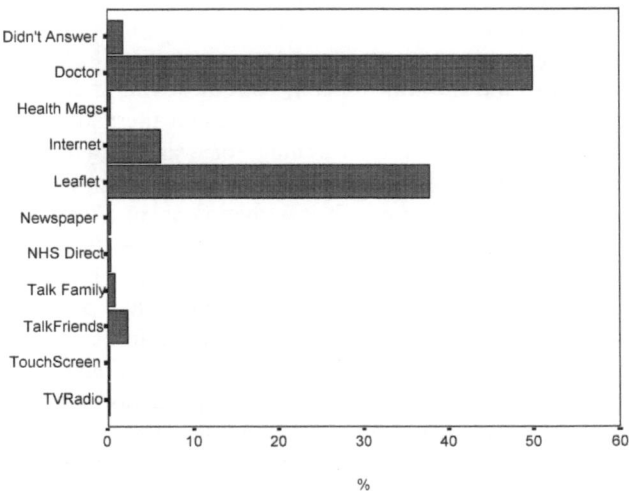

Figure 4.11 SurgeryDoor – first information source sought

Doctors were also the second most important information source (28%). However, the Internet emerged as the second most consulted information source, with 26% of respondents saying that they used it second. Overall, fifty percent of respondents listed the 'Internet' as one of their top three information sources. Friends also featured strongly, with 19% of respondents saying they consulted them second. Interestingly, the family seemed not to be considered as either a first or second source of health information.

Respondents were further asked about the Internet as an information source, how many sites they had visited (in addition to SurgeryDoor) and when they last used the Internet to search for health information. Just under a third said that they visited just the one site, suggesting that these users were core users of the SurgeryDoor site and trusted the site sufficiently not to visit other sites for their health enquiries. Seventy percent of users said that they had visited more than one site. For these information seekers visiting a number of sites was probably a way of checking the authority of the sites.

There was also evidence to suggest that the younger the users the more likely they were to exhibit a promiscuous form of behaviour. Forty-six percent of those aged under 34 visited three or more sites compared to 41% of those aged 35 to 54 and 22% of those aged 55 and over. Those aged 55 and over were most likely to visit just one site.

The same questionnaire provided an explanation of why so many sites were being visited. Respondents were asked to rate SurgeryDoor in regard to the breadth and depth of content and trust in the information. The number of health sites visited was found to be correlated to a scoring over the three attributes derived by factor analysis. Importantly, a relationship was found between the respondent's score in regard to content and the number of health sites visited. As the number of health websites that the user visited increased so the user's rating of content depth, breadth and trust declined. This suggests that users who visit a number of sites were not as worried about the content attributes of an individual site as these attributes were maximised by visiting a number of site. Alternatively, they realised that all sites lack content attributes and that content attributes can only be maximised by visiting many sites. What we are witnessing here then is the kind of remote-flicking channel behaviour that children exhibit while watching television.

Nearly all respondents (92%) who visited more than one site said that they did so to compare health information between sites. Nicholas *et al* (2003a) found that the greater the number of sites visited the greater the likelihood of a healthy behaviour outcome. This provides support for an information model that argues that not all sites will present the information in the same way, detail or in the same design. Users 'benefit' from collecting information from a number of sites, partly because they find the information easier to digest on some sites than others. Partly also because the process of jumping from site to site means that users can compare and contrast information and this says something about how users become knowledgeable.

NHS Direct Online

It was not the intention to provide equal treatment with SurgeryDoor for NHS Direct Online because the latter was evaluated largely to provide comparative performance data in some key areas of performance and use.

'NHS Direct' is the name given to a remote health care service for patients mediated firstly through the telephone (launched March 1998), and accompanied later by the Web version – NHS Direct Online (December 1999). Both services have been reasonably well received, if we exclude criticisms emanating from the British Medical Association. Thus Munro *et al* (2000), monitoring the telephone service, found that call rates to the telephone 'hotline' were continuing to rise, doubling during the first year of operation. Equally positively, press reports (e.g. Internet magazine 2000) claim that over one and a half million people visited the website on the day it launched.

The purpose of NHS Direct Online was to provide the general public (rather than medical professionals) with information about aspects of health and medical care. This included advice for those facing a surgical operation, attempting to give up smoking or simply desirous of leading a healthier lifestyle. The site also featured a health consumer magazine and latest health news. As Gann and Sadler (2001) put it in a letter to the BMJ, NHS Direct Online acts both as a source of original content (including the NHS Direct Healthcare Guide, which offers algorithmic guidance on a number of common health problems), and as a gateway to a wide range of other health information websites (through the Conditions and Treatment section). A multidisciplinary editorial board of doctors, nurses, pharmacists and consumers review content.

The site was menu-based with search facility options. At the time of the research, there were ten main content items on the site,[10] which were: Health features (NHS Direct Online's magazine), Healthy living, About NHS Direct Online, Healthcare guide, A-Z guide to the NHS, Conditions and treatment, Frequently asked questions, Listen here, Site guide, Feedback on the site, International Partner Organisations.

There was no menu hierarchy on the home page – sub menus were given on the page at which the main menu item opens. The search facility on the site was unusual. Every main topic entry included this, but in each case it only searched the section of the site currently open. In other words, activating the facility from 'Health Features' resulted in a search only of that section. The 'Conditions and Treatment' topic was interesting in this context, as there was three ways to access information. The first of these was a 'Body Map', which, as its name implies, was an image of the body, the various parts of which could be activated. This may be useful for a problem that can be pinpointed to a part of the body, but not appropriate for symptoms that manifest themselves throughout the body – chronic fatigue, for example. To help retrieve information on these general topics, a Keywords browsing facility was available.

---

10 The site has changed considerably over the past year – introducing a webmail enquiry service and a 'My Healthspace' personalised information service, for example. The description given in this report is that pertaining to the site at the time of the various analyses (2000-2002).

Users could choose a letter and scroll down a list of topics (That for 'A' begins: Accidents, Acne, Addiction, Adolescents, Adults, Ageing, Aids ...).

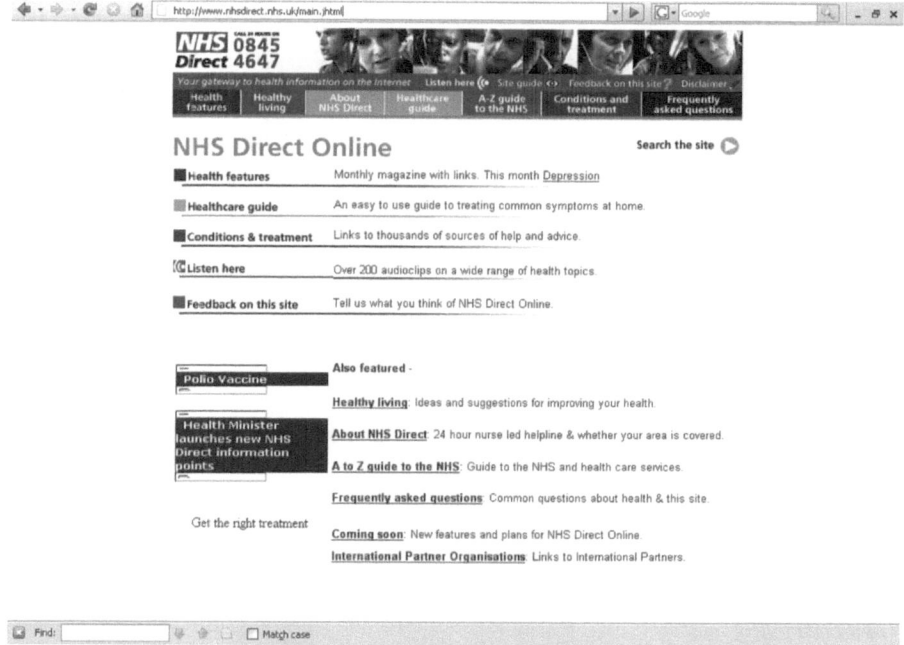

Figure 4.12 Homepage of NHS Direct Online

Users and use

During November 2000 NHS Direct Online attracted 41,510 individual visitors (separate identifiable IP addresses), saw 68,955 search sessions conducted and 879,344 pages viewed. By contrast the SurgeryDoor website attracted approximately half the number of visitors (20,611), 30,157 sessions and about 15% of the page views (138,862). Figure 4.13 shows the comparative daily record of visitors for the month for the two sites (excluding robots).

The NHS site attracted considerably more users than SurgeryDoor. Monthly figures clearly shows a marked weekly pattern of use with a low number of users on both sites occurring on Saturdays and Sundays and high numbers occurring in mid-week.

Table 4.2 provides a breakdown of the pattern of returns over the month for the site. For NHS Direct Online 84% of users visited the site once only. For SurgeryDoor this figure was significantly higher – 89%. Of course, sites maybe revisited more often because the information contained on a site changes so regularly that users are compelled to return frequently to up date their knowledge.

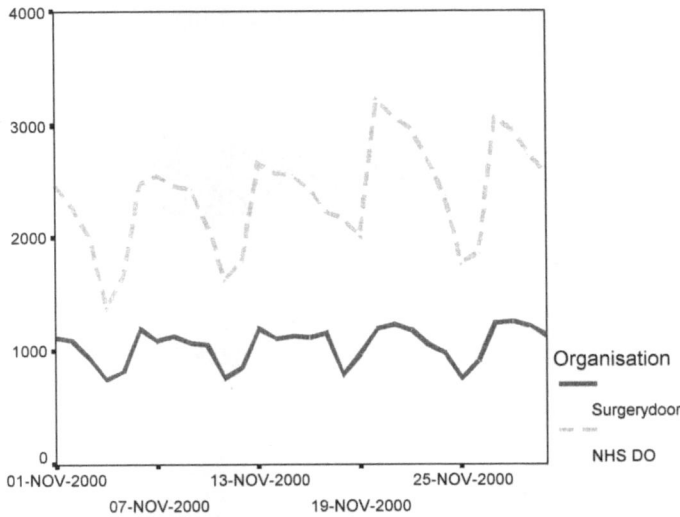

Figure 4.13 NHS Direct Online v SurgeryDoor – daily number of user visits during November 2000

Table 4.2 NHS Direct Online: number of visits within a month (November 2000)

Visit once	84%
Visited 2-5 times	12.4%
Visited 6-15 times	2.3%
Over 15 times	1.2%

(Excluding Robots).

Interestingly, users visiting both the sites were far more likely to revisit at least one of the sites – in fact, three or more times as compared to users who only visited one site. Those visiting only one site were less likely to be repeat visitors. Sixty percent of users who had visited both sites once came back and re-visited at least one of the sites again. However this was only true for 11% of NHS Direct only visitors and 4% of SurgeryDoor only visitors.

A further study compared returnees for a number of health sites, including NHS Direct Online and, again, this was determined by questionnaire. Figure 4.14 displays the results. In terms of repeat use Yahoo! Health performed poorly and saw the least percentage (24%) of users coming back three or more times to the site; SurgeryDoor, on the other hand, performed particularly well by this metric. About half of its users returned to the site three or more times, suggesting it had the most loyal audience. Sixty-three percent of respondents had visited the NHS Direct Online site just once or twice, 29% three to nine times and 8% 10 plus times; so placing the NHS site in the middle according to the 'loyalty' metric. However, this particular study was, by its method of sampling, biased towards readers of The Guardian newspaper.

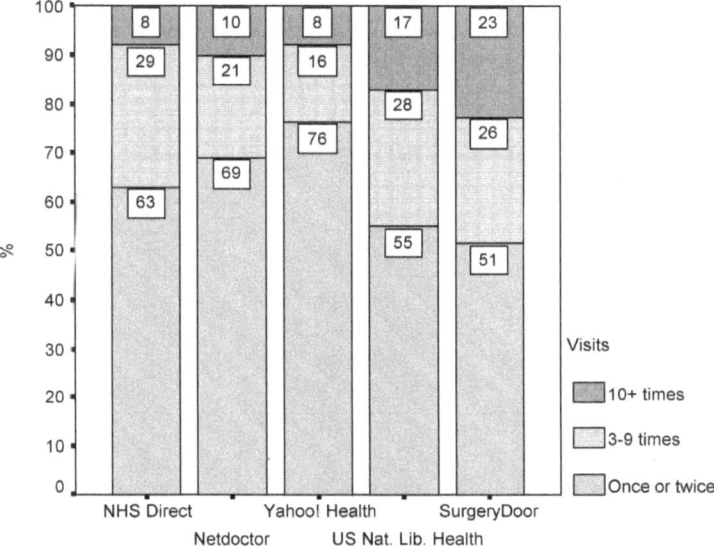

Figure 4.14 NHS Direct Online – number of times visited for five health websites

It is useful to distinguish between three types of user session – single page sessions, single daily sessions and multiple user sessions in a day. Single page sessions are those where the user only views one page during their visit. In these cases no session time, or indeed page view time, can be calculated, as the Internet provides no log-off signal. The first and last entry times of these users are therefore the same. Single daily sessions are relatively straightforward – single visits, but ones in which more than one page is viewed. The calculation of session time for these users is also relatively straightforward, except that the last page viewed in the session is discarded. The last group 'multiple user sessions in a day' describes that type of users who make multiple (repeat) visits to the site in the same day. The calculation of session time for these users is more difficult as there is no clear distinction between sessions, no demarcation line as to when a session ends and when a new one begins. For our purposes the ending of a session and the beginning of a new session was identified by a lapse of time between two recorded page uploads, deemed by the researchers to be 'significant'. For this particular study a time gap of five minutes was tested. Data for the three group types across the two sites are provided in Table 4.3.

There proved to be significant differences in the sites, with users of SurgeryDoor undertaking a far higher proportion (43%) of single page sessions than NHS Direct Online users (14%). The latter were far more likely to undertake multiple sessions in a day: 42% were of this type, as compared to 21% for SurgeryDoor. It was possible to determine why. As noted, SurgeryDoor attracted more 'Single page session' users;

this might partly reflect caching in that if a user requests a multiple page file they can investigate a number of pages without requesting further pages from the server. Alternatively, SurgeryDoor has been identified as attracting more individual evening users than NHS Direct Online, and these users may have greater time constraints in that they are paying for their online searches (telephone costs) and were likely to move on if they could not find what they wanted quickly.

Table 4.3 NHS Direct Online v SurgeryDoor – accesses to the site by type of daily session

	NHS Direct Online	SurgeryDoor
Single page sessions	9,638 (14.0%)	12,835 (42.6%)
Single sessions	30,372 (44.0%)	10,957 (36.3%)
More than 1 session conducted	28,985 (42.0%)	6,365 (21.1%)
Total	68,995 (100%)	30,157 (100%)

An alternative to the number of pages viewed in a session metric – and one not subject to caching – is session duration time. Session time is defined as the time difference between the first and last page uploaded to the client's machine. It is not subject to caching because it records the session rather than individual pages. To obtain this data IP addresses were sorted by day of the month, IP number and time and session time found by computing the difference between the first and last time entry for that IP address.

The session time for all users was between three to four minutes. This is significantly less than session time estimates typically provided by proprietary software of seven to eight minutes. However, proprietary software tends to estimate session time without addressing the problems associated with a skewed distribution and hence are considerably biased and unreliable. Furthermore, session time estimates were significantly more than that for other consumer digital health information systems.

By the session time metric SurgeryDoor performed as well as, if not slightly better than, NHS Direct Online. The session duration of users on the SurgeryDoor site was 19% longer than that recorded for the NHS Direct Online site, respectively 227 seconds and 191 seconds. In this case session time gives a more accurate idea of the extent of use of a site compared to the number of pages viewed in a session and the number of pages viewed.

The overall estimates suggest that SurgeryDoor users spent about three times as much time viewing a page as NHS Direct Online users – 67 seconds compared to 22 seconds, but viewed only one third the number of pages – 6.6 pages compared to 2.2 pages. The data would suggest that NHS Direct Online users tended to be quick readers, viewing a large number of pages, while users of SurgeryDoor looked at only a few pages but spent a longer time looking at them. This could be a false supposition and shows the dangers of relying wholly on Web logs. As indicated above, SurgeryDoor users were making use of cached pages stored on their hard disk. The server does not record these views and hence the view time of these pages were added to the previous server recorded page.

The density of information on a page may effect delivery time, and it is to be expected that the denser the information is on screen the longer the download time. A metric of information density can be computed by dividing the estimated number of page views into the total number of files uploaded. This would give the number of files uploaded on the client's computer per page view. It could provide another use metric or it could be used in conjunction with another metric (like time) to improve its accuracy. We discuss it here in that context.

Table 4.4 NHS Direct Online v SurgeryDoor – number of files downloaded per page by site

	Total Files uploaded (Nov)	Estimated page views (Incl. Robots)	Number of files per page view
NHS Direct Online	7,688,862	1,083,363	7.10
SurgeryDoor	1,638,719	177,896	9.21

SurgeryDoor uploaded approximately two more files per page view compared to NHS Direct: 9.21 files per page as compared to 7.10 (Table 4.4). However, this metric also reflects differences in the architecture of the site.

For the SurgeryDoor site, as of November 2000, content pages were single HTML pages containing information on a number of topics with a menu structured as internal links at the top of the page. There were up to two higher level menus. However, there were a variety of links from the opening page that went directly to a multiple page view HTML page. Depending on how users entered the site it was highly likely that they would have cached a multiple topic information page and a menu page by downloading just two pages. They could then access the cached information and menu pages 'exploring' a number of related topics without requesting further pages from the server. The architecture of the NHS Direct site matched separate HTML pages to menu items. Hence the user would have requested a number of HTML files from the server by employing the menu structure.

Caching creates a false picture in that it impacts on the metrics page view time and the number of pages recorded in a session. The SurgeryDoor site metrics, particularly those related to page view statistics, cannot be safely compared to that of NHS Direct Online, as users of the SurgeryDoor site were accessing multiple page files from their cache and these page views are not recorded by the server. Hence the server under records the actual pages viewed and estimates of view time on the pages that are recorded will appear long than merited. Comparisons between the two sites were limited because architecture differences result in a significant difference in the number of pages cached.

Caching further creates a false impression when comparing pages viewed. Comparing the two sites by the number of pages viewed, as already stated, implies that SurgeryDoor attracts just 15% of the use that NHS Direct does. This is a false picture that arises as a result of the extensive caching of SurgeryDoor multiple page files on to user's cash. When comparing the sites by user numbers a different picture emerges and the SurgeryDoor site attracts approximately 50% of visitors compared to NHS Direct Online.

SurgeryDoor attracted more evening users (7pm to midnight) compared to NHS Direct Online, respectively 22% and 17%. NHS Direct had slightly more users logging on for the first time during morning office hours (10am to 2pm) – 36% compared to 30% for SurgeryDoor. This would argue that there was greater use of the NHS Direct Online site during business hours, while SurgeryDoor attracted more evening users – home and non-business use. Perhaps, it is more acceptable to search a Government site at work?

In terms of day of the week, the distribution was remarkably similar for both sites. Sundays attracted a smaller number of users compared to the other days of the week, and SurgeryDoor attracted slightly more users on Sundays, but only by 1%. Wednesdays seemed to be the most popular day of the week for users of both sites, attracting almost 20% of all users.

Categories of user

Figure 4.15 shows the country from which visitors came from, as indicated by their IP address. SurgeryDoor attracted proportionally fewer visitors with an UK registered IP address, 15% as compared to 26% for the NHS site. Conversely, SurgeryDoor had a higher international appeal with more users having either a US or an IP address located in the rest of the world. This is perhaps surprising given that one might have expected the NHS to have higher international brand awareness.

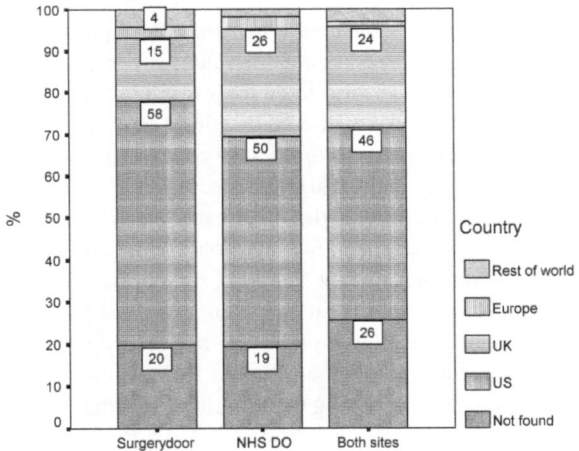

Figure 4.15 NHS Direct Online v SurgeryDoor – geographical location of users (logs) (excluding robots)

It was found that nearly all respondents came from the U.K, 95%, compared to 5% who said that they came from outside the UK This is very different to the geographical distribution indicated by the transaction logs from the web servers. An analysis of the of Internet protocol (IP) numbers that had logged on to NHS Direct Online in November 2000 showed that 26% of resolved numbers could be tracked back to UK ISPs while 49% of could be tracked back to ISPs in the US (Figure 4.16).

Clearly, some of the difference can be accounted for by a proportion of UK users signing-up with US ISPs. It is also possible that only UK tax payers felt they had the right to reply, or felt it was in their interests, to do so.

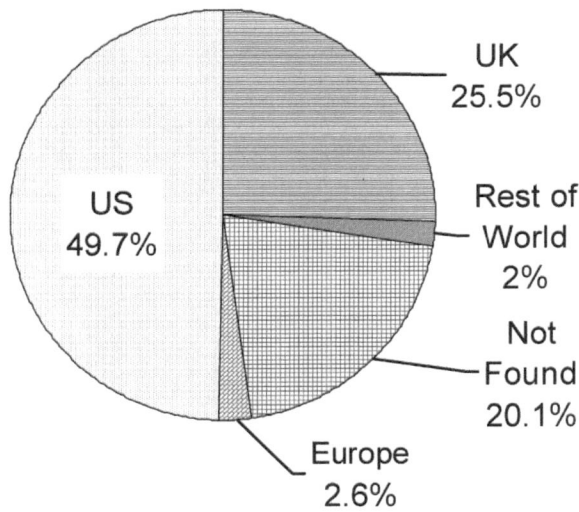

Figure 4.16 NHS Direct Online – geographical location of users (IP address)

An analysis was conducted for each site of the type of organisation from which visitors came from. The IP number also provided this information. The NHS Direct Online site attracted a greater percentage of commercially registered users: 52% compared to 43% for SurgeryDoor. However, NHS Direct Online had a smaller percentage of users connecting via Internet providers like AOL online, 17% as compared to 26% for SurgeryDoor. Individuals were more likely to connect to the Internet via an Internet provider and this argues that SurgeryDoor attracted a higher percentage of individual users. The greater use of the NHS Direct Online site by commercial users argues that the site is more subject to proxy server caching and this will have an impact on the total page view and user count.

Questionnaire respondents were asked from where they had searched the NHS Direct Online site. By far the largest number, of respondents (67%) accessed the site from home, and a further 28% of from work. Those coming from academic institutes accounted for 6%, and 1% each came from libraries and public access terminals.

Accessing from a home computer increased significantly with age. While only 49% of the under 18 years of age accessed the site from home, 65% of 35 to 44 year olds, and a high 95% of 65 to 74 year olds did so.

Access and proximity to computers also determined use. For example, young people aged below 18 and between 18 and 24, accessed the site from academic institutes, while users of working age (25 to 64) did so from work. Those aged between 25 and 34 were most likely to log on from a work computer as compared to other age groups – 37% of this age grouped logged onto the site from work.

Thirty five percent of those people aged over 75 used public access and library terminals. As a proportion public access machines were important to the over 75 and this appeared to be an important access point for medical information for this age group.

Health topics sought

NHS Direct Online was split into seven main sections (not including 'Frequently Asked Questions'): NHS A-Z, About NHS Direct, Conditions & Treatment, Healthcare Guide, Health in the News, Healthy Living and Listen Here. People were asked which sections of the site they had visited.

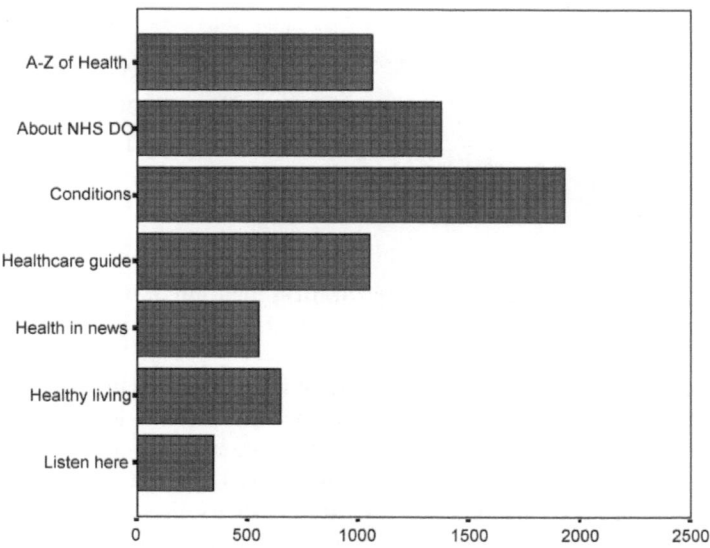

Figure 4.17 NHS Direct Online – health sections visited (questionnaire)

Forty three percent of respondents said that they had visited just one of the sections, 23% had visited two sections and 33% said that they had visited three or more sections. Figure 4.17 gives the number of users visiting each of the sections. The most popular section appeared to be Conditions and Treatment followed by About NHS Direct and then A-Z of the NHS. Sixty percent of users said that they had visited the Conditions and Treatment section, but this percentage decreased over time with 63% saying that they had visited this section in the first quarter and 57% in the fourth quarter. While Health in the News, increased from 16% to 20% from the last week of 1999 to January 2001,[11] there was suggestive evidence that over time users will not revisit a source that they know does not change quickly, and this is clearly a case of tactical information seeking.

Looking at the numbers of people accessing pages from these sections on an average day, it turned out again that Conditions & Treatment was the most popular by far.

Table 4.5 lists the top 15 pages and directories viewed. Internet pages are stored in directories and it was decided to list this information as well. Page names and directories are often obscurely labelled.

For this analysis it was decided to exclude pages used to get to an information page. Anthrax, a featured topic from the main menu page, made up about 2% of the information pages viewed. This was during a period when anthrax featured prominently in the world press and the use to this page reflected interest derived from such media reports. Other important pages include Depression (1.6%), Haemorrhoids (1.2%), Thrush (1.1%), Hypertension (1.1%) and Back Pain (1.1%). These top five pages made up about 7% of all the information pages viewed.

Table 4.5 NHS Direct Online – page topics and directories viewed (excluding menu pages)

Page name viewed	%	Directory	%
anthrax	1.9	Conditions	11.4
depression	1.6	Search	8.1
haemorrhoids	1.2	Pages	5.2
thrush	1.1	Lower_abdome	5.1
hypertension	1.1	Audio_cache	3.9
back_pain	1.1	Healthcare	3.9
joint_pain	1.0	a-z	3.6
urinary_tract_inf	1.0	head_brain	2.7
chlamydia_infecti	0.9	abdomen	2.4
influenza	0.8	faqs	1.9
accidents	0.8	EnqForm	1.8
body_mass	0.8	Skin	1.6
dizziness	0.8	About	1.6
diabetes	0.7	Upper_body	1.6
		Bones_joints	1.4

---

11 chi=24.57, 3, p=0.000.

Health interest (or demand) can be shown by the search terms people enter into the system. Table 4.6 gives the top ranked 25 search terms used on NHS Direct site for November 2000. The website had a search option that allowed users to search for information. The top 25 search terms accounted for 15% of the total number of search expressions used. There were 8,006 different search expressions in all.

Table 4.6 NHS Direct Online – health terms/expressions used to search the site using the internal search engine

Top 25 search terms used	As % of terms used	Top 25 pages viewed	As % of total number of pages viewed
Information	1.7	Anthrax	1.4
Depression	1.3	haemorrhoids	1.3
NHS	.9	depression	1.2
Piles	.8	joint_pain	1.2
Pregnancy	.8	thrush	1.1
Shingles	.7	back_pain	1.1
Diabetes	.6	hypertension	.9
Thyroid	.6	urinary_tract_inf	.9
Asthma	.6	dizziness	.9
Chickenpox	.6	allergies	.9
Cholesterol	.6	body_mass	.8
Body	.5	diabetes	.8
Contraception	.5	pregnancy_childbi	.8
Scabies	.5	chlamydia_infecti	.8
Cancer	.4	testicular_cancer	.8
Dermatomyositis	.4	ireritable_bowel_	.8
Impetigo	.4	risk_factors	.8
panic+attacks	.4	accidents	.8
chlamydia	.4	contraception	.7
chronic+fatigue+synd	.4	worms	.7
menopause	.4	breast_cancer	.7
testicular+cancer	.4	influenza	.7
gout	.3	bowel_cancer	.7
smoking	.3	cystitis	.7
stress	.3	shingles	.7

Nearly all the search expressions used were medical words that are common and well used, only 2 words seemed to be difficult medical words (Column 1); these were Dermatomyositis and Impetigo. This suggests that users were not referencing medical text or leaflets when they searched the site, and that the searching represented a first point of contact in their pursuit of medical information. Column 3 provides for comparison the ranked use of health pages. Interestingly, only one topic figures in the top ten of both lists – depression.

Table 4.7 classifies search expressions by health topic. For instance, in the case of the column headed blood and bleeding groups all search terms that mention either blood or bleeding are included there. The Table offers an insight into common terms used to search NHS Direct Online. In all cases non-medical terms were used.

Table 4.7 NHS Direct Online – ranked top 15 search terms or each group of search terms

Blood and bleeding	Aches, pains and sores	Swelling, bumps and lumps	Rashes and itches	Fevers and sweats
blood+pressure	chest+pain	lump	rash	glandular+fever
bleeding	back+pain	swollen+glands	itching	temperature
high+blood+pressure	leg+pain	swelling	itch	fever
blood	pain	lumps	blisters	scarlet+fever
anal+bleeding	headache	swollen	rashes	chest+infection
low+blood+pressure	neck+pain	swollen+ankles	itchy	kidney+infection
blood+clots	abdominal+pain	lump+on+head	skin+rash	sweating
nose+bleed	stomach+pain	swollen+ankle	twitching+eye	infection
rectal+bleeding	muscle+pain	swollen+eyes	itch	ear+infection
nosebleed	kidney+pain	swollen+and+face	itchy+spots	hot+flushes
bleeding+and+rectum	shoulder+pain	swollen+stomach	mouth+blisters	viral+infection
blood+in+urine	headaches	swelling+ankle	blister	night+sweats
low+blood+sugar	sore+throat	swollen+anus	vaginal+itching	temperature
vaginal+bleeding	backache	lumps+in+the+back	heat+rash	respiratory+infection
blood+in+stools	groin+pain	swollen+face	nappy+rash	urinary+tract+infection
				urine+infection

Pregnancy and babies	Colds and flu	Burns and accidents	Women's and men's health	Heart
pregnancy	flu	burns	thrush	heart
pregnant	throat	burn	penis	heart+palpitations
childbirth	influenza	fallen+arches	cystitis	heartbeat
baby	sore+throat	cuts	periods	heart+rate
children	cold+sore	scalp+cut	testicles	heart+attack
babies	hot+flushes	acute+bronchitis	urine	heart+beat
nappy+rash	cold	cut	period	heart+burn
pregnancy+sickness	cold+feet	sunburn	cervical+cancer	fast+heart+beat
pregnancy+symptoms	cold+sores	cerebroaccident	hepatitis	enlarged+heart
palpatations+and+children	common+cold	small+cut+on+the+sc	vaginal+discharge	irregular+heartbeat
pregnant+and+itch	fluid+retention	alp+of+t	cervical	heartburn
genital+problems+in+	fluid	roaccutane	hepatitus	heart+bi+pass
babies	gastro+oesophageal+	drop+in+center	ejaculation	heart+irregularities
a-z+childhood+illnesses	reflux+d	wound+care	sex	suspected+heart+attack
pregnancy+test	food+sticks+in+throat	acute+tonsillitis	vagina	missed+heart+beat
pregancy+and+sickness	throat+conditions	drop+in+clinic		

Ease of use/usability

The usability of the NHS Direct Online website was tested by questionnaire and usability study. It is worth noting that since the evaluation described here, the NHS website has undergone a major restructuring. It is, however, still worth discussing the findings as they provide a context for the log and survey findings and inform the development of health information sites for the future.

The majority of questionnaire respondents found that the home page 'confusing' and with 'too much information'. They said that the text and images were structured in such a way that it did not help the user to focus on content. More specifically, eight respondents complained about the duplication of the menu items – a problem also highlighted with regard to the SurgeryDoor site.

Body map and ease of use Sometimes a more visual approach to information retrieval is more effective, especially in a field like medicine where terms are difficult to spell (for entering a search) and routes to topics therefore not provided in layman's terms. Given the problems already mentioned in regard to more traditional search avenues one would have expected the body map provided on the site to be used as a route to information retrieval. The questionnaire included a question about this feature. Surprisingly, 30% of all respondents did not even know it was there, and over a quarter (27%) felt it was no help at all. Just 8% felt it helped a lot. It may be that many users required information that was not specific to a particular part of the body – such as advice about exercise, information on insomnia etc.

Links and navigation Another problem was that participants in the usability study had difficulty in recognising which entries were hyper-links. This was observed during one task in which subjects did not realise that the heading 'Lupus' was a hyper-link and thus missed information, and also when people were consulting the site guide. In this case it took time for participants to realise that the sub-headings under each listed section were hyper-links. In both cases this was because the hyper-links were not highlighted.

Navigation: Interviews and observation results from one study showed that, surprisingly, none of the participants realised that the NHS Direct sign at the top of the page was a link to the home page. The back button was the method used to find this, except for four users who ran their cursors over the NHS logo and found it was a link. In fact, the 'home page' itself is not labelled as such, which was disorienting for some users.

The duplication of menu items was not well received. Observation with the usability session participants showed that they tended to look at the same menu entries twice, as they were confused, and it took them time to realise that the menu entries below were the same as the ones at the top of the page.

Apart from problems with the duplication of menu items, almost all of the 19 participants in the usability study found the navigation 'straightforward', 'easy' or 'no problem'. Particularly liked was the ability to search the whole site from the home page with the help of the main navigation bar at the top of the site. They also liked the fact the main navigation menu bar was apparent in every page.

Menu nomenclature and usability The labelling of the various menu options was also a topic explored with respondents of one of our studies. Comments included that the sections 'aren't clear'; 'the URL isn't intuitive', and the use of multimedia was 'inappropriate'. Regarding the latter:

One final point regarding navigation is that users missed information because some significant links were below the bottom of the screen and required scrolling.

NHS Direct Online questionnaire respondents also commented generally upon navigational issues although only in very vague terms. One comment was that the navigation was 'easy', whilst another claimed it to be 'hard' – both without any accompanying explanatory text. Broken links were, however, mentioned specifically, with three users complaining about problems in accessing 'A-Z of the NHS', and two others mentioned external dead links.

As previously noted the search facility on the NHS Direct Online site was unusual at the time of the evaluation, in that each section on the site (Health Features, Healthy Living, About NHS Direct, Healthcare Guide etc.) had its own search facility. In other words, the search engine only searched that particular section. Only the search engine found on the home page looked for pages on the whole site. This caused much confusion, with users assuming that if their searches achieved poor results that this applied site-wide, not just to that section. Problems of this nature were largely to do with the way the site was put together – it was assembled from existing material, quickly pressed into service together with a few new sections or topics, commissioned as 'one-offs'. The Healthcare Guide and A-Z sections were effectively separate, self-contained sites. They were located on different servers and used different software, which is why a consistent search across all parts of the site could not be conducted. In technical terms, the facility was not actually a search engine at all – most of the page content was held in an Oracle database with pages generated on the fly – the search is effectively searching database fields and is fairly crude. Multi-word searches defaulted to logical OR – hence sore throat retrieving throat cancer. In response to criticisms of the search facility NHS Direct have now changed the organisation of the site, and an across-site search engine is now functioning (although most searches retrieve results from a new online health encyclopaedia).

Searching the site was shown to be problematic for people across the different target groups. A third of respondents said that the search facility helped a lot. However, as with the target groups, a worrying number (28%) said it was of no help. Thus, more than a quarter of all respondents felt that a key function on the site was of little benefit to them.

Generally, the following can be inferred from this:

- The search system on the original site was fragmented and confusing and resulted in poor or misleading searches.
- The modular architecture meant that information on a single topic could be spread across several modules making it difficult to find but also risking duplication of information.
- The lack of cross-referencing between information on the same topic maintained by different organisations meant that users could have the impression of partial coverage of that topic.

Purpose and reasons for using website

In a national study of health sites, users were given a list of topics and asked to indicate if each was a topic about which they had searched. Respondents were grouped by whether they had:

- never used NHS Direct Online,

- only used NHS Direct Online
- used NHS Direct Online with other site(s)

Almost all of the UK respondents (97%) who had accessed the Internet for health information had done so in order to look up information about a particular illness and condition. Fifty-seven percent had gathered information regarding a visit to the doctor and 52% had used the Internet to look for information or advice about nutrition, exercise, or weight control. Just under half of this sample had looked for information about alternative medicines. Further, 44% had looked for information about a sensitive health topic which it was difficult to talk about. This is significant in that many of these respondents would not go on to talk to a medical professional about these issues. Forty percent looked for information about a mental health issue like depression or anxiety and 34% looked for information about innovative or experimental treatments. Only 23% of respondents sought to diagnose or treat a medical condition on your own, using information from the Internet, without consulting your doctor.

In terms of what information people sought, those only using NHS Direct Online appeared not to make as much use of information on mental health, alternative medicine, new treatments and prescription drugs as compared to either respondents who never used the NHS (they used other sites) or those who made use of additional sites as well. For each of these topics, the percentage of NHS Direct Online use only respondents was less than that of those who never used NHS Direct Online and those who used NHS Direct Online in combination with other sites. The largest difference was recorded for new treatments. Only 23% of those who only used NHS Direct Online went to the site for this topic, compared to 31% of those who had accessed this topic but had never used the site, and 41% of those accessing this topic but using a combination of sites. This may reflect on the characteristics of those people who use NHS Direct Online. Alternatively, it may reflect a weakness in how these topics are covered by NHS. The NHS Direct site seemed to cover the following topics well: on a particular illness or condition, information about doctors and hospitals, information on sensitive health topics and information about doctor appointments.

An online questionnaire examined use and reasons for use. The roles of people using the Internet for health included:

- Patients
- Professional (nurses, journalists etc.)
- Intermediaries (i.e. to research information on behalf of another)
- General consumers

Some respondents used the Internet in connection with more than one of these roles, indicating both usage when ill (i.e. as patients), and in good health, for general interest reasons. Using the Internet in terms of information seeking naturally depended on the role and context of the information seeker and the following uses were elicited:

- Self-care, including self-diagnosis (i.e. as a substitute for visiting a medical professional)
- Complement to information from a health professional
- Peer support (i.e. patient to patient)
- For professional reasons (in users' roles as health professionals, journalists and others)
- General interest
- As a reference guide (i.e. to medical location addresses, opening times etc.)

Patient use (1): Self care Many respondents (74%) indicated that they had used the Internet in their role as a patient (i.e. to solve a health problem of their own). Self-care, including self-diagnosis (i.e. as a substitute for visiting a medical professional) was a major attraction for these respondents.

Patient use (2): Complementary information source In addition to self-help, respondents also mentioned using the Internet as a complementary information service to that obtained from medical professionals.

Patient use (3): Peer-support Peer support (i.e. patient to patient), often put forward as a great advantage of the Internet, was not a reason given by many respondents for using the Internet. However, it must be remembered that the questionnaire being referred to was posted on to a specifically health *information* website – there was no patient to patient section on NHS Direct Online at the time. Nevertheless, one website which did include a message board system for people to offer mutual support, describe personal experiences and ask questions from their peers, SurgeryDoor, only attracted 127 messages on its 'Medical' message board in a year (2002). The site was visited by an estimated 20,000 unique IP addresses per month, so, clearly, a surprisingly low proportion seemed to be interested in this facility – maybe a case of early days and if we investigated today we might find things had changed.

Professional use A minority of respondents (10%) indicated that they were health professionals.

General interest use General interest browsing was not an activity undertaken by many respondents. In fact, only 12% described activities that could be coded as 'general interest', and even one of these – a journalist – used the Net in this way for professional reasons, to research for possible stories. A minority of people (8%) said they use the Internet as a kind of directory or reference guide – to find, for example, medical addresses, opening times etc.

Intermediary use Using the Internet in the capacity of an intermediary – that is, researching topics for other people – was mentioned by several (20%) respondents. Specifically mentioned were 'family members who asked', one's children, partners and friends.

Benefits/satisfaction/trust/outcomes

Many questionnaire respondents answered a question on why they turn to Internet information in terms of the advantages or benefits of the Internet over other sources of information. The most popular advantages of the Internet over other systems and services were thought to be convenience and anonymity.

With regard to the convenience of the system, much was made of the facility to research from one's own home. As a childbirth educator and freelance health writer put it: 'It is open 24/7 and right in my own home. I don't even need an appointment. No waiting!'

Issues relating to anonymity were mentioned alongside the convenience of having information provided in one's own home. It may be that 'convenience' may be interchangeable with 'anonymity' for some respondents, in the sense that the anonymity is, itself, one of the conveniences.

Surprisingly, few people mentioned currency as an advantage of the Internet over other sources. Maybe the assumption was that digital information, almost be definition, was up to date, a dangerous assumption of course. Perhaps, also surprisingly, the depth and breadth of information on the Internet was not cited by many as a good reason for using it for health information. It may be that this aspect of the Internet is so well known and accepted that it was not considered worth mentioning. Those who did mention the quantity of information were impressed that one could 'search on wide range of topics – much more than local library' and also that this breadth made it possible to consult 'a range of sources and perspectives'. There was some indication that this gave the patient or enquirer more power in what a minority appeared to view as an adversarial encounter with a health professional. No having to rely on 'industry' sponsored leaflets at GP's surgery was also a plus.

When given the opportunity to comment on any aspect of the site the majority (81%) of people mentioned the quality of information content. Just fewer than 50% of all comments asked for more information, just over 10% provided positive feedback about the site, and 7% noted errors on it.

Looking into users' feedback over time showed that, on average, there were just under six (5.91) negative responses per week and just over six (6.29) positive responses per week. Only 10% of all responses included some negative feedback about the site. Comments to open questions were gathered from the first 200 questionnaire returns collected. They were grouped by theme and analysed to provide additional evaluative data. By far the greatest number of comments concerned the omission of condition-specific information. No fewer than 33 respondents (16.5%) complained that there was 'no information' on a particular topic, or that they were unable to find any information.

As previously mentioned, a major issue when considering information found on the Internet is, of course, that of its quality and accuracy. Respondents were asked: 'How do you look at the issue of 'information quality' regarding material you find on the Internet? Does it make any difference to you where you get the information from?' Of course, it needs to be stressed that the very act of asking people about quality may itself prompt them into thinking about an issue about which they may not hitherto have been overly concerned.

Unsurprisingly, medical professionals had a good deal to say on this subject. Their comments were concerned with problems inherent in 'informal' and unregulated sites, but also, perhaps surprisingly, with issues regarding 'authoritative sites' too. The problem of 'unofficial', non-authoritative sites was summed up by the health psychology student: 'I think that most people realise that there isn't any particularly effective restrictions in place as yet on the Internet, therefore, anybody can set up a website containing false, misleading, incorrect or offensive content.' She looked at the issue also from the viewpoint of her studies: 'From an academic perspective I have to be especially careful which information to trust from the Internet as it could be the difference between a pass or fail'.

An 'Independent Consultant Nurse' raised the issue of authoritative sites being at fault. She said: 'Quality is so important and sometimes one gets the impression that the search for 'innovation' is prized by the DoH above everything else. Some nursing sites can be misleading when innovations are mentioned, but are not evaluated, so who knows if they're any good?' This is interesting as it suggests that not even so-called 'authoritative' sites are always correct. This is evidenced in the literature too. Coulter *et al* (1999), for example, point out that even 'official' information published by the NHS and other government bodies can be of dubious quality. Her research indicated a multitude of problems: much of the information was inaccurate and out of date, technical terms were not explained, and few materials provided 'adequate' information about treatment risks and side-effects.

The 'general public' also showed a great concern over the issue of quality and authority, although, as mentioned above, the extent to which this was as a result of prompting is not clear. A retired 71 year old summed up what appeared to be a general feeling: 'obviously I would tend toward a reputable organisation to provide … information.' In total, 36% who responded to this question indicated a preference for accessing information from 'official', 'reputable' or 'well known' sites. One person cautioned, however, that, 'any information that you are unsure about should be checked with your GP/ Dr and should not be the basis for important decisions'.

Another respondent commented that: 'I prefer sites, which are written by Doctors for Doctors [sic]. I also like to see references to the research papers that back up articles'. This phenomenon of exploiting the Internet at a deeper level than that which might be expected of a lay user reflects a trend noted by various health information providers and researchers. Dr. Jack London, for example, an expert on the application of computer and telecommunications technology to cancer clinical trials, was instrumental in the design of the academic cancer website, Kimmel Cancer Centre (at www.kcc.tju.edu). This has pages for healthcare professionals and general scientific researchers, as well as those targeted at the lay public. He quickly found that 'our database listings of currently open clinical trials, targeted at cancer physicians, were frequently accessed by members of the lay public' (London 1999). Following this discovery, the site developers began to include lay descriptions in their trial listings. Similarly, Eysenbach *et al* (1999) found that even a dermatology website intended for medical practitioners was accessed more by lay consumers than healthcare workers.

Of course, perceptions of quality and authority often depend on the viewpoint and beliefs of the information seeker. One of the journalist respondents was candid enough to say: 'if someone doesn't share my philosophy or just gives me a bad feeling, I don't really listen. It definitely matters who gives the information'. Of interest to the authors were people who took or approved of so called 'alternative' medicine, as they may have regarded the NHS as not being an authoritative voice when it came to this kind of treatment. In a questionnaire survey posted on the SurgeryDoor website, we found that alternative medicine users were more likely to use information found on the net to replace a visit to the doctor, perhaps indicating disenchantment with orthodox remedies and perhaps even with the NHS itself. Indeed, work (reported elsewhere in the book) undertaken in evaluating health initiatives on digital interactive TV indicated that those interesting in alternative medicine were less likely to trust the NHS than other groups.

There was some indicative evidence to support this contention. Thus, a respondent claimed: 'I guess I never just trust what the NHS says', having offered her view that 'western medicine in general is myopic in its approach to the matter of health. Basically I feel there is too much of the notion that current medical practices can "heal" you and too little on the concept of responsibility for one's own state of health; mentally, physically and spiritually. I guess you could say that I fall into the category of people who really do subscribe to the notion of a holistic approach to life. What the NHS offers is just one part of the whole. … I always research their diagnosis as well as their proposed remedy before using it.'

Another of the 'alternative medicine' users looked at quality in terms of trust. She was selective in her 'trust' for the NHS, indicating it was 'trustworthy in the sense that the information present will be accurate on the whole but biased in the sense that there is an economic consideration with healthcare provision and the NHS is representing the DoH policies and may not promote treatments that are not available widely on the NHS or new research'.

Tactics for validating information (and here those advocating alternative medicine adopted the same measures as other information seekers) were elicited from those answering an open questionnaire on the NHS Direct Online website. They included checking the organisation responsible, in one case to see if it is 'transparent and not hiding anything about their credentials or the sources of the info they provide', and in another to see 'whether it is a recognisable source'. Of course, for those interested in alternative remedies, particular kinds of orthodox treatments, or in specific conditions these 'recognisable sources will be different'. Further work is required to delve into this topic at a deeper level. One person, a freelance researcher, wrote the criteria she uses almost as a checklist:

- 'who is paying for this website?'
- 'what are they doing it for?'
- 'are they selling something?'
- 'do they agree with what others say?'
- 'do they give any evidence?'

Respondents in the UK National Internet survey who said that they had found misleading information were additionally asked what lead them to question the reliability of the information. Eighty-eight percent of respondents said that the source appeared to be unqualified to furnish such information. Equally as important was the fact that the information contradicted other information found on the Web (87% said this). Eighty one percent said that the fact that there was no identifiable source connected with the site resulted in them questioning its reliability. Other reasons for questioning reliability were that the information contradicted their own experience (63%), came from a drug company (53%) and, least importantly, that the information found had contradicted that given by their doctor (29%). Clearly, users were using multiple methods to check reliability. There was some evidence from a further survey that users felt that NHS Direct did not quote their sources and this lead some respondents not to revisit the site.

Although there was no specific question on trustworthiness in our questionnaires, it was an issue that came out in the replies to questions on authority and quality and, in one case, in reply to a question on the sites visited. 14% of respondents gave answers that were de-coded as being related to 'trust'. These people were generally supportive of the NHS. One said: 'In terms of published information, I have a positive view of the NHS (i.e. I trust the information they publish). In other areas, such as trusting my health or that of my family to the NHS, I have a balanced view based on realistic expectations and personal experience (both good and bad)'. A similar view was expressed by a respondent describing him or herself as a 'health professional', who said 'I trust the info [sic] provided by the NHS. However, like treating any other ... sources, I usually check up a few other professional websites for the same info [sic], so I get a more complete picture of the subject, instead of relying completely on ... one source'. Others mentioned trusting the NHS 'to a large extent' or 'on the whole', but, 'also look elsewhere for the information'. This echoes a constant theme of Internet usage – that people will look at several Internet sites (and therefore, consult several organisations) for information. This appears to be true even when people 'trust' one site, or when they go to predefined site types, such as 'academic' etc. The ease of information access has made Internet users into information connoisseurs.

Another important issue was raised regarding trust. One respondent considered that the information was 'Trustworthy in the sense that the information present will be accurate on the whole', but went on to say that it was, however, 'biased in the sense that there is an economic consideration with healthcare provision and the NHS is representing the DoH policies and may not promote treatments that are not available widely on the NHS'. This may be a view held by others who also elect to seek corroborative information from elsewhere. This emphasis on the NHS providing information favourable to its own or wider government policies was articulated most starkly by a female (age 30-40 years) who supported homeopathic medicine. She went so far as to say 'I guess I never just trust what the NHS says. I always research their diagnosis as well as their proposed remedy before using it.' This was because, 'western medicine in general is myopic in its approach to the matter of health. Basically I feel there is too much of the notion that current medical practices can "heal" you and too little on the concept of responsibility for one's own state of health; mentally, physically and spiritually. ... What the NHS offers is just one part of the whole'. This subject takes the debate to a new level, where trust is withheld because the information provided fits a philosophy of health and treatment at odds with that of the information seeker.

People can be expected to obtain a variety of benefits as a result of using health websites to achieve healthy outcomes. Figure 4.18 looks at a variety of outcomes broken down by respondents who had never used NHS Direct Online, those who used NHS Direct Online only and those that had used a combination of sites. This study is biased towards broadsheet readers and these users were more likely to be NHS Direct Online users.

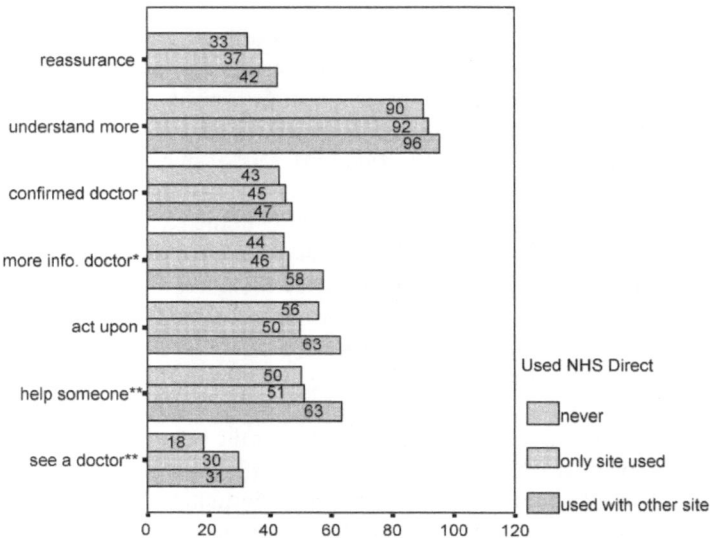

Figure 4.18 Perceived benefits of Internet health information by websites used

Ninety-three percent of respondents said that the information found had helped in understanding more about an illness or injury and a relatively high 57% of respondents said that the information found was sufficient for them to improve their health. Fifty-eight percent said that information found enabled them to help someone else, while 51% said that it gave then information that the doctor had not given them. Forty-six percent of respondents said that the information found had confirmed what the doctor had told them, while 38% said the information found had given reassurance about recovery from an illness or injury. Twenty-six percent said that the information found had affected their decision about whether to see a doctor.

In general, those respondents who visited a combination of websites that included NHS Direct Online reported better outcomes. This was particularly true for the following outcomes: finding more information than the doctor had given them, finding information that helped someone else and finding information that affected their decision about whether to see a doctor. There was no difference in outcome between those who used NHS Direct Online only and those who had never used it in the cases of finding more information than provided by the doctor and finding information that helped someone else. Those using NHS Direct Online only reported the same outcome as those using this site in combination with others. In the case of finding information that affected their decision about whether to see a doctor, both groups had a better outcome compared to those that never visited NHS Direct. Respondents who had used NHS Direct Online only reported a lower outcome than either those who had never used NHS Direct Online or used it in combination, in the case of finding sufficient information for them to improve their health. However the difference was not significant. Generally, those respondents who had included the NHS site as a visited site reported better outcomes compared to respondents that had never used NHS Direct. But the outcome difference was small and suggests that further research in this area is needed.

Respondents were also asked if obtaining health and medical information on the Internet influenced them in changing their health-related behaviour. We broke down the results by respondents who had never used NHS Direct Online, those who only used NHS Direct Online, and those who used a combination of sites.

Nearly half the respondents (45%) said that information found had caused them to think about the things they eat. Forty percent said that information found had made them more aware of the need to live a healthy life while 38% had said it encouraged them to take more exercise. Just under a third said that the information found led them to eat more fruit and vegetables while 26% said that it had encouraged them to relax more. Internet information seems to have the least impact on smoking and drinking habits with only 4% of respondents saying they were influenced to give up smoking while 11% said that the information found had influenced the amount of alcohol consumed. Six percent said that the information found had caused them to 'go for regular health checks with my doctor'.

Again those who used NHS Direct Online in combination with other sites were more likely to find information that resulted in a change in behaviour. This was most true in connection with finding information that resulted in health lifestyle changes: 50% of respondents using a combination of sites reported this compared to 30% of those that just used NHS Direct Online and 34% of those that never used it.

Impact on health professionals

Material to inform this issue was obtained from studies principally concerning kiosks. In addition to views being sought specifically about the kiosk, medical professionals were asked about the impact on them of the availability of consumer health information on the Internet.

Results suggested that health professionals used the Internet to obtain a large amount of information. If it had not impacted on their work with patients, it certainly had with regard to their own professional development and information requirements. Doctors indicated that, in the comparatively rare occasions when patients came to the surgery with complaints that required research on the part of the medical professionals, the Internet – in the shape of online medical journals and other resources mentioned above – made the job of diagnosis and patient advice a lot easier. Not surprisingly, none of the respondents indicated that they consulted the

Internet during a consultation, but undertook their research in time for a following appointment.

Of more direct interest to this study is the impact of the Internet on health professionals with regard to their dealings with patients. One development seems to be the encouragement by health professionals for their patients to use the Internet – despite the claim in a recent British Medical Journal editorial that some doctors have gone so far as to warn their patients, 'Whatever you do, don't go on the Internet.' (Ferguson 2002). In one case this encouragement was for them to 'use, in particular, NHS Direct', in this case for self-care and other information. This represents an interesting development following the well publicised phenomenon of patients using the Internet to challenge or complement information provided by the GP (see, e.g. Rumbelow 1999). Of course, the particular sample was Internet-using respondents, so there might be a natural propensity amongst this group to champion the system.

When asked specifically about patients bringing in Internet printouts or discussing information they had acquired through this medium, the prevailing view was that, in fact, it was not the Internet per se which had had an impact on their work, but what one called the 'Information explosion'. He continued 'we are inundated with half heard or understood fragments of information from the television or half read magazine articles'. Another said that 'quite often someone will come in with something in their head grabbed from Radio Four that morning'. As previous literature indicates (e.g. Potts and Wyatt 2002), the main impact of patients seeking information prior to consultations, is that those consultations are longer, a result that was not considered a positive development, owing to the time constraints under which doctors operate. There was some debate about whether the information obtained by patients at least made the consultation better, albeit inconveniently long. The general view seemed to be that 'in some cases' it helped going through any accompanying literature, but that 'usually the doctor has to allay fears or iron out misconceptions'.

Published research suggests (Pergament *et al* 1999; Friedewald 2000; Poensgen and Larsson 2001), there are indications that there might be a somewhat bigger impact in the future. One respondent complained that 'I can see the time when people are steaming in with bits of paper to wave at me from God knows what dodgy Internet site'. Another, in a more sober assessment, said that information was gradually 'permeating' everybody's lives, and that it would become more and more important for health care and health consultations for patients to be better informed – a view that, although not mentioned, was articulated in the recent report on the future of healthcare by Wanless (2002). Others, too, indicated that as the Internet and digital television became more and more available, so health information – as with all other forms – would become, as one put it, 'unavoidably imbibed'. This would affect consultations, 'largely to the good', although there might be implications regarding consultation time allocations.

Patients and the general public were also asked about the impact of the Internet in their dealings with medical professionals. There was some indication that the Internet had enhanced the doctor-patient encounter.

Use of other health information sources

Respondents were asked about the extent to which (if at all) the Internet had replaced other sources of information. At first this might seem a straightforward issue. However, as with other aspects of the impact of the Internet, the situation is more complex than meets the eye (see, e.g. Menou 2000). The key to this question was highlighted by a 20-30 year old female respondent, who said: 'it is difficult to know whether I would have used other sources if the net was not around or whether my interest in health info developed in line with the availability on the net'. It might be, then, that a respondent who says the Internet has not replaced any other information sources may nevertheless use the system very heavily, undertaking research that might not otherwise have been considered. One person hinted at this by saying that 'I would not have known where to find books or magazines on my condition'. It may also be that someone claiming that the Internet has replaced other sources to a great extent is simply looking for more information now that it is so easily accessible. Similarly, as another respondent pointed out, 'generally the Internet provides information that just wasn't available before to normal (i.e. non-medical) people'. With these caveats, then, the results indicated that for these respondents at least, the Internet has replaced other sources quite dramatically. Of the 36 people who addressed this question, 22 (61%) gave answers indicating a major displacement (as evidenced by use of phrases such as 'by far', 'totally', 'almost completely', and actual percentages – one person, for example, claimed that, for him 'The Internet has replaced 80% of all information media').

A minority of responses to this question either gave reasons for any displacement, or indicted what media were being displaced. In one case, actually mentioned earlier with regard to the impact on dealings with the medical profession, one person claimed to visit their doctor less often. In other cases the displacement was of books or surgery pamphlets. Those who gave reasons for displacement mentioned:

- Convenience and accessibility (a journalist wrote, 'Its so convenient – I never phone organisations for freebie leaflets any more'; and another respondent that 'it has totally replaced books, Information is much more easily accessible',
- Interactivity (a childbirth educator said that 'it's overtaken other methods by far. It's far more interesting and I can't interact with a book or magazine'),
- Currency (according to a company director 'Books are too out of date relating to medical matters'. Similarly, another respondent felt that 'you will always be able to access the most up to date information on the Internet, whereas a library may not have it available).

The Internet appeared to have displaced some sources by moving up in the ranking of sources consulted. Several respondents stated that the Internet was now the first source consulted, and that other sources are only consulted 'when I can't get what I need from the Internet'. This is true even for one correspondent working in a location where there was a medical library: 'I usually first try to find relevant info on the net, because it is easier than getting hold of hard copies of the same or similar info. If the net can't offer enough, then I will try to get the information from medical library at work'. Conversely, another claimed to still use books, but 'only because I haven't had a look at what is on the Internet yet'. This respondent is interested in alternative medicines and it is possible (although she did not respond to a follow-up email) that she has her own hardcopy collection, which may be as convenient to consult as going online.

Interestingly, one respondent felt that the Internet had replaced other sources 'too much in some ways!'; explaining that 'It's great, for what it is. But too many people forget its limitations, and the fact that a lot of these pages are posted up by well meaning but incorrect people!'

With regard to exactly what has been displaced, quite a few respondents mentioned particular media (but no-one mentioned specific sources such as a particular reference book or video series etc.). For all of these subjects, it was hardcopy media that was being displaced (e.g. 'I am not purchasing as many alternative health references books as I used to.' ... 'It has largely replaced book based material'). Although, as covered in a different question, there were some remarks in answer to this question to suggest that information was being used as a substitute for visiting a doctor, the scale of this seems to be very low. The observation made by some respondents in the present study that they now looked for information whereas in the past they might not have, indicates that as the Internet has been instrumental in facilitating the availability of information, it might, in the longer term, actually lead to a small displacement in seeking information from doctors to the use of electronic sources.

Categorising users of NHS Direct Online and SurgeryDoor

It is evident that different user types might be attracted to different types of health sites. A 'one-size, all-purpose' health site that fits all user types and interest of users is unlikely to exist. People may be attracted to a site for style differences as well as site attribute factors and content differences. Also, old and young users may distinguish themselves by adopting different site visiting behaviour. We can look at user differences revealed between SurgeryDoor users who have visited different combinations of health sites. Here we will look at site attribute, topic interest and user characteristic differences between SurgeryDoor users who also used NHS Direct Online and with SurgeryDoor users who also visited NetDoctor. The aim of the analysis is to see whether these differences revealed any information about the profiles of users for the various consumer health sites.

Twenty nine percent of SurgeryDoor questionnaire respondents said that they visited just one site for their health information, 71% visited two or more sites and 39% visited three or more different sites.

Looking at which site people visited first and which ones they additionally used, it was found, not surprisingly perhaps, that about nine in 10 users said that SurgeryDoor was their first choice. NHS Direct Online, NetDoctor (http://www.netdoctor.co.uk), Medicdirect and Health in Focus were also mentioned as a first choice but the percentages were insignificant, between 1% and 4%. These four sites however were significant as second sites visited. NetDoctor and NHS Direct Online were clearly important, each attracting around a third of responses as a second site preference.

In comparing NHS Direct Online users to other users, salary was found to be an important distinguishing factor. There was an increased incidence of a person being a NHS Direct Online user as income levels increased. NHS Direct Online seemed to attract the more wealthy users. Of course, the wealth variable here may be an indicator of other variables that relate to it, for example the user's education and class. The NHS Direct Online site might appeal to this type of user. Hence NHS Direct Online may well be perceived to be a more upmarket or a traditional, safe and conservative site – a broad sheet rather than a tabloid type of health site. However, as noted above, a quarter of respondents found out about the site via press advertisements and users of broadsheet newspapers may respond better to press advertisement than tabloid readers. NHS Direct Online users were also, significantly more likely to rate general health, and to a lesser extent medical news information. as important or very important.

Users identified as wanting to stay fit and healthy do differentiate between the sites. Thus the 'staying fit and healthy' user type tended to be more likely to be also an NHS Direct Online user and less likely to be a NetDoctor user. Those who used both SurgeryDoor and NHS Direct Online were more likely to be a 'staying fit and healthy' type user, while those SurgeryDoor and NetDoctor users were less likely to be. This type of user seemed more attracted to NHS Direct Online and less attracted to the NetDoctor site. This says something about the type of user; the variable itself 'staying fit and healthy' may indicate a type of seriousness about health. Perhaps NetDoctor users are not so interested in staying fit and healthy but are more interested in the health limitations and implications for their life style? This may also say something about the content difference between the two sites (NetDoctor and NHS Direct Online) and how each site markets itself.

In a survey conducted of UK Internet users, which sought to find out whether people had used health websites and which ones they had used, the most accessed site by some margin proved to be NHS Direct Online. More than two-thirds (64%) of all UK respondents had visited this site, a very high proportion indeed when you consider the sheer choice of sites on offer. The next most visited sites, by some distance, were NetDoctor (25%) and Yahoo! Health (24%).

However, this result cannot be comfortably generalised to the UK population of online users searching for consumer health information. This is because the sample was heavily biased towards readers of The Guardian newspaper, who it was discovered (see below) were just under twice as likely to use NHS Direct Online as other newspaper readers.

Just over a third of respondents (35%) had visited just one of the above sites, 53% had visited between 2 to 5 sites, 10% had visited between 6 to 10 of the sites and 4% had visited 11 or more of the sites.

Here we shall compare the characteristics of those respondents who had used NHS Direct Online with those who had not used it. In all, 36% of respondents had not used NHS Direct Online. Variables found not significant in the analysis were gender, ethnicity, the respondent's health rating, where the user accessed the site from (home or work) and occupation; NHS Direct Online users do not appear to be different from non-NHS Direct Online users in these respects. Variables found significant for this study were the respondents' age, marital status, the newspaper the respondent read (Sun, Guardian and Independent), and whether the respondent was just browsing for no site in particular.

This study found that NHS Direct Online users were likely to be younger compared to respondents who had never used it. Those respondents who were living with a partner or married were about twice as likely to be NHS Direct Online users compared to single or widowed or separated respondents. Respondents who read the Sun were about half as likely to be an NHS Direct Online user, while Guardian readers were just under twice as likely to use the service. Independent users were about one-third less likely to be NHS Direct users. This confirms previous results that found that the NHS Direct Online site attracted users with a wealth profile. Those just browsing were unlikely to find NHS Direct Online. These respondents were, in fact, only half as likely as other groups to have found the site.

Medicdirect

The Medicdirect evaluation was somewhat different to that of the two other website evaluations and the chief concern was to discover how a doctor-lead service performed as compared to the commercial (SurgeryDoor) and government (NHS Direct Online) services. A description of the key attributes of the site follows.

Site construction Medicdirect's homepage was split into three sections longitudinally down the page (Figure 4.19). On the left-hand side were the login features for registered and new users, there were also general links to information about the site included are a site guide and press releases. The main sources of information were located in the middle of the page, which contained the 'Contents' and 'Features' section. These areas contained links to the full repository of information that Medicdirect publish. The right hand side of the page contained a shortened navigational menu with a series of links to news topics, videos, contacting a specialist, a medical A-Z, other resources, feedback facility, and the opportunity to join the mailing list of the site. Below this was the 'Health Focus' area dedicated to raising the awareness of specific health themes. The home page was spread over two screens so only the Contents section, part of the Features section and the right hand menu options were immediately visible prior to any scrolling down.

Information sources Health care professionals wrote the information provided on the site. Their backgrounds covered a wide range of specialist areas including doctors, surgeons, dentists, nurses, and hygienists. Each contributor was contractually obliged to review the information they wrote every three months and make updates where necessary. The Medicdirect editorial board reviewed these updates prior to any implementation on the site.

Personalisation Medicdirect allowed users to personalise the home page with topics that were of interest to them. In order to use this functionality, users were first required to register, using their email addresses. As well as providing information in text format, the site provides videos showing operations and patient information. Users could also email questions to the site, and get feedback from the relevant health practitioner.

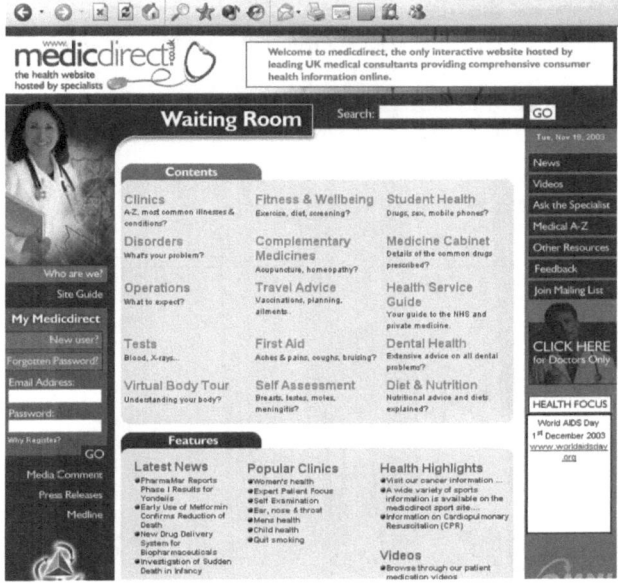

Figure 4.19 Medicdirect home page

Use and users

Table 4.8 gives the overall metric of use for the study period October – December 2003. There were approximately 1000 user sessions per day. The average number of pages viewed in a day was about 9,500. Over the period approximately 500 robot or user agents visited the site and these were excluded from the analysis. Sessions lasted on average just over four and half minutes and individual page view time was about 12 seconds.

Table 4.8 Key Medicdirect use metrics

Metric	Daily average
Average daily number of users per day	961
Average daily number of pages viewed per day	9,565
Average daily number of pages printed per day	61
Average session length (seconds)	282
Average page view time (seconds)	12.2

Note, the Medicdirect site was unusual in enabling the researchers to determine whether pages were printed or not.

Figure 4.20 shows the daily number of users for the three month period October – December 2003. Daily user numbers varied from about 800 to 1400 users in October to 600 to a 1000 in December. A noticeable decline in daily user figures can be seen through out the period and this decline is typical of Internet use that tends to dip over the seasonal break period. Over the three month period surveyed most users (89%) only visited the site once, 10% visited two to five times and 1% visited six or more times.

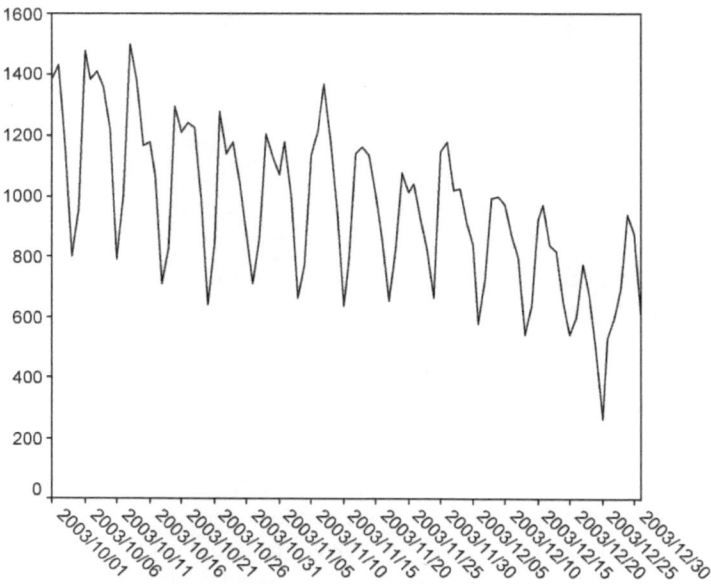

Figure 4.20 Medicdirect – daily number of users (October-December 2003)

In terms of using Medicdirect's 'print this page' online option those returning more regularly to the site were more likely to use this facility (Figure 4.21). This could be a function of familiarity or simply be a reflection of the fact that if you return you must obviously think there is data worth returning for, and printing out is another manifestation of interest/relevance. Well over a third (38%) of those returning more 15 times had printed, compared to 9% who returned six to 15 times and 2% returning between two to five times. This is a useful metric. Overall, it was found that approximately 1% of all pages were printed using Medicdirect's 'Print this page' option. The possibility of people using the browser print option to print might explain this very low figure. Of course, it was possible that the promiscuous user had seen all they wanted and had moved on, without bothering to print.

Daily use varied from about 8-9000 to 12 to 13,000 views. A decline in daily use figures (similar to the decline in users) occurred from about the middle of November and this decline is typical of Internet use which tends to dip over the seasonal period.

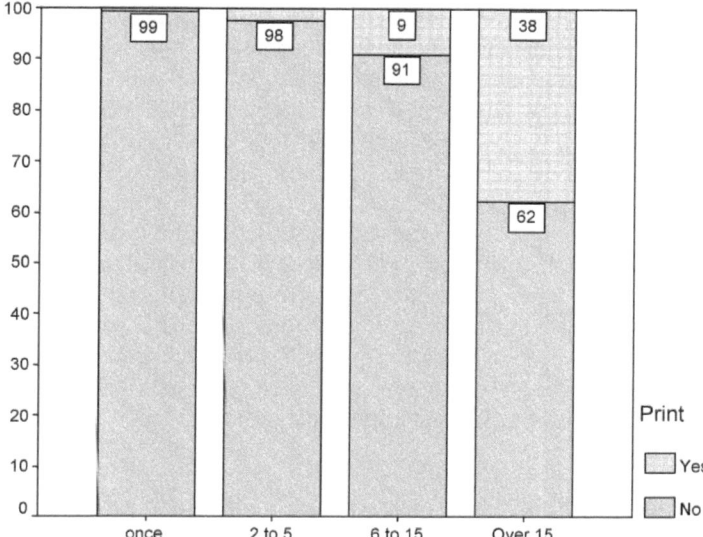

Figure 4.21 Medicdirect – distribution of pages printed by number of visits

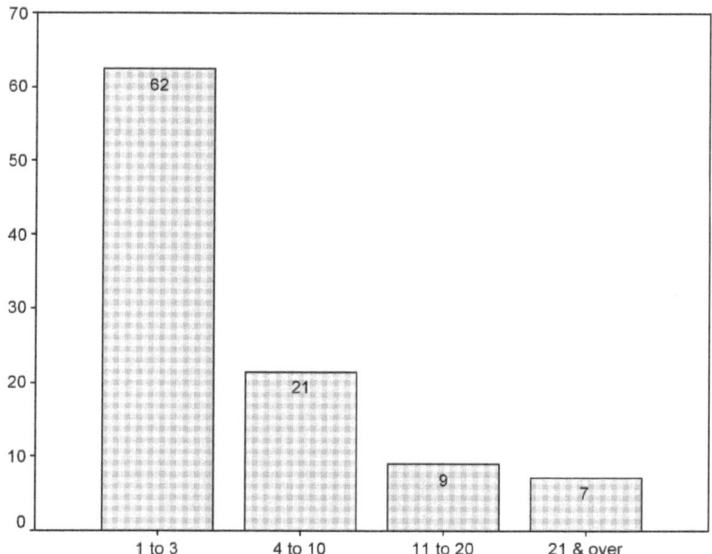

Figure 4.22 Medicdirect – system page penetration – the percentage distribution of pages viewed in a session

In terms of the number of pages viewed in a session, 62% saw just one to three pages viewed, 21% viewed between four to 10 pages, 9% 11 to 20 pages, and 7% of session viewed 21 or more pages (Figure 4.22). It was estimated that users spent approximately 12 seconds viewing a page. In terms of the time spent viewing different subject pages, the longest time was recorded for 'monitor' pages, and users spent on average 43 seconds looking at this page. Other pages/sections that also recorded a long page view time were diet (22 seconds), medical A to Z (25 seconds), newstuff (32 seconds), search (26 seconds) and specialist (21 seconds).

The use pattern of day of week was similar to that recorded for SurgeryDoor. A low weekday use was recorded for Fridays (respectively, 13% and 14%) and a high use recorded for Mondays and Tuesdays (16% and 17%), while Sundays for both sites had a higher use than Saturdays (13% and 12% compared to 11% and 10%).

Use throughout the day increased from a low point at 7am and peaked at about 1pm; the decline after 2pm was steady with a blip increase between 6 and 7pm. Use was lowest between 3 to 6am. Medicdirect and SurgeryDoor peaked at the same time; however Medicdirect had a higher peak compared to SurgeryDoor. Almost 12% of its use was recorded at about 1pm and this compared to about 6% for SurgeryDoor at the same time.

Topics viewed/ Health concerns The top 15 sections accounted for about 91% of all views. The most popular section was diseases (22%), followed by clinics (18%) and the homepage (8%).

Table 4.9 Medicdirect – top 20 pages viewed

Pages	%
Downloadable Videos – Operations	2.0
Virtual Body: Woman	.6
Biographies – Medicine	.6
Virtual Body: Man	.5
Advertising and Sponsorship With medicdirect.co.uk	.5
Doctors Speak	.5
Dental Abscesses	.5
Stress Saving Strategies	.4
A-Z of Homeopathy	.4
Links	.4
Mouth Ulcers	.4
Who are we?	.3
Bowel Cancer (Cancer of the Colon and Rectum)	.3
Peptic Ulcer Disease (Duodenal Ulcer: Gastric Ulcer)	.3
Weight Reducing Diets	.3
Laparoscopy Operation	.3
Testicular Self-Examination	.3
Tonsillitis and Glandular Fever	.3
Osteoporosis	.3
Bladder Cancer	.3
Accounts as a % of all page views	9.3

Medicdirect had 1,843 content pages in all. The top 20 accounted for just below 10% of all content viewed (Table 4.9), suggesting that interest was quite widespread. The most viewed documents were, Downloadable Videos – Operations (2%), Virtual Body: Woman (0.6%), Biographies – Medicine (0.6%). Interestingly, videos appeared more popular here than they did on the NHS Direct Digital/Communicopia service. It could be to do with the quality or subject difference of the videos. Of special interest is the popularity of the page 'Downloadable Videos – Operations'. This reinforces the popularity of health videos argument.

Characterising users

Most users, 58%, had a USA IP address and only 24% had a UK address, this as we explained before can be biased because many UK users may register their Internet IP address in the US. In terms of organisation type nearly 44 percent of users accessed the site via a commercial institution while 30% accessed it from an educational institution and about 23% via a net provider (home users perhaps). Looking just at academic and government users to get a more accurate estimation of the geographical location of the user, it was found that between 51% to 57% of Medicdirect users were actually located in the UK, 24% to 36% were located in the US, about 12% were located in Australia, and 8% in Canada.

The referrer link gives for each user the site address of the last site visited. This information is useful for identifying those users coming from search engines, and who might be different in character from those people coming via different routes. For this study, four referrer groupings were identified: Other link, Other ISP link, External link and a link via a Search engine.

- Search engine links were those user sessions that were identified as coming from the following links: Lycos, AOLsearch, Ask, Google, MSN, Yahoo or Your dictionary.
- External links were assumed to have come in via a Medicdirect hotspot advert link (i.e. aol.medicdirect), these include: Tiscali, GMTV, AOL or medicdirectsports.
- Other ISPs include those users coming in via one of the following: supanet, doctordirect, ntlworld or ifeelyuk.
- Other links are all those links that could not be easily grouped.

Over one third of sessions (38%) came into the site via an external (hotspot) link, 24% via a search engine, a third (33%) via an ungrouped link and 6% via an other ISP link.

The following Table (4.10) gives the top 13 referrer links. The top links account for a high 85% of all sessions. The most popular three being: gmtv.medicdirect.co.uk (14%), tiscali.medicdirect.co.uk (13.4%) and aol.medicdirect.co.uk (9.6%). Hotspots were plainly a popular means of finding the website. This is further evidence of the browsing, promiscuous user.

Table 4.10 Medicdirect – top 13 referrer links

Referrer link	%
google.com gmtv.medicdirect.co.uk	14.2
tiscali.medicdirect.co.uk	14.0
aol.medicdirect.co.uk	13.4
medicdirectsport.com	9.6
medicdirect.co.uk	9.0
ntlworld.com	3.6
supanet.com	3.3
uk.search.msn.com	2.6
search.yahoo.com	2.4
uk.search.yahoo.com	2.1
yourdictionary.com	1.0
ask.co.uk	1.0
mic.ki.se	.8
Accounts as % of all sessions	85.3

In terms of session time those coming in via an external link recorded the longest average (median) session time. Those coming in from an external link were estimated to have spent approximately 7 to 8 minutes on a session and this was unexpected, given that they did not view considerably more pages than the other groups. Perhaps those coming in from external links were subject to a load wait time, maybe as a result of a recording of the event by such organisations as Adclick. Those coming in from other ISP links also recorded a session length in excess of seven minutes. However, this should be expected as this group also recorded a particularly high number of views in a session. Those users coming in via a search recorded the shortest session of about two minutes.

Although well over a third (37%) of users came in via a search engine, these users were far more likely to view a smaller number of pages in a session compared to other users. About three-quarters viewed just 1 to 3 pages and then left, compared to 57% of those coming in via other links and 29% of those coming in via other ISP links. Search engine users consequently recorded shorter sessions. They were estimated to have had a session length of about two minutes; those coming in via another link recorded a session length twice as long, while those coming in via other ISP link recorded sessions three times the length. Furthermore, those coming in via a search engine were far more likely just to visit once and not return.

Chapter 5

Health Digital Interactive Television (DiTV)

DiTV, sometimes referred to as interactive digital TV (IDTV), combines television content with some of the interactivity we are now used to on the internet such as clicking on links. Interactive digital TV channels are supplied onto a television set through a 'set top box', which sits on or near the TV. The interactive element comes from the channels having what is known as a 'return path' – a means whereby the user can send their own signals back to the broadcaster. This allows the user to request different pieces of information, still images or video clips, within a browser environment similar to but less sophisticated than a web browser.

In this exciting new world of modern interactive communications technology, digital television has been regarded as having greater potential than the internet because television is already a well-established medium. Nearly every household in the UK has at leas one TV set and they are all to be digital by 2012. In 1997 White Paper, The New NHS (Department of Health 1997) identified the Internet and digital TV as key media through which public access to the NHS could be improved. It was envisaged that new interactive communications media could empower patients to take more care of their own health as well as improving the efficiency of health provision in the UK In June 2000, Gisela Stuart, the (then) Parliamentary Under-Secretary of State for Health, announced that the DoH would fund a series of pilot projects exploring possible health applications of DiTV. The aim was to provide patients with easy and fast access at home to health advice and information. What is presented in this chapter is a description of the characteristics of these DiTV services and the results of evaluative studies undertaken on these services.

In particular we wished to:

- determine whether digital interactive television 'worked' in a consumer health context. Did it, for instance, deliver the numbers, the particular audience profile, the ease of access and the hoped for health outcomes?
- evaluate and compare the four DoH contracted consortia's approaches to the delivery of health information on DiTV, to establish which approaches worked, with whom, and which of the approaches worked best?

The key evaluative criteria used to evaluate the DiTV services were similar to the one's we have used for the other platforms covered by this book, but, as the services were more varied than with the other platforms (i.e. including transactional services; real-time video conferencing; on-demand videos etc.) there were a few differences in how each element was explored. We were interested in:

- volume and pattern of use;
- users' experience and perceptions of the service;
- the range, quality and appropriateness of the services offered;
- co-ordination with other health services available;
- impact on NHS of supporting the service;
- impact on users' use of health services;
- impact on users' health status;
- impact on their perceptions of the NHS.

The four DiTV pilots offered distinctive services, although there were some overlapping features. The distinctive qualities included the type of platform on which a service was transmitted, the amount and nature of content, the presentation formats used, and the degree of interactivity involved in each case. The four consortia were: Communicopia, Flextech Telewest, Living Health, Channel Health and dktv (A Different Kind of Television). The latter two services where narrower in scope and ambition, and also provided little in the way of logs – our principal evaluation tool, to help us evaluate them. As a consequence, and to maintain the standardised evaluation adopted throughout the book, we cover these services in somewhat less detail.

Communicopia Productions – NHS Direct Digital

The service, developed and provided by Communicopia Productions, with content supplied by the NHS (and hence the brand name 'NHS Direct Digital'), aimed to extend the reach of the NHS Direct telephone and online service onto digital television. It was launched in November 2001, to an audience in Kingston upon Hull and the East Riding of Yorkshire via Kingston Interactive Television's (KIT) local ADSL (telephone) network. It was later also launched on Video Network's HomeChoice platform, as a pilot to viewers in London, in February 2002. The service enabled TV viewers to access key sets of data from the NHS Direct Online website, including details of over 400 illnesses and medical conditions, support organisations, and advice about living a more healthy life. Utilising a mixture of existing text-based material and specially produced video clips, the service provided users with over 20,000 pages of information, and video-on-demand offering both the perspective of medical professionals and that of patients. The service also provided users with interactive options such as health quizzes and an SMS text messaging reminder service for children's vaccination dates. This service was transmitted to 10,000 KIT subscribers, and The HomeChoice service was available to all those subscribing to the HomeChoice service at the time – 10,900 households.

Communicopia offered a similar information service to that of Living Health. The main menu offered the following options (Figure 5.1):

- Not Feeling Well? This part of the service allowed the viewer to choose a part of the body (head and chest; abdomen; limbs, or skin) and to choose from a list of possible symptoms, or to choose from a full list of all 54 symptoms. The viewer then had to answer yes or no to a series of questions which led them to a possible diagnosis and suggested courses of action (e.g., see GP; telephone 999 – the emergency services).

- A-Z of conditions. This section listed 274 conditions, more than the Living Health service, which listed a total of 157 conditions and operations. The section contained 3,661 pages of information. For each condition, information was typically given on symptoms, causes, prevention etc.
- First Aid. This section contained information on the recognition and treatment of following common problems such as bleeding, scalds, choking, heart attack etc.
- Medicine Cabinet. This was another searchable A-Z index of 149 medicines – fewer than the Living Health service (360). Brand name synonyms were helpfully included, e.g., Lisinopril/Zestril. There were also links to mini-menus of generic terms such as 'cream' and 'lotion'. Typically information was given on use, dosage, effect and duration etc.
- Healthy Living. This section covered topics such as Eating for Health, Getting Active and Quitting Smoking. Some quizzes were also included.
- Local Information. Information was provided on blood donation (including a video) and details of local doctors, hospitals and pharmacies. It was possible to search for currently open pharmacies.
- About This Service. Information was given about the pilot service and those involved in its production and content provision, including an FAQ section and a privacy statement.

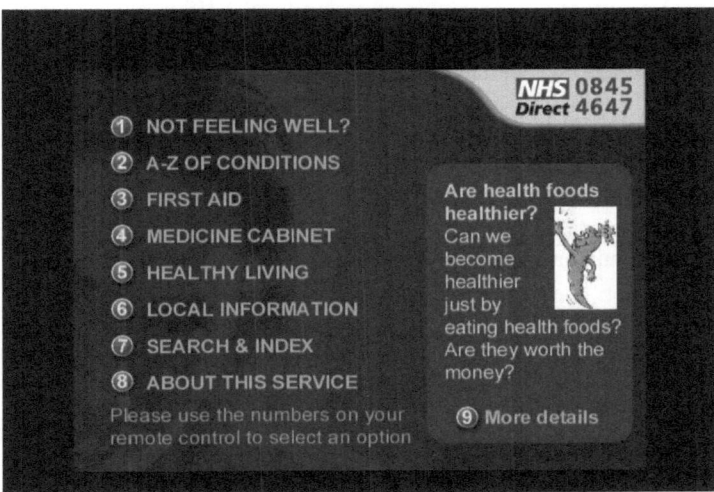

Figure 5.1 NHS Direct Digital: screenshot

The service had a hierarchical structure with users having to click through up to four hierarchical menus before arriving at the final information content. The content pages listed the other menu options at the same hierarchical level for that particular topic. Unlike the Living Health service, the DiTV service to which it bore the closest resemblance, menu pages also contained some introductory content. It was possible to read this text only and gain at least a rudimentary level of information, and so not have to proceed further to content at the next level. This additional text also meant that some menus spanned two screens.

The coverage of this service differed from that of Living Health (see below). There was a greater concentration on conditions and treatment and less on healthy lifestyles and practical advice. The content was more focused on medical information than on information on coping, self-help and the emotional aspects of life. Unlike Living Health, the content was not targeted at specific groups (i.e., men, women and children). The information was also largely accessible only through a search menu system. In addition to the text content there were 95 videos, linked to the topics outlined above. There were videos on, for example, MMR, Exercise for Older People, Baby Resuscitation, Adult Resuscitation, Blood Donation, and Eating for Health.

Flextech Telewest – Living Health

Flextech Living Health Ltd. and partners launched a pilot service featuring a range of digital TV health applications in June 2001, to a potential average audience of 45,000 in the Birmingham area via the Telewest cable network. The applications included the very innovative NHS Direct InVision (talking to and actually seeing a nurse), a system for booking an appointment with a GP through the TV and a wide range (over 22,000 pages) of information services covering local NHS services, healthy living, health conditions and treatments and a database of medicines. The pilot ran for six months and was then extended by Flextech Living Health for another six months.

The Living Health service received a number of media awards including two awards at the New Media Age Effectiveness Awards, best interactive TV service at the International EMMA (Electronic Media) Awards in 2001 and best project for Government Services to Citizen award at the 2002 Government Computing Innovation Conference.

The information service on Living Health consisted of eight sections (Figure 5.2). These were:

- Today's health news: consisting of current news stories having a health angle.
- Healthy Living: consisted of a large number of subheadings including Calculate Your Alcohol Intake, Alcohol, and Drugs.
- Men's Health: included sub-headers on, for example, Men's Sexual Health Sports Injuries (which activated the same link as a submenu item on the Healthy Living pages).
- Women's Health: included Antenatal Tests and Pregnancy and Birth.
- Children's Health: included Child Care and Development, Immunisation and Minor Ailments.

- Illness and Treatment: included Alternative Medicine, Being Prepared for an Emergency, and Common Illnesses. The latter opened to a submenu with 75 conditions listed, from AIDS to Wisdom Tooth Removal.
- Local Health Services: included a local directory of Chemists, Dentists, Doctors, etc.
- InVision: This opened the sequence leading to the online nurse consultation service, a one-way video (two way audio) link to a nurse at an NHS call centre.

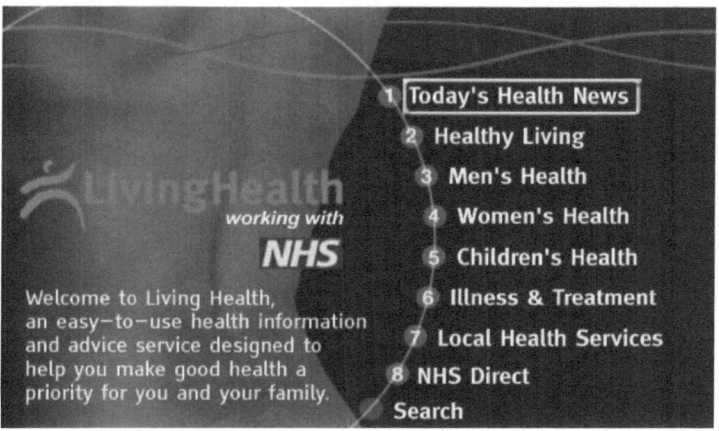

Figure 5.2 Living Health: screenshot

The hierarchical menu structure had up to six levels but most sections used four or five. Today's Health News simply gave a sub-menu of current topics of interest which lead directly to content, but in most sections the viewer needed to go step-wise through two to four menus before arriving at information content. The first sub-menus under sections two to four (Health Matters) were something of an exception to this. Selecting, for example, Men's Health Matter, took the viewer-user directly to content. From there, there was a link back to a menu listing the topic already viewed, and others.

Channel Health

Channel Health piloted a series of broadcast TV programmes (called Bush Babies, as it featured pregnant women from Shepherds Bush) to a national audience of over five million, with linked interactive services. The programmes dealt with health, social and financial issues relevant to pregnant women and the interactivity enhanced and supplemented these by providing a range of text-based pregnancy and maternity related information. Channel Health presented a text-based information service linked to special broadcasts in its regular schedule on the Sky Digital platform.

It experimented, on a local basis, with a package of other interactive services for pregnant women comprising mainly email support links between users and health professionals.

This service was predominantly a broadcast programme, Bush Babies, which told the stories of seven women, in varying stages of their pregnancy. Each expectant mother was said by the Channel Health website guide to represent different ethnic and social groupings. The programmes filmed their progress through the different stages of pregnancy.

Each programme provided Fact Files, which were short information segments that contained up-to-date information and advice on many aspects of pregnancy (Figure 5.3). An example of a Fact File was:

'Pregnancy: some of the signs:
*   increased vaginal discharge
*   feeling tired
*   strange taste in mouth
*   going off certain things'

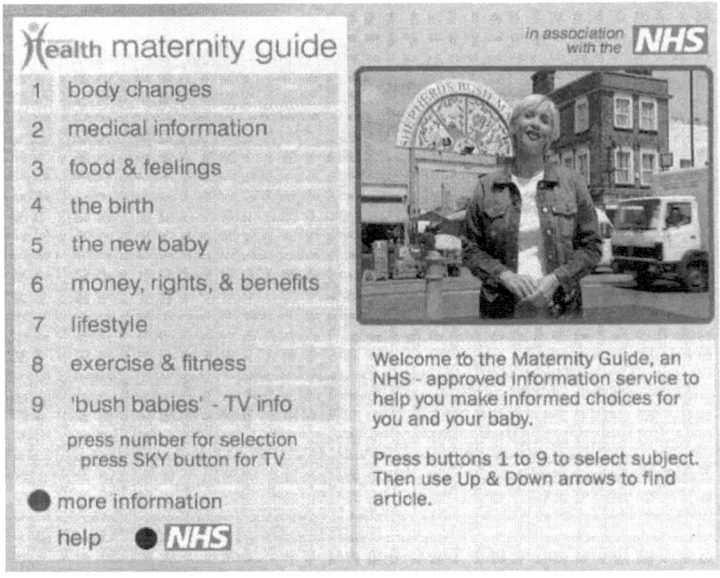

Figure 5.3 Channel Health Maternity Guide: screenshot

An 'enhanced' service consisted of information pages about pregnancy, covering such topics as benefits, medication, symptoms etc.

As the evaluation concerned Bush Babies and not the entire health output of Channel Health, where we have referred to the service as 'Channel Health' this should be taken to mean the channel's Bush Babies series unless otherwise stated.

dktv

Developed by dktv for the HomeChoice platform and launched initially to Newham residents, this service aimed to work together with public sector organisations to provide national and local interactive television content. The service relied on the HomeChoice video-on-demand, enabling users to select and find out more about the local services on offer to them. The video clips were presented by local service employees and provided users with the option to press a button to forward their details to local service providers. Originally intended to be rolled out on cable TV and broadband platforms in London, in the end only the broadband version of the service was launched by dktv and evaluated. This service was transmitted to approximately 500 potential users on Video Networks Limited's HomeChoice service in Newham.

The Health information service, which we evaluated could be found under a Family Services subheading on the main menu of the service (Figure 5.4).

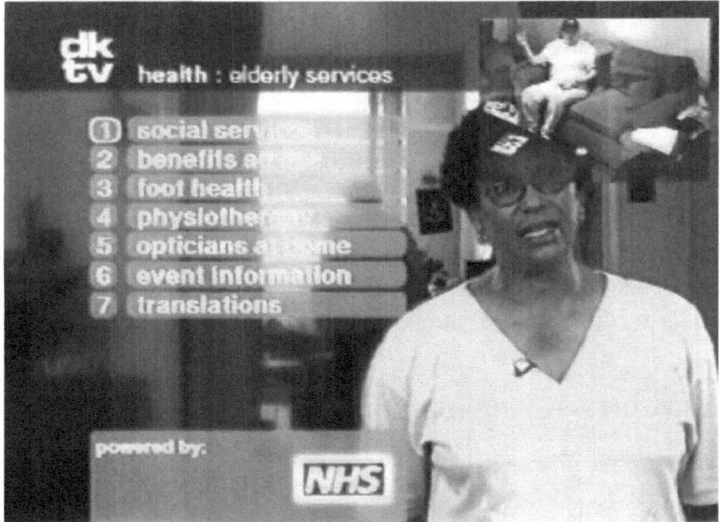

Figure 5.4 dktv: screenshot

In the context of health information, the dktv service was vying with a separate link to NHS Direct Interactive from the Leisure section of the Home Choice main menu. Health was just one of seven options on dktv's main menu. Other options included Local services; Housing; Learning etc. Accessing the main Health menu triggers a short video of a woman explaining the contents of the section. People who wanted to access two or three pages in each section had to view this each time they went back to the main menu.

The Health section covered five common topics, – heart health; smoking; stress; diet; drinking. Each topic consisted of a video of just over a minute's length and details of useful contact numbers and/or NHS Direct Online. Each video employed a mixture of voiceover and/or 'talking head'. There was a Further information option available from each topic, leading to the statement: '[Name] – your details are about to be forwarded to NHS Direct and dktv. Press OK to confirm or step back to cancel.' You would then be sent an information pack, although this was not stated. Further health related community information was available in the Social Services section. The six videos here were slightly longer, at around 1m30s. The scenes were all appropriate to the topic, showing the people running the services going about their business, e.g. delivering meals, giving someone a health check, doing someone's shopping. Voiceovers were mostly used, but in this section some clients were also interviewed, e.g. a man and a lady talking about the aids that have helped them in their home (disability section). Service providers also contributed, e.g. a home help.

Use and users

Table 5.1 gives the overall metric estimates of use for the Living Health Service and Communicopia (NHS Digital). Living Health had a higher average number of users and page views compared to NHS Direct Digital. The service attracted on average 235 daily users and 7,266 page views compared to 31 daily users and 1,112 pages views for Communicopia (NHS Direct Digital). Part of this difference can be explained by differences in the potential user base or audience. The potential user base that could receive Living Health was approximately four times that of NHS Direct Digital – 40,000 compared to 10,000 potential users (KIT households). We would therefore expect Living Health figures to be larger. However, Living Health appeared to have attracted a higher multiple, as on average, it attracted seven to eight times as many users as NHS Direct Digital. However, half of this difference is accounted for by differences in the subscriber base of the two services.

Table 5.1 Key DiTV usage metrics

Metric	Living Health	Communicopia (NHS Direct Digital)
Average daily number of users per day	235	31
Average daily number of pages viewed per day	6,878	1,112
Average daily number of pages printed per day	N/A	N/A
Average session length (seconds)	279	484
Average page view time (seconds)	12.64	14.96
Potential user base	40,000	10,000

Note: Calculated over a 5 month period.

The average page view time of the Living Health service was about 13 seconds and the average session duration was just under five minutes. The figures for the

NHS Direct Digital service were slightly different. For this service, on average, users spent 15 seconds viewing a page and over seven minutes on a visit (session). The figures were higher for the NHS Direct Digital service. There could be two reasons for this: (1) the NHS Direct Digital service did include an option for the user to download and watch videos; (2) the user could not start the first session (in a day) without watching an introductory video. Clearly both of these factors would have added to the session time estimate.

Over the 12-month pilot period the four DiTV pilots were made available to a potential combined audience of five to six million households, equating to an estimated 11.5 to 12 million individual viewers.

Living Health was available to 40,000 subscribers. Over the period monitored, 13,718 different households used the system. Based upon this figure it is estimated that 30% to 34% of potential subscribing households accessed the service during the period – a healthy figure by any standards, especially considering that viewers had so much choice as what to view (sport, soaps, news etc). Note that reach is a function of the service period over which the figure is calculated. The longer the period over which reach is calculated the higher the reach figure will be. However, the rate of increase in the reach figure declines as the period over which the figure is calculated is lengthened, as returnees make up a bigger share of total users.

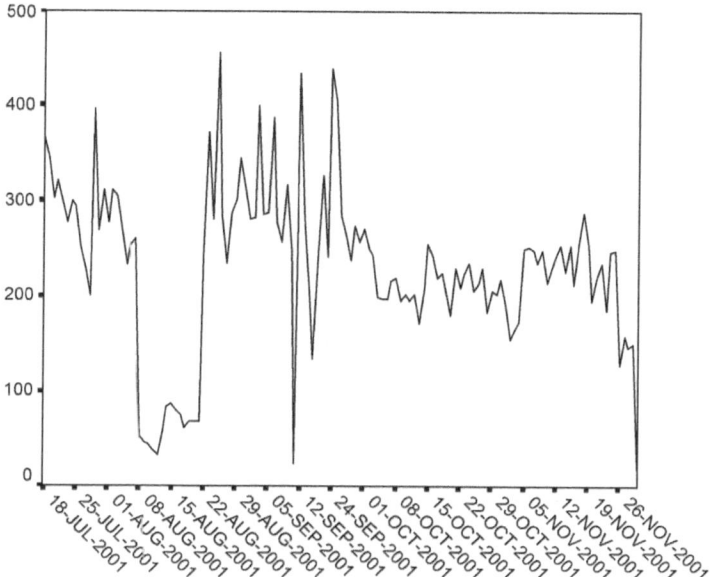

Figure 5.5 Daily user numbers – Living Health

Figure 5.5 shows the pattern of users over time. As for any new service use was volatile. The falling trend in use, the initial surge, and then decline may well be due to novelty value and early marketing efforts, and is probably unlikely to signify long-term stagnation. The potential for growth may be there, with well over eight in ten (84%) questionnaire respondents saying that they would be either fairly likely to or very likely to access Living Health if the service continued to be broadcast. Living Health interviewee respondents were equally enthusiastic: 'It will definitely become a prime source of information for me if it carries on – and if it doesn't I will be disappointed'.

NHS Direct Digital, delivered via KIT, was available to approximately 10,000 potential homes. During the period from January to the end of May 2002, the service was seen by around one in five (20%) of KIT subscribers (1,965). That is, the reach figure was estimated as 20%.

In terms of audience reach, Living Health performed much better than Communicopia/NHS Direct Digital, the service with which it had most in common. It should be noted that there are fundamental differences in the nature of video as opposed to text-based information delivery, and the lower reach figure for the former need not necessarily imply that the text service is 'better'.

In the case of dktv, during the two-month survey period 142 users availed themselves of the service, out of the 403 to 513 households receiving it – a reach figure of about 35%.

The only nationwide service, Channel Health, attracted aggregated audiences of around 2.8 million to episodes of its 'Bush Babies' series over the duration of its pilot. BARB data indicated that 'Bush Babies' episodes aggregated (across their repeat showings) audiences of over 300,000 in the first (6-week) phase, over 200,000 in the second (5-week) phase, and 2.3 million in the final (3-month) phase. By way of context, Channel Health calculated that 160,000 out of 700,000 annual births in the UK could occur in Channel Health receiving homes. Channel Health is estimated to have a monthly reach figure among Sky viewers of approximately 15%. Given a Sky Digital audience base of around 5.7 million households then the audience of Bush Babies was estimated to be about 200,000 homes. According to self-report survey data, 27% of Channel Health viewers watched Bush Babies. This is quite impressive, given that the target audience was pregnant women, not only a low percentage of the population as a whole, but, presumably, a low number even of Channel Health viewers.

It is estimated that between 250-300,000 people availed themselves of one or other of the digital television health services, a reach figure of 2%. At first glance this might appear to be disappointingly low. However, why the reach figure was so small overall is because most of the base population of approaching six million was contributed by Sky, and the reach of Channel Health in percentage terms was small (though it reached the largest potential audience overall). On Channel health, 30% of respondents who had identified themselves as viewers of 'Bush Babies' reported using the maternity guide – the enhanced text service that supported the 'Bush Babies' programmes. Hence, the much healthier reach figures for Living Health and Communicopia were significantly diluted by the performance of the service on Sky. The specialised nature of some of the services (i.e. pregnancy information) and the short time-span of their availability also needs to be taken into account in any reach calculation.

For Living Health just over 59% of people visited the channel just once in the operational period – meaning that a high percentage (41%) visited the service again (Table 5.2). For NHS Direct Digital the figure was quite similar: 65% of users visited the service only once and 35% visited the service again. The NHS Direct Digital service did not appear to attract so many repeat visits.

Table 5.2 shows the pattern of return visitors for the Living Health and NHS Direct Digital channel.

Table 5.2 Return visits within three months for two DiTV services

Number of days visited	Percentage frequency of users – Living Health	Percentage frequency of users – NHS Direct Digital
Once	59.0	67.1
2 to 5	35.0	28.7
6 to 15	5.4	3.8
Over 15	0.6	0.4
	100%	100%

Estimates based on a three-month use period.

The metric is however sensitive to differences in the time period over which the figure is calculated. Furthermore, the large number of users at the service inception who had a look to see what it was like, but had not returned to use it, may have thrown out this figure.

An alternative approach to take is to calculate returnees between periods of time. The number of new users attracted by NHS Direct has dropped substantially from one month to the next and in March the service attracted only about a quarter (167) of the January figure (708).

The situation at Living Health was quite different as the number of new users had remained almost the same from one month to the next (Figure 5.6).

The percentage share of returnees in the second period for each service was similar – 29% for NHS Direct Digital compared to 23% for Living Health. However, in the third period, returnees from periods one and two to NHS Direct Digital made up 50% of users, while for Living Health, this figure was 34%. In part this is explained by the fact the NHS Direct Digital was not attracting new users, thus weighting the percentage share towards returnees. In the third period, NHS Direct Digital recorded more returnees from period one compared to period two, 35% compared to 15%. During this period NHS Direct Digital visibility on the KIT main menu was reduced. That is, it was moved from the main menu first to a second level menu then to a third level menu. The reduced digital visibility of the services impacted on the attraction of new users. This argument, and the concept of digital visibility, is fully explored in Chapter 6.

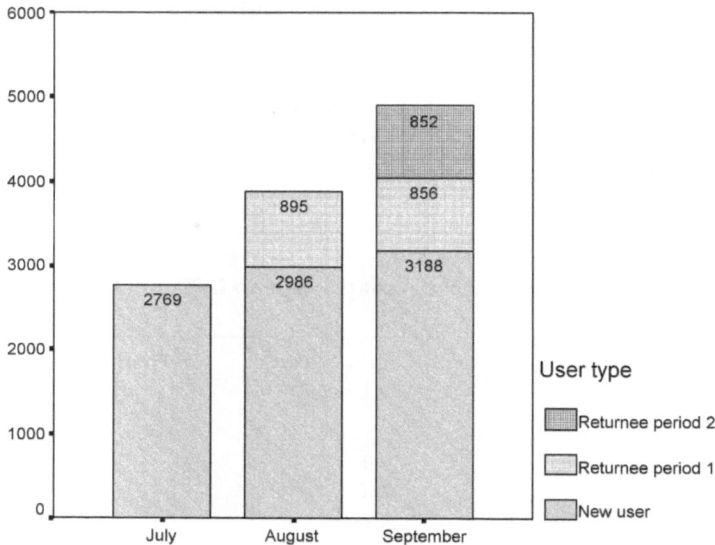

**Figure 5.6 Numbers of new users and returnees between months –
Living Health**

Use of NHS Direct Digital showed a massive initial peak in use of 15,000 page views per day during the first week after launch. Putting aside the first six days after launch date, the service recorded an average of around 1500 page views per day during the period analysed. April was quite a strong month in terms of demand and reflected the use increase as a result of the questionnaire that we sent to all KIT users.

The same volatility was shown in use figures for Living Health. Figure 5.7 gives the number of pages viewed per day. Use at the beginning of the period, 14 July, stood at approximately 14,000 page views a day. This represented a peak in use and from September use stabilised and fluctuated within the range of between 7,300 to 7,800 daily page views. There was a fall off in use during August 2001 due to sever problems. The peak in use in September reflected the use increase that resulted from the questionnaire that was sent to all Telewest subscribers who could receive the Living Health service. There was a sharp decline in use in the last week of November again as a result of server problems.

During a visit to Living Health users typically viewed 19 pages. For NHS Direct Digital, they viewed 23 pages. However, this service was a menu-heavy service and had a number of menu screens associated with both the video and text service. For both services there was evidence that once people had found the service they showed a significant degree of interest in it. In the case of Living Health, for example, 39% of users viewed more than 20 pages during a visit. Similarly, in the case of NHS Direct Digital, 44% of users viewed more than 20 pages (Table 5.3). Users viewing just one to three pages were unlikely to have accessed an actual information page and can be termed 'bouncers'. By contrast, users viewing over 20 pages can be described as heavy users or 'burrowers' with a good understanding of how to jump between pages and to use the technology to find the information they seek. Light users stay long enough to view a couple of pages and as a result show more interest and commitment than bouncers. Medium users have clearly an understanding of the service and have penetrated it to a limited depth.

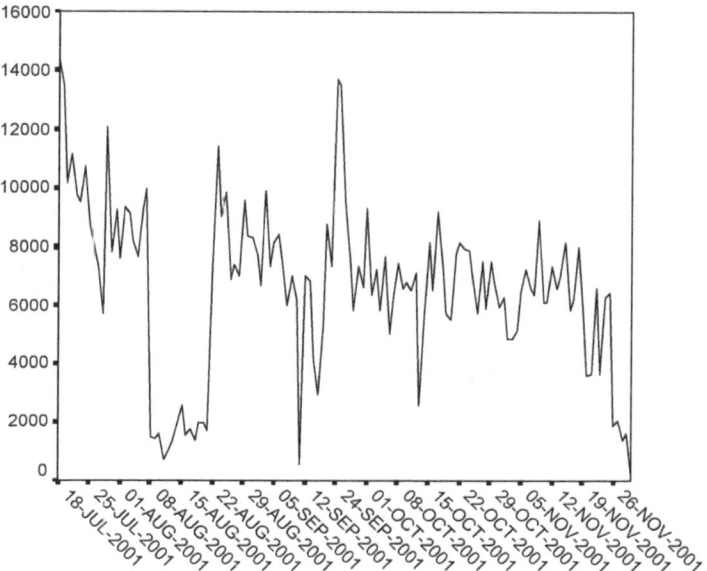

Figure 5.7 Living Health – daily use

Table 5.3 System page penetration for two DiTV services

User type	Number of pages viewed in a visit	Percentage frequency of users (Living Health)	Percentage frequency of users* (NHS Direct Digital)
Bouncers	1 to 3 pages viewed	18.9	19.0
Light users	4 to 10 pages viewed	23.0	20.4
Medium users	11 to 20 pages viewed	18.9	16.8
Heavy users	Over 20 pages viewed	39.2	43.9

* excludes video views
Estimates based on a three-month use period.

The figures were very similar for both services – approximately 19% of users on both services were bouncers. Bouncers were unlikely to have found anything of interest. The bouncer rate for DiTV was significantly less than for the Internet. This is probably because Internet users have much more choice and they avail themselves of this choice.

For the InVision service logs revealed that only 12% of those accessing the service actually completed a session (i.e., engaged in an online consultation with a nurse). These figures may provide evidence that early users were 'checking out' the system for future reference, not having an immediate need.

Table 5.3 may not give an accurate picture of service penetration. The NHS Direct Digital figure does not include views to the video service. Videos were of two kinds: introductory videos on how to use the service and parts of the service, and content videos. There was an introductory video to the whole service and each section of the service included an introductory video. Every viewer saw an introductory video either on entering the service or when selecting a section of the service. The ordering and downloading of videos necessarily entailed the user viewing considerably more menu screens.

Table 5.4 gives the number of menu screens and content objects (video or text) for each service. Over two thirds (68%) of views to the NHS Direct Digital services were made to menu screens: 56% for the text service, 3% for menus related to the video service and 9% to introductory video views. This compares to 44% of views that were made to menu screens for the Living Health service.

Table 5.4 Number of menu screens and content objects (video or text) for each service

	NHS Direct Digital		Living Health	
	N	%	N	%
Menu Screens for text service	45,474	56	285,071	44
Menu screens for video service	2,757	3	-	-
Introductory videos viewed	7,011	9	N/A	-
Content text screens viewed	25,208	31	368,327	56
Content Videos viewed	618	1	N/A	-
Total views	**81,068**	-	**653,398**	-

Estimates based on a three-month use period.

Given the views to menu screens, NHS Direct Digital viewers accessed approximately one content object (video or text) for every two menu objects. That is, only approximate one third of views related to pages with content. For Living Health this view ratio was better. There was approximately one content object view for just less that one menu screen and 56% of objects viewed relate to content views.

However, this impression given can be misleading. A content screen is a single screen or page of text information on a topic and there may well be number of pages for each topic while for video it is a stream of images. Clearly watching a video is similar to viewing a number of pages, in that information is being sought in each case, though there is no simple conversion. Specific points of information can only be serially accessed on a video (although DVD format, not available on this service, will make random access easier; and one might speculate that the type of information required may be different – one may, for example, watch a video for a general overview and to get a 'feel' for the topic, whereas consulting a page of text on DVD may indicate a more specific and formalised information need).

Page view and session time were furnished for Living Health in Table 5.5. Using Huber's robust M-estimator the average page view time was about 13 seconds and session duration was over four minutes.

Table 5.5 Average page view time and session time (in seconds)

	Living Health		NHS Direct Digital	
	Page view time	Session duration	Page view time	Session time
Mean	16.8	421	30.5	1079
Median	12.0	248	14.0	427
5% trimmed mean	14.2	351	16.1	655
Huber's M-estimator	12.6	279	14.9	484

Note: Calculated over a 5 month period for Living Health and over a six month period for NHS Direct Digital.

More time was spent online to NHS Direct Digital (Table 5.5): users spent around 15 seconds viewing a page and over seven minutes on a visit (session). Thus NHS Direct Digital users spent approximately 50-100% more time on a visit as compared to Living Health users. This difference was thought to be due to the viewing of videos by NHS Direct Digital users – video viewing is more time-intensive. An analysis of the distribution of use, pages viewed by day of the week shows that health viewing went on throughout the week but that Mondays and Thursdays were the busier days for both services. In terms of time of day, generally afternoon (1-3pm) and evenings (7-9 pm) were the key viewing times.

Categorising users

The proportional use of health information by men tended to increase with age, a phenomenon also found with kiosk usage. For NHS Direct Digital younger male respondents were more likely to use the text service as opposed to the video service, compared to older and female respondents. Men aged 55 and under were just over one and half times more likely to use the text service compared to women 55 years and under. The relationship was also true of the video service. Furthermore, men over the age of 55 were just about twice as likely to use the service compared to women under the age of 55. As for service preference, men reported a preference for videos over text.

In the case of the InVision video-conference nursing service, men and women used the service equally, although for different reasons – women tended to do so on behalf of others (particularly children) whilst men wanted answers to their own health problems (maybe the privacy of the home was the incentive).

Not surprisingly given the nature of the Channel Health service (i.e. pregnancy information), those aged over 45 were four times less likely to use the service than younger viewers. Women were twice as likely to use the service. This still represented an encouraging interest in the service on the part of males. Interviewees all confirmed the interest of their partners in the programme and, indeed, how the content and information helped them understand and manage their situation: 'we watch the programme together whenever we can – where (partner's name) is at work, he watches on his own later – or I watch it a second time, with him'.

There was a high level of use of Living Health in areas where there was a higher incidence of 0-14 year olds. This finding could not be confirmed among users of NHS Direct Digital or for those using Channel Health's Bush Babies service. Interestingly, the researchers found high levels of usage of other health information services (especially touch-screen kiosks), among the under 15s.

DiTV appeared to attract low-income users. This was encouraging in that it supports the DoH held view that DiTV threw an ICT health lifeline to those who had been excluded from the digital revolution – the less well off and potentially socially excluded. Living Health respondents living in an area with a low incidence of £20,000+ income earners were more likely to use the service. Respondents from wealthier areas were half as likely to use a DiTV health information text information service, as were those people who came from less well off areas. In addition, users from lower income areas were more likely to say Living Health was useful compared to users from higher income areas. It was the same for Channel Health users using the Bush Babies service too. Those in social class D and E were two and three quarter times more likely to have viewed Bush Babies compared to those in social class A and B. Those in social class A and B were least likely to have viewed the service. In the case of NHS Direct Digital, people from postcode areas with a low incidence of £20,000+ earners were about twice as likely to use the service as those in higher income areas. Again this argues a greater use among low-income households.

Topics viewed

What health topics consumers decided to view or what medical conditions they wanted to look up is plainly of major interest to health information providers everywhere. However, we need to interpret these data carefully, as choice is determined by a number of factors – what content is provided, how visible or accessible that content is, what health topics interest users and from what medical conditions they – or their family – may suffer. Comparisons between channels are difficult because of differences in the content, media, audiences and interactive services provided. The indications were that users turned to DiTV health services to address real information/ health needs rather than to browse or surf.

Living Health

The sections that users were most interested in were the 'Illness and Treatment' section followed by 'Women's Health' and 'Men's Health' (Figure 5.8). The Illness and Treatment section accounted to 36% of all pages viewed. The most popular topics in the Illness and Treatment section were Back Pain, Depression, Impotence, Aids, and Irritable Bowel Syndrome (Table 5.6).

Popular topics under Women's Health were: Orgasm problems, dyspareunia, thrush and cystitis. Popular topics under 'Illness and Treatment' were Back Pain, Depression and Anxiety. For 'Men's Health' these were: Impotence, Premature Ejaculation, Sexual Infections, Gay Sex and Sexual Health Help. Clearly, the privacy of one's home appears to be the ideal environment in which to explore issues that may be too intimate or embarrassing to research via a publicly placed information terminal.

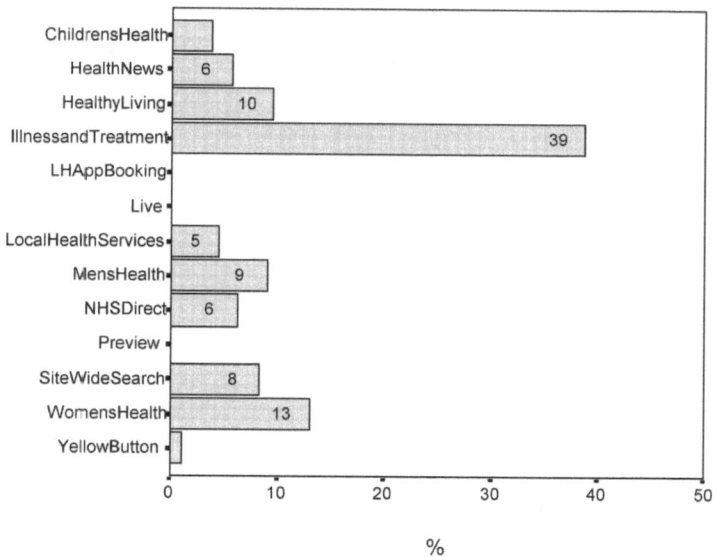

%

Figure 5.8 Living Health – general health sections viewed

Table 5.6 Living Health – pages viewed by health section (ranked by age)

Children's Health	Women's Health	Men's Health
ToothVaccineKids	Orgasmproblems	Impotence
UnderstandingChildDiff	Dyspareunia	Prematureejaculation
Chickenpox-WhatIsIt	Thrushandcystitis	SexualInfections
TrackingDevelopment	Vaginismus	GaySex
MMRVaccine	STIs	SexualHealthHelp
LearnDifficultySpecifi	Findoutifyouarepregnan	Preventingprostatecanc
Treatingchickenpox	Prevention	Flatulence
AttnDefctHyperactivity	CervicalSmears	Injurytreatmentprincip
Babyeczema	Hairtransplant	SaferSex
BehaviourConductDisord	BreastCancerChecks	PenisEnlargement
LearnDisabilityGeneral	Cervicalsmear	Delayedejaculation
CutsBruisesGrazes	Idontwanttogetpregnant	Benignprostatichyper
InsectBitesStings	Metabolism	Dwarrior
FoodAllergies	WomenBaldness	HIVAIDS
Swimming	BreastFood	BloodPressure
30.3% of information section pages	*32.3% of information section pages*	*49.4% of information section pages*

Health Living	Illnesses and Treatment	Health News
Keepyrsexlifeingoodsha	NoContent	NHSDirectLaunch
Practisingsafersex	Backpainhowdoesitoccur	FolicAcid
SheddingPounds	backpainhowisittreated	NHSDirectInVisionLaunc
MainMeals	backpainwhydoesitoccur	SkinCancer
Overweight	Depressiontreatinvolve	KidneyPainkillers
Healthyweight	Anxietytreatmentinvolv	CancerSalad
Breakfast	Backpainduringtreatmen	Panicattackgene
IwouldExercisebut...	Impotence-HowDoesOccur	HeartWeekend
Avoidingpregnancy	Aidswhatisit	ProstateCancer
StartingActivityProgra	backpainwhatisit	FishHeart
GeneralFoodSafety	Depressionwhatisit	Lincoln
Ready-madeMeals	IrritableBowelSynd-Tre	BowelGene
Headaches	bowelcancer	ElecToothbrush
Take-aways	Anginatreatmentinvolve	CancerGenes
Snacks	Impotence-HowTreated	AsianChew
31.7% of information section pages	*10% of information section pages*	*9.1% of information section pages*

NHS Direct Digital

The 'A-Z of Conditions' was the most popular section on NHS Direct Digital by some margin and accounted for 57 percent of text pages viewed (Figure 5.9). The second most popular section was 'Not Feeling Well', and accounted for 13 percent of pages viewed. Interviewees and questionnaire respondents tended to stress their desire to avoid visiting a doctor: 'If I find out that the problem is not serious I can avoid going to my GP. You have to make an appointment, it's a long way, and the doctors are over-stretched anyway'.

An established pattern of topic viewing emerged in the 'A-Z Conditions' section from about February with diabetes, lower back pain, asthma, mellitus appearing in the top ten of subjects viewed in each of these months. For topic videos over which the user had a choice to view, the most popular were the 'Foray for health', 'Diabetes' and 'Coronary Heart Disease'. These three videos accounted for 42% of topic videos viewed. Each topic was represented by a series of videos that the user could view independently. For topics where only one video was available, Hypertension (downloaded 54 times) and MMR (Measles, Mumps and Rubella) inoculation videos (downloaded 44 times) were the most watched. There were no views of videos on Ulcerative Colitis or Testicular Cancer. The latter might be considered disappointing to the DoH, as there was some concern that men were not undertaking regular self checks to spot this condition early. This raises the issue of whether topic positioning in the digital service should be used strategically to help ensure important topics are viewed.

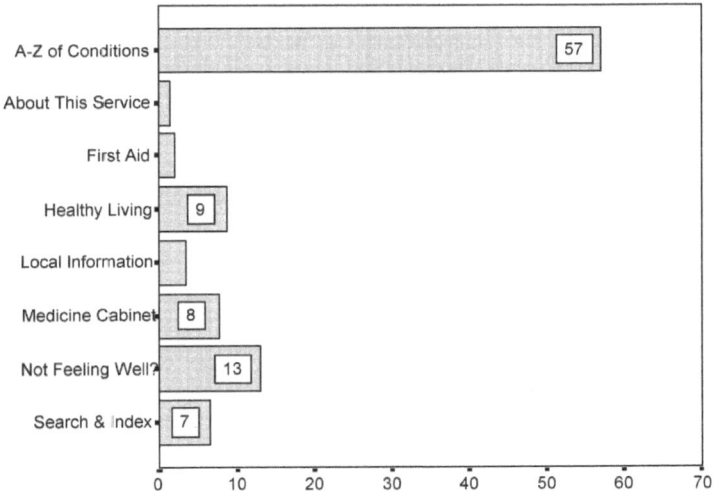

Figure 5.9 NHS Direct Digital: health section accesses under main menu titles as a percentage of all pages accessed

Table 5.7 shows a detailed breakdown of topics viewed for three sections of the NHS Direct Digital service: Medicine Cabinet, Healthy Living and First Aid sections for the period December 2001 to April 2002. About 6% of views to the Medicine Cabinet were for Ibuprofen (Brufen) and 4% to Atenolol (Tenormin – a blood pressure-reducing drug). During the survey period 149 different health pages were viewed, although the top 25 pages (16% of all pages – listed in Table 5.7 – Medicine Cabinet) accounted for two-thirds of page views.

Table 5.7 NHS Direct Digital – use of Medicine Cabinet, Health Living and First Aid sections (December 2001 to April 2002)

Medicine Cabinet	%	Health Living	%	First Aid	%
Ibuprofen (Brufen)	5.7	Eating for Health	23	Resuscitation (DrABC)	28.6
Atenolol (Tenormin)	4.3	Getting Active	20	Bleeding	11.1
Ranitidine Hydrochloride (Zantac)	3.6	Health Quizzes	16	Broken Bones	11.1
Thyroxine Sodium (Eltroxin)	3.6	Maintaining a Healthy Weight	10	Heart Attack	10.2
Bendrofluazide (Aprinox)	3.5	Managing Stress	7.9	Burns and Scalds	10
Simvastatin (Zocor)	3.1	Quitting Smoking	7.4	Strains and Sprains	9.6
Amitriptyline Hydrochloride (Trypti)	3.1	Vaccinations	4.9	Fainting and Unconsciousness	5.5
Paracetamol (Calpol)	2.9	Thinking about Drink	4.8	Head Injuries	4.1
Fluoxetine Capsules (Prozac)	2.9	Keeping Your Teeth Healthy	3.4	Drowning & Electric Shock	3.5
Amoxycillin (Amoxil)	2.8	Staying Healthy at Work	3.1	Poisoning	2.7
Amlodipine (Istin)	2.4			Eye Injuries	2.3
Nifedipine (Adalat)	2.2			Shock	1.3
Aspirin (Nu-Seals)	2.2				
Diclofenac Sodium (Voltarol)	2.2				
Salbutamol (Ventolin)	2.1				
Ipratropium Bromide (Atrovent)	1.9				
Metformin Hydrochloride (Glucophage)	1.8				
Co-Proxamol (Distalgesic)	1.8				
Ispaghula Husk (Fybogel)	1.8				
Lisinopril (Zestril)	1.7				
Sildenafil (Viagra)	1.6				
Omeprazole (Losec)	1.5				
Lansoprazole (Zoton)	1.5				
Gaviscon Liquid	1.4				
Co-Codamol (Tylex)	1.4				
149 topics viewed	**78**		**100**		**100**

Eating for Health accounted for 23% of the Healthy Living section page views. Getting Active accounted for 20% and Health Quizzes 16%. There were sub topics available for this section. For example under Eating for Health popular sub-topics were Improving Your Diet, Balance of Good Health and Glossary of Nutrients – these three topics accounted for three-quarters of Eating for Health page views. Improving Your Diet subsequently broke down into page views – Health Meals, Fats, Fruit and Vegetables etc. Pages on Resuscitation were the most popular for the First Aid section and accounted for 29% of this section's use.

Video versus text

The DiTV pilots featured a range of digital formats – text and video based services and interactive and transactional services. The relative popularity of each type of service was assessed. In the case of those viewing Bush Babies on Channel Health, 70% of respondents just viewed one of the 'Bush Babies' programmes, 23% reportedly viewed text and a video, while 7% just viewed the text. In the case of NHS Direct Digital, people used both. Forty-one percent of those who had used the service claimed that they only used the text service and that they had not requested a video; 6% said that they had only used the video service and 54% said that they had used both text and video. Text, however, was the more popular. Sixty percent of NHS Direct Digital users said that they preferred the text service while 38% said that they preferred the video service. There was evidence that men aged under 36 preferred videos. Focus group interviewees felt that some information presented in video form would have been better as text. It was suggested that information on medication, for instance, could have been better presented in tabular form. Young men preferred videos. Sixty-three percent of men aged under 36 said that they preferred to watch videos rather that read text, compared to 26% of females in this age group who said so.

Users of NHS Direct Digital were also asked to rate the importance of the health video and text service formats. The average scores were similar, though there is some evidence that videos were easier to understand (3.4) compared to text (3.3) and that videos are more interesting (3.3) than the text service (3.1). Focus group interviewees tended to be of this opinion: 'Of course, it's not just the information – if it is boring or dull, people won't take it in. Watching a video is at least a little more interesting'. Only 34% of NHS Direct Digital users, however, agreed with the statement that watching a health video was a big improvement on reading the text. One third disagreed and one third had no opinion. Men aged between 36 and 55, and men and women aged over 55 were more likely to say that watching a health video was an improvement. Forty-two percent of this group agreed compared to 31% of females in the 36 to 55 age group, only 20% of those aged under 36 (male or female) agreed with this statement.

Transactional services

These services were important as they explored the potential of DiTV as a two-way medium where the user becomes an information sender as well as receiver. Such applications represent more advanced forms of interactivity and require a different mindset on the part of users who engage in a customised activity geared to addressing their specific problems rather than ones of a more general nature. These are genuinely new applications of DiTV. The applications tested in the pilots included visual interpersonal communication with an NHS nurse (InVision), online appointments booking with one's GP, and the maintenance of personal medical details online, in this instance personal immunisation records. In addition, one consortium (Channel Health) tested a small-scale email support service for a specific group – pregnant women.

InVision   Despite the obvious warmth with which the service was received – by both consumers and nurses – relatively few people chose to use it. One hundred and sixty three users from a potential audience of around 42,000 subscribing households in four months appeared low. Four possible explanations suggest themselves: (1) a small potential user population; (2) the discouragement, by the channel in its publicity, of casual users; (3) the lack of publicity for these services; and, possibly, most importantly, (4) the novelty and unfamiliarity of the services. Nonetheless, the number of people (1,380) who activated pages leading to the 'point of no return' connection button indicates much potential interest. The issue was how you converted these 'lookers' into users.

Living Health – GP Surgery Bookings Service   Use was plainly very low, with just 30 people making an online appointment with their doctor over a period of six months. This was partly to do with the fact that there were only three surgeries in the pilot, and one did not appear to show any interest in the service. It was also partly to do with the fact that surgeries did not 'sell' the service sufficiently to their patients. Given the amount of work that would have been involved to fully sign-up to the project and that it would only be available for a period of six months, this was probably unrealistic. An open-ended (time wise) rollout might have produced different results.

NHS Direct Digital   Views to the vaccination service accounted for 0.14% of use; approximately 28 people used it. The service consisted of a reminder of when a jab was needed and users had to enter all relevant, personal details. The take-up could be regarded as disappointing, but one has to question the value of this to a consumer when they know that it will only be in place for a short period of time.

Ease of use/usability

Data were obtained from user reaction surveys, follow-up qualitative interviews and usability lab research carried out by the commercial organisation 'Serco'. DiTV is thought to be an easy-to-use health information medium. In practice, however, ease of usability of the pilot services was found to vary with the individual user and the nature of the service being used.

Twenty eight percent of Living Health respondents said that it was 'very easy' to find the information. Just under half found it either OK, hard or very hard to find information on the channel. Interviewees complained of the number of screens required to navigate ('there is hardly any information on a page – even the shortest of topics has six or seven pages to it'). Most participants in Serco's dktv usability sessions were unclear about where to find the dktv service within the HomeChoice menu on a broadband platform.

Some services proved almost trouble-free. The interactive service linked to the 'Bush Babies' television series on Channel Health was universally described as being easy to use, although even here there was some concern about using arrow keys and sub-menus. Interviews with users of the email service indicated that they experienced difficulties using this service, even though the principle of it was highly regarded. 'It wasn't Channel Health – it was the email service that didn't work very well.'

In an investigation of the menu position of NHS Direct Digital on KIT, it was found that the service became more difficult to access as its sign posting became ever more removed from the television service's opening menu; this lead to the proportion of new visitors (as a percentage) of all users declining alarmingly. New users did not come through because of the increasing difficulty of finding the service. Those people who battled through to find the service, however, showed their tenacity by making more extensive use of the channel when they arrived.

In laboratory-based usability tests, Serco found other instances of poor positioning leading to a lack of use – dktv's 'further details' button, for example, was missed by several viewers engrossed in the video content of the channel. In sum, the number of clicks to obtain content is a critical feature with DiTV interactive services.

Regarding gender and age differences, women were less likely to find the Living Health system useful 'all of the time' compared to men women were also more likely to say that the information offered was full of medical jargon. The elderly were a source of particular concern. The age of the respondent was found to impact on how easy the user found it to understand Living Health. Users over 66 were more likely to report that they ran into difficulties. Furthermore, older NHS Direct Digital users, particularly women aged over 55, found the service difficult to use. Focus group sessions in which Communicopia/NHS Direct Digital videos were shown to elderly people revealed some anxiety about the march of information technology. Older participants felt that they would not have access to digital television in their lifetime and would be unsure of how to use it even if they did: 'I can't even use a video [recorder] these days – it's got so complicated'.

Not surprisingly, users with a greater experience of technology were more likely to find the navigation and menu structure of Living Health easier. Users reporting that the general KIT DiTV service was easy to use were more likely to have used the NHS Direct Digital service provided by Communicopia. Many interviewees who had used Living Health, or used the Bush Babies interactive service, or viewed the videos on NHS Direct Digital tended to use these in concert with a variety of other sources – Internet, books etc. These information hungry respondents were used to various menu systems, indexes and different information configurations, and found it easy to adapt their skills to the medium of DiTV.

The DiTV services were meant to be consumer friendly, obviously. Nevertheless, there was a tendency amongst health professionals to underestimate the consumer.

Thus nurses, who watched the NHS Direct Digital, videos felt that the language and terminology used was often too difficult for the lay viewer. However, information professionals, general consumer interest groups and others all felt there was no problem in this area whatsoever.

Usefulness and trust

Seventy seven percent of Living Health viewers said that the service had been useful all the time (23%) or most of the time (54%), while 17% said that the service had not been useful some of the time and 2% said that the service was not at all useful. From this, it appears that when DiTV is rolled out nationally there may be significant health gains. Interviewees echoed the questionnaire findings, by indicating that the service was very useful, enabling them to, for example, avoid visiting the doctor, research a condition for a friend, and check information about medication.

The InVision service went down extremely well with the (relatively few) people who used it and comparisons between this and the telephone service were instructive. Respondents rated the InVision service either very satisfactory (76%) or satisfactory (24%) – 100%, versus 97.8% (combined totals) for the NHS Direct telephone-only service. Similarly, 100% of InVision customers polled said they would use the service again and/or recommend it to friends/family, compared to a figure of 97.8% for telephony. Finally, 88% of those who had used both InVision and the telephony service preferred InVision (the rest had no preference). These results suggest that the nurses were able to offer an equivalent service in satisfaction terms while having to engage the camera and operate the image retrieval system in addition to the normal CAS (Clinical Assessment System) software. Interviewees all rated InVision above the telephone only NHS Direct – enthusing about the facility to see the nurse (rather than about how images could be sent to them): 'It was so good to see the nurse – it was obvious she was interested. With the telephone service you cannot tell how much she is paying attention'.

The average satisfaction score for dktv indicated that these respondents were only 'quite satisfied' with the service – the 35 respondents who claimed to have viewed or used dktv were asked to rate their overall satisfaction with dktv on a four-point scale from very satisfied to not satisfied at all. Two respondents were very satisfied, 21 were quite satisfied, seven were not very satisfied and one was not at all satisfied. The remainder did not know.

Most people thought that the Bush Babies series quite useful – 60% said so. Those in Social Class D/E were less likely to say that the information would be useful for them; 17% of this group said the information would be useful for them, compared to 40% from other groups. Furthermore, those living with a partner said that the videos were useful to them: 56% said this compared to 37% of married and eight per cent of single users.

In the case of NHS Direct Digital, people generally found what they were looking for. Fifteen per cent of viewers agreed and 69% disagreed with the statement that in general users could not find what they were looking for on the service. Eighty-one per cent of users said that if they needed health advice that they would consult health information on KIT. Carers (informal and formal) were less likely to say that they would consult the service compared to non-carers. This however needs further research, particularly as it is contrary to what one might expect.

Today people can use a variety of information sources to help them keep healthy or tackle a particular ailment. With an ever-increasing range of sources available, many now in a digital form, we might expect that people will be using a wider array of sources. What we wanted to determine was how they rated these sources comparatively, and where digital interactive television (DiTV) was ranked among these sources. KIT and Telewest subscribers were surveyed to see how DiTV viewers rated a variety of information sources, including information from the doctor, health books, the web and television. Scores were given out of four, where four indicated the information source to be very important. The two sources that scored highest for both groups of subscribers were their own doctor and the practice nurse. The scores for both KIT subscribers and Telewest subscribers for information from the doctor were identical – 3.7, and for the practice nurse near identical – 3.1 (KIT) and 3.2 (Telewest). We might expect the doctor and nurse to be considered the most important information source – the medical equivalent of the horse's mouth. More surprisingly perhaps, the order of importance of the remaining sources was different between KIT and Telewest subscribers. KIT subscribers rated Friends and Family (2.8) and the NHS Direct telephone line (2.6) as the next two most important sources, while Telewest subscribers placed information via DiTV provided by Living Health (2.9) and NHS Direct telephone line (2.9) as next highest rated sources. The web was the rated the least important source of information by both sets of subscribers and scored just 2 by KIT subscribers and 2.2 by Telewest subscribers.

Comparing the two DiTV health information services, NHS Direct Digital on KIT scored 2.5 while Living Health delivered by Telewest scored 2.9. This result suggested that Living Health subscribers were happier with their DiTV health service than KIT subscribers were with theirs. This difference might have occurred because of the differences in either the demographic profile of Hull and Birmingham users, because of poorer marketing of the KIT service, or as a result of differences between the services delivered.

There was a difference between how people used the two digital TV health services. When the service ranking was correlated against health interest the coefficients recorded for Living Health were higher than those recorded for NHS Direct Digital. Table 5.8 gives the coefficients for each service and difference, as a percentage of the NHS Direct Digital figures. The correlation is between the users' rating of each information service against their ratings for their interest in health. The idea here is that users with a health topic would have used the service and the service's delivery on their topic would impact on their rating of the service. The analysis argues that the NHS Direct Digital information service on KIT was found to be an important source for prescription drugs (r=.31) and new treatments (r=.35) Furthermore, that the Living Health service was an important information source for medical news (r=.39), new treatments (r=.38), general health (r=.37) and prescription drugs (r=.36).

The largest differences in the correlations between the services were recorded for the use of Healthy Living information. Living Health recorded a score on Healthy

Living that was 72% higher than that for the NHS Direct Digital service on KIT. Furthermore, Living Health's score on diet was 64% higher on general health. It was 42% higher and on medical news 34% higher. These results suggest, perhaps, that either KIT subscribers were not replacing their existing sources with the information provided by NHS Direct Digital in these areas or that the service needed to be improved in these areas. It also implies that neither service got its exercise or diet health information content right. This is suggested by the relatively poor correlations here (0.14 for NHS Direct Digital; 0.23 for Living Health) and indicated that users were using other sources of information for these areas (mainly books and magazines). Perhaps these users prefer books and magazines for this type of health topic.

Table 5.8 Correlation values between interest in a health topic and how important Living Health and NHS Direct Digital is as an information source

	NHS Direct Digital	Living Health	% difference
Prescription drugs	0.31	0.36	16%
New treatments	0.35	0.38	9%
Healthy living	0.18	0.31	72%
Medical News	0.29	0.39	34%
Alternative medicine	0.25	0.31	24%
Diet	0.14	0.23	64%
Specific condition	0.24	0.30	25%
Medical Research	0.27	0.31	15%
General health	0.26	0.37	42%
Exercise	0.20	0.24	20%

Authority, trust and branding

DiTV is a very new platform for health information and issues over trust, and whether the NHS brand was visible and what it meant were of some concern. Clearly matters were complicated by the fact that, with so many parties involved with the content, production and distribution of the digital services, ownership and responsibility are far from clear.

Thirty eight percent of users on Telewest's Birmingham cable subscribers said that they would trust the health information found on DiTV. Sixty percent said they trusted the information for most things and only 3% said that they did not trust the information found. Just under half (42%) said they would not use the service should the NHS not be involved, and a large majority (81%) thought the NHS should be involved with digital television, a finding echoed in interviews: 'I just assumed the NHS was involved – it's a public service isn't it?'

For certain kinds of people the NHS brand really meant something. DiTV subscribers who had either used the Living Health service, which carried NHS branded health information, or had heard of the service were more likely to say that the NHS was a symbol of trust than DiTV subscribers who had not used the service. There were, however, digital users who did not buy into the NHS brand. DiTV users visiting the doctor less frequently and those less interested in health information were less likely to accept the NHS as a symbol of trust, were less likely to recognise the NHS symbol, and were less likely to say that the NHS branded information could be trusted. Younger respondents were also less likely to recognise the NHS as a symbol of trust compared to older respondents.

NHS Direct Digital users were asked to rate the trustworthiness of health information sources out of five. Sources where the NHS appeared in the name performed well – NHS Direct telephone and the NHS Direct service available on KIT scored respectively 3.9 and 3.8. This score placed these services below doctors and nurses (4.5 and 4,2) but well above medical magazines and books (3.0).

Around half of those who had viewed Bush Babies and surveyed for their reactions to its service were aware of NHS involvement and their reactions to this were largely positive. NHS branding was seen as offering more authority and credibility to the content ('It was nice to know that this was real information from a proper source. It was obvious the programme was helped by the NHS'). The more respondents had viewed the 'Bush babies' TV series, the greater their awareness of NHS involvement became.

Outcomes

Two-thirds of Living Health users (67%) said that the information they obtained had either helped or helped them a lot in becoming better informed about their condition confirmed this, with respondents enthusing about having health information so easily to hand: 'It has given me a whole new source of information, and right there at home.' Most users (90%) of NHS Direct Digital said they felt better informed about a condition after having used the service. Pre-launch focus group interviewees felt that people would be, as one put it: 'much better informed about health matters'.

Well over half (55%) of Living Health users queried the service for information about their consultation with the doctor either before or after, or both before and after their consultation. Forty percent of users felt that the information they found had helped or helped a lot in their dealings with the doctor. This was also a theme among depth interviewees: 'I now go to the doctors with a much better idea of what's wrong with me, and what I can ask about'.

Seventy-three percent of NHS Direct Digital users felt that the information they found had helped a little or helped a lot in their dealings with the doctor. Just over one in four NHS Direct Digital users, 27%, said that they would use the service to look for information that they would not want to discuss with their doctor. Plainly this might be an important role for DiTV health services.

Bush Babies interviewees felt that they were far better prepared when they met their GPs, midwives and obstetricians, and praised the 'Bush Babies' series for giving them an excellent knowledge base regarding their condition: 'It gave me so much information that I know I wouldn't have got elsewhere – I don't go fishing for information in books – and it's easy to forget what the doctor tells you'.

Fifty three percent of Living Health users confirmed that they had used information they found to replace a visit to the doctor. Certain types of people had a predilection to do so. Those reportedly using the Living Health service were just under twice as likely to use information found as an alternative to seeing the doctor. Older users and men, however, were less likely to use information in this way. NHS Direct online, health books and magazines and the Internet generally were also significant sources used as an alternative to seeing the doctor. The younger the respondent the more likely they were to substitute information for a visit to the doctor. Those aged over 55, were half as likely to use information found on Living Health as an alternative to a doctor's visit as compared to younger people.

People interested in general health, prescription drugs, healthy living and alternative health, were more likely to use an information source as an alternative to seeing the doctor. This was strongly apparent in interview data as well as questionnaire returns ('I maybe know more about my health than the average person, and have a good idea about when I need to go to the doctors. I always do some research first now I have an extra resource.') Indeed, subscribers considered Living Health as important, if not more important, as a source of information compared to the NHS Direct Telephone line. This has to be regarded as justification for the decision to rollout digital health to the nation.

Information on NHS Direct Digital also impacted on whether viewers used information as a substitute for a visit to the doctor. Those using the service were just under one and half times as likely to use information found in this way. This result was only significant at the 10% significance level. It was found, however, to be the least important information source compared to medical magazines and books, NHS Direct telephone line and the web. This suggested that the impact of this service was not as important as these other sources, probably because of its relatively limited content base.

One-third of Living Health users said that the information found either helped or helped a lot in improving their condition. Whether the service improved the user's condition or helped in understanding the condition depended on the extent to which people understood the nature of the Living Health service. Generally, those finding the service easy to use were most likely to say there were health outcomes. This points to the importance of design, navigation and documentation, and possibly also, digital literacy training. There was one surprise result – whether the user found the system easy to read impacted on whether the person expressed a positive health outcome as a result of receiving digital health information, but the relationship was the inverse of what we might have expected. Those finding the system easy to read all the time were less likely to say that using the service had improved their condition. This may well reflect a type of user who prefers other text based information sources, such as the Internet or health books or magazines.

Forty percent of users felt that the information they found had helped (20%) or helped a lot (20%) in their dealings with the doctor (Figure 5.10) and one in five said it had helped a lot. Reflecting the findings of earlier studies (Cyber Dialogue,

2000) most people said they felt better informed about a condition after having used the service. Sixty-seven percent of Living Health users said that the information had either helped or helped them a lot in becoming better informed, nearly half (47%) being helped 'a lot'. Nearly one third of Living Health users (31%) said that the information found either helped or helped a lot in improving their condition. Overall these findings provide grounds for optimism on the part of Government.

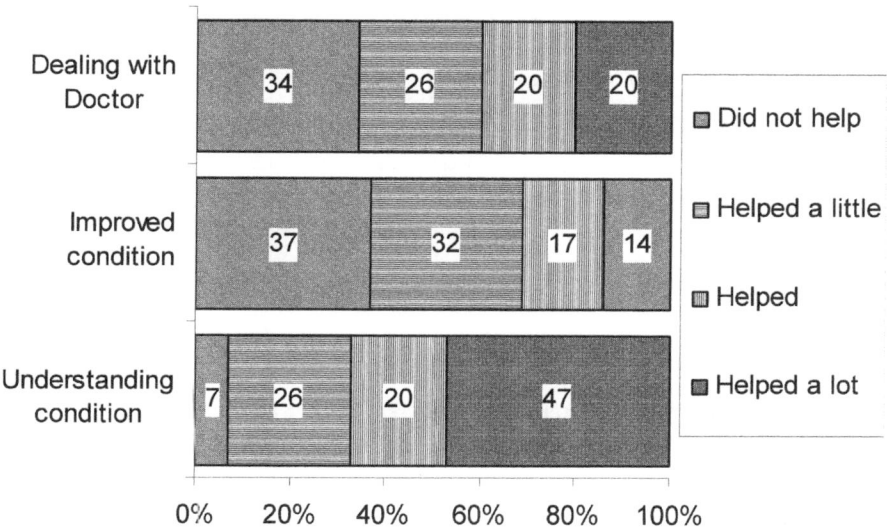

Figure 5.10 The amount of help given by information found on Living Health

The same question was asked of NHS Direct Digital users in Hull. Nearly 62% of NHS Direct Digital users said that the information found either helped a little or helped a lot in improving their condition and 15% said that it had helped a lot. Seventy-three percent of users felt that the information they found had helped a little or helped a lot in their dealings with the doctor (Figure 5.11) and one in five (22%) said it had helped a lot. As with the Living Health users, 90% of NHS Direct users said that the information had either helped a little or helped them a lot in becoming better informed (understood condition), over half (55%) being helped 'a lot'. Nearly 62% of NHS Direct users said that the information found either helped a little or helped a lot in improving their condition and 15% said that it had helped a lot. Overall these findings provided grounds for optimism on the part of Government and NHS Direct producers.

Respondents were asked if they had ever used health information from 'any source' as an alternative to seeing the doctor. In terms of information sources, the use of the NHS Direct telephone line, the digital television services, the web and medical books were found to be significant predictors in both models. Other sources such as family or friends, leaflets in the surgery and other TV programmes did not emerge as significant predictors of the outcome.

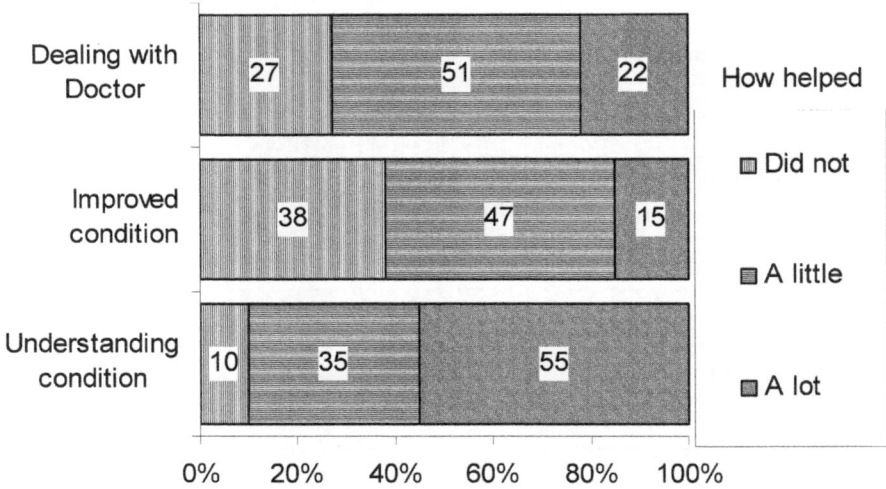

Figure 5.11 The amount of help given by NHS Direct Digital

For both models, medical books were the most important factor in terms of an information source that a user might utilise as a substitute for a visit to the doctor. Telewest users who were very interested in this information source were three and half times more likely to use information found as a substitute for a visit to the doctor compared to those not at all interested.

The second most important source for Telewest users was the Living Health service. Respondents who had used the Living Health service were just under twice as likely as non-users to say they would use medical information sources as an alternative to seeing the doctor. Bivariate analysis showed that while 52% of Telewest subscribers who had not used Living Health had substituted information found for a visit to the doctor this was true of 69% of Living Health users – approximately 40% more. This is a significant indication that health information delivered via DiTV had an impact on this outcome. The finding was also true of KIT users viewing the NHS Direct Digital service, but the result was only rated at 10% significance. This suggested that the impact of the NHS Direct Digital health information service was lower on this outcome variable compared to the Living Health service.

Use of NHS Direct telephone line also had an impact on this outcome. Respondents who had used the service were about one and half times more likely than those who had not used it to say that they had used information found as an alternative to seeing the doctor. The estimated odds ratios between Telewest and KIT subscribers were surprisingly similar, 1.47 compared to 1.54. The telephone help service appears therefore to provide a functional alternative to seeing the doctor with approximately the same effect in Birmingham as in Hull.

The use of the web was also significant in both regions. Those users who said they were very interested in the web were about twice as likely to use information found as a substitute for a visit to the doctor as were those users who did not use the web as an information source. The estimated odds ratios between Telewest and KIT subscribers were again similar, 2.06 compared to 2.03. This suggests that the impact of the web was much the same in Birmingham as in Hull – we might expect this as there would be little difference in what the web offers between the two locations.

In terms of personal characteristics, age and gender of the respondent were also significant. Those aged 56 and over were about half as likely to use information from sources found as an alternative to a visit to the doctor compared to younger age groups. Surprisingly this was less true for KIT subscribers as Telewest subscribers. This finding was consistent with previous research on the use of consumer health information on the Internet. Gender was also significant, with women being just under twice as likely to use information found as an alternative as compared to men, but this was truer of Telewest subscribers than of KIT subscribers.

With regard to outcomes related to Channel Health, three out of four women who used the enhanced Bush Babies text service, supporting the broadcast programmes, said that they found its information reassuring. Bush Babies interviewees tended to say that the way they approached their pregnancy was healthier because of the programme contents: 'My diet was better, I exercised, I felt better about what was happening. The programme helped me in all of these things'.

Discussion

The pilot exercise was designed to test the efficacy of different platforms, formats and health information transmission strategies in delivering health information and advice to the public and, more especially, NHS patients. There were a number of key issues that the contracted consortia were expected to address and design services that would deliver pertinent outcomes. Some of the key questions asked of digital interactive television as a health platform are listed below and summary answers provided on the basis of the research completed here.

Did DiTV deliver?

The question is whether DiTV worked in a consumer health context. Specifically, did DiTV:

1. Deliver significant numbers of health consumers?
2. Draw in a new audience for health information – people who have not traditionally used health information services?
3. Have the added 'magic' pulling power for health over other platforms and sources, in that it provides better, more acceptable, more interesting health information and advice?

4. Help to take the pressure off hard-pressed primary health services – like GP surgeries and hospitals, because the information and advice provided helps people to help themselves?

Did DiTV deliver health consumers?

The basic answer to this question was 'yes', in that significant numbers of potential users of these services did utilise the health pilot programmes to some degree during the 4-6 months duration of each pilot. The key figure here, given the limited time window, is 'reach'. This represents the total number of individuals with access to a service who used it at least once over a given period of time. The meaning and significance of such a figure, of course, must be qualified in terms of the size of the subscriber base and type of platform on which a service is being delivered.

With Living Health, perhaps the most developed and comprehensive of the pilots, the reach figure – derived from digital log data – achieved an estimated level of over 30% and it is estimated that 13,718 households tuned in to its service on Telewest cable in Birmingham (subscriber base averaging 42,000) over its six-month pilot run. If this figure is projected up to cable subscribers across the UK, it indicates a potential nation-wide reach of nearly three-quarters of a million people who would tune in at least once over a six-month period.

Channel Health offered a different prospect from Living Health in that Bush Babies was transmitted on the Sky Digital platform, which during the pilot period had a potential audience averaging 5.8 million subscribing homes, containing 11.5 million adults. Data obtained by Channel Health from BARB indicated that viewing of its general programme service attained an average per series episode of 307,000 adults (aged 16+) during the first six weeks of the service, 216,000 adults during the next five weeks, and 2.31 million adults during the next three months of the pilot period. These figures are based on aggregating over the audiences for repeat-showings of specific episodes. Self-report survey data indicated that 27% of respondents claimed to have watched the Bush Babies series.

With NHS Direct Digital, the service was transmitted on a different platform – a broadband network. The test service was presented to a modest-sized subscriber market in Hull of just 10,000 subscribers to Kingston Interactive Television. Over a five-month pilot period, log data indicated that 20% of KIT subscribers used NHS Direct Digital's service (1,956 households). Although not comparing a period of precisely the same length (five months versus six months), it can be seen, nonetheless, that this service did not achieve the reach of Living Health. The explanation for this difference in performance is not unequivocal and may be due to critical features of the reception platforms or formats. During the NHS Direct Digital pilot, for example, there was some experimentation with the placement of the NHS Direct Digital service in the KIT TV-on-demand environment. This was observed to have an impact on overall user levels and repeat use. Also the NHS Direct Digital service was arguably not as comprehensive or detailed as that of Living Health.

Turning to dktv, this service was transmitted on a broadband platform, but to a tiny potential user base of 513 households in the Newham area of London for whom digital log data were available for 403. Its service reached 35% of these logged subscribers to the HomeChoice TV-on-demand service over a monitored period of around three months.

In sum, digital interactive television health services – from a standing start – can (and did) deliver significant numbers of occasional users.

Did DiTV draw in a new audience for health Information?

The evidence was that DiTV might prove effective at reaching and attracting those communities that other technologies may not reach. Furthermore, it may also attract user groups who traditionally do not engage in self-care.

The Living Health service, for example, attracted more male than female users, and the gap between genders was especially pronounced among the over 55s. In comparison with use of touch-screen kiosks, another technology platform that has been used in the rollout of digitised health information, DiTV performed well in this pilot in attracting older male users. The Living Health service was also more widely used by individuals from poorer households – another major target group for the NHS. Finally, respondents with children were more likely to be users.

With Channel Health on Sky, the target audience was more targeted. The programme and associated interactive services were aimed at pregnant women and new mothers. Audience figures showed that the service was successful in attracting this target audience. Nearly seven in ten adult viewers (69%) of Channel Health's broadcast programmes were women, with a slightly larger proportion (71%) falling into the category of 'housewives'. In the BARB audience measurement system, 'housewives' are not exclusively women, but the person in the household responsible for the main weekly shopping. One in five Channel Health programme viewers were housewives with children (aged under 16) at home.

From the survey data on Bush Babies use, it emerged that there was also a social class factor at play, with less well-off households with pregnant women or new mothers being more likely to tune in. Despite this, young single mothers reportedly found the service less useful than did mothers or mums-to-be who lived with partners.

NHS Direct Digital, although offering a service that overlapped in type and content with much of that offered by Living Health, attracted a younger user profile, especially among males. Despite this, there were consistencies with Living Health in that older men were bigger users than older women, and poorer households were also more likely to tune in than better-off households.

With dktv, a small base size of users and limited log data meant that few lessons could be learned about the demographic profile of users of health information through this channel.

Overall, DiTV attracted low-income users. Respondents living in an area with a low incidence of £20,000+ income earners were more likely to use Living Health service and the NHS Direct Digital services. Those from middle and lower social classes were two to three times more likely to have viewed Bush babies on Channel Health. This supports the idea that DiTV may help provide a service to people who might otherwise be excluded from other sources of health information and advice.

Did DiTV attract users from other platforms?

DiTV complemented certain other information sources while being used instead of others. The users of Living Health and NHS Direct Digital's services were more likely to have used NHS Direct in the past year compared with non-users. In respect of Living Health, however, DiTV did not emerge as a substitute for the Internet as a health information source. By the half-way point in the Living Health pilot, survey respondents who considered the web important as a source for health information were more likely to have heard of Living Health, but not used it compared to those who did not consider the web as important for health.

DiTV, in the form of the service offered by Living Health, was used instead of printed media by some users. However, web users were less likely to cross over to DiTV to find health information.

Can DiTV take the pressure off primary health services?

The simple answer to this question was that after just six months of piloting, it was too early to judge, although early evidence suggests that DiTV may make some inroads here. It is worth considering some of the suggestive evidence that emerged from this research.

DiTV did seem to provide information that is valued by users, especially by ones who reportedly suffer from a medical condition. This finding emerged among users of Living Health and NHS Direct Digital. Many users acknowledged the usefulness of having information on their TV to prepare them for when they visited their doctor. Some liked to consult television information before seeing the doctor, and others afterwards.

The role played by DiTV as a health information source was dependent upon need and circumstance. For some people the service acted as an alternative to seeing the doctor. For others, the information was useful as an aid for their consultations. Thus, DiTV (Living Health) was found to be the second most important source of health information used as an alternative to seeing the doctor. Users of Living Health were just under twice as likely to use health information found as an alternative to seeing the doctor. Over half of Living Health users had used the DiTV service to query information for their consultation. Further three-quarters of users felt that the information had helped in dealing with their doctor and two thirds said that the information found had helped in improving their condition. Use is clearly beneficial. This self-report data was backed up by the logs in that they plainly showed people were using the service, not just saying they did.

With the more specialised service provided by Bush Babies, many users said they obtained reassurance from it. But, it was not seen as offering an acceptable substitute for going to the doctor. Face to face contact with health professionals was still regarded by mothers-to-be as essential.

Two consortia offered interactive services that went beyond the provision of text information or videos-on-demand, offering more personal information and advice. Living Health operated an appointments booking service with GP surgeries in Birmingham and the groundbreaking InVision service, in collaboration with NHS

Direct, provided the services of a televised nurse in the home. Both services attracted a modest level of custom during the pilot period. Eighty-one people registered for the GP appointments booking service and 30 appointments were made by 18 of these patients over six months. With InVision, 163 people used the service over four months. There were 1,380 Living Health users who activated the InVision page, however, but who did not follow through. Perhaps this figure points to the level of potential or future demand. Interestingly, and perhaps significantly, the intention of those surveyed and interviewed was to use the service instead of seeing their doctor.

Is the NHS a visible brand on DiTV?

DiTV is a very new platform for health information and a major issue was whether the information could be trusted, and whether the NHS brand had any impact. It was found that the presence of the NHS was viewed positively. For example, a large majority (81%) of Living Health users thought the NHS should be involved with digital television. Indeed, three out of four Living Health users (77%) regarded the NHS as a symbol of trust. An even larger proportion (83%) agreed that they trusted the information because the NHS was involved. However, there is also a degree of trust attached to television as a medium and many Living Health respondents (68%) said they would carry on using the service even if the NHS was not involved.

Overall, people who used the health information services or the health service itself were more likely to accept the NHS as a symbol of trust, than those who did not avail themselves of these services. NHS Direct Digital/Communicopia users rated the NHS brand below doctors and nurses, but above medical magazines and books as a source of trusted information.

Among self-identified viewers of Channel Health's 'Bush Babies' TV series, a positive association emerged between how much of this series was watched and belief that the NHS was involved.

Conclusions

DiTV had the potential to attract a large audience. This audience comprised an extensive number of occasional users rather than a large regular audience, but that probably reflects the nature of the health need. Reach figures indicated that significant numbers of people who had access to these online services would use them from time to time. Encouraging take-up figures suggest a viable future, and evidence showed that when people used the services once, they were likely to do so again, albeit on an ad hoc basis.

Health is a popular topic likely to attract viewers to watch regular television programmes, but it can also encourage viewers to use television more interactively. People maybe more prepared to search for information that is of use to them or their families. It should be noted, however, that they may not be prepared to search as much for health information as Internet users. Hence, interactive TV sites must be easy to use and enable users quickly and efficiently to reach the information they seek, and the content has got to be worth seeking.

What was also encouraging was that the digital health services appeared to reach groups that the DoH had targeted because they have proved that can be difficult to access via other methods. Furthermore, DiTV has achieved a different demographic profile of users from that of other platforms, which showed that a suite of online technologies was needed rather than all the investment going to a single, supposedly convergent technology.

As well as low-income groups, DiTV reached older users, especially older male users. There was also evidence that it encouraged younger male users who are noted for not checking up on their health. It can also be effective at reaching specific groups with specific conditions, e.g., pregnant women.

Low take-up of Living Health's InVision and online GP bookings services suggested unfamiliarity and an uncertainty with transactional services. The level of use recorded for Communicopia/NHS Digital Direct's immunisation records service reinforces this point. This may point to a need both for user-friendly interface designs and possibly also training designed to promote interactive TV literacy. Alternatively, it may also indicate that some applications, such as an appointments booking service, where a degree of negotiation and flexibility are required among patients and health service providers, are more difficult to transfer into the online environment.

People appeared to be selective in their use of different media. Pages and topics accessed via DiTV were different from those accessed on the Internet or a publicly located touch-screen kiosk, due to considerations of privacy, time availability and the amount of choice offered. With regard to format, video appeared to be less consulted than text services. However, it might be a case that while the absolute number of videos consulted was less than the absolute number of text pages examined, users spent more time with videos than text, so overall distribution of time to these formats might work out about the same in the end.

Once again, there is the issue of 'application effectiveness'. This means finding the most appropriate, effective and acceptable format for a particular type of application. Focus group interviewees suggested that text was more appropriate for certain kinds of information (e.g., basic facts), and more easily consulted than having to run through a video to find a particular item. Video has a different psychological functionality for users. Text is factual, while videos can succour emotional needs too. This point is important both in respect of the construction of online libraries of health information, and also in relation to 'live' transactional links. There is mounting research on the use of computer-mediated communications – outside the health sphere – that has shown that the rules of interpersonal communication online may vary from those that prevail in face-to-face communication. This research may have important implications for the design of user interfaces and decisions about the types of formats that could most effectively be applied to facilitate online health-related communications.

Considering that there was no facility (i.e. printer) to copy information, time spent perusing pages has to be regarded as minimal. Further work is needed to examine how information is assimilated and used by DiTV subscribers. For instance some users may feel better informed by video, but absorb less factual information than they would from text.

The health topics viewed, whilst differing across platforms and formats, nevertheless suggest the services were used very much for consultation/reference with regard to specific conditions, rather than for general browsing or recreational use, which one might have expected. Users of Living Health acknowledged that this was a primary reason for using the service. Digital health services provide support for a number of specific functional needs on the part of NHS patients and members of the general public. Future research should attempt systematically to map out these needs and determine the delivery platforms, formats and content that will effectively satisfy them.

The information retrieved appears, for all services, to have made some impact on dealings with doctors, and there is some evidence to suggest that people are using it as an alternative to making GP appointments. Our data provide support for the belief that digital health services could help the NHS in terms of reduced demand or economies in relation to certain offline services. Furthermore, and in a broader sense, if online health information can cultivate greater self-care and adoption of preventative 'medicine', further economies may be felt in an over-stretched NHS.

Self-report data indicate that having information does help one manage medical problems, in a conditional way. The degree to which this occurs also depends on the type of user. For example, Living Health users stated that the type of service it provided could help them in relation to consultations with a doctor. There was further evidence that it could serve as an alternative to information from a doctor – though non-users indicated that they preferred getting medical information straight from the doctor – whether spoken or in writing – than any other information source.

For the pregnant women of Channel Health, the TV/interactive service was seen mostly as a supplement to seeing health professionals. With their particular condition, it was still essential to have physical diagnoses and checks with doctors and nurses, etc. There was some indication that a service such as Channel Health's interactive elements could be used in relation to reminders of appointments – as endorsed by health professionals. But as the Living Health experience demonstrated, there is a relatively slow take-up for an actual online appointments booking service.

Summing up, the DiTV online health service pilot delivered mixed results across a variety of services. Early audience uptake of these services indicated that a market for digital health does exist. The public were likely to welcome an online health information service sourced by a trusted brand. Health-related programmes, especially on themes of special interest to niche audience groups, will attract viewers, as will health-related videos on demand, provided they are of good production quality. Enhanced information services that lie behind familiar broadcasting will also be accessed, provided the user interface is not overly complex. More sophisticated interactive services that invite two-way flows of information between the user at home and health service provider are likely to take longer to become established. In popular parlance, television is a 'lean back' medium that has not traditionally invited its users to actively engage with it. In contrast, the personal computer is a 'lean forward' medium that has always encouraged a high degree of interactivity on the part of its users.

Different technologies are associated with distinct psychological dispositions on the part of their users. This distinction must not be forgotten when considering television's potential as an interactive technology. Over time these two technologies may become largely indistinguishable as will the psychology of users in each case. Until then, any application of television as an interactive health information medium must be mindful of these distinctions and take them into full consideration when determining the nature and form of digital health services on the box.

Postscript

As a consequence of the pilot evaluations the DoH put out a tender for a consumer health television channel. None of the pilot services were selected, instead it was decided to establish in 2004 a new television service called NHS Direct Digital TV (http://www.nhsdirect.tv/). The service is run by MMTV, a company specialising in interactive television applications. It is intended that £15 million will be invested in developing and running this interactive service over a period of 3 years. Content includes:

- NHS services (such as directories of GPs, dentists, pharmacies etc.
- An encyclopaedia of illnesses and conditions, tests, treatments and operations.
- Self-care advice on treating common health problems.
- Advice on healthy living.
- Hot topics on current health issues.

This information will be supported by useful images and video clips.

The service so far appears to be a disappointment in regards to what it might have achieved given the lessons learnt in the pilot services. In truth the current service is very flat and pedestrian and certainly is a long way from the heights achieved with the 'broadband nurse'. Maybe it will improve with time.

Chapter 6

Digital Platform Comparisons

This chapter is an important one as it looks at characteristics and issues that cut right across the individual digital health platforms and makes comparisons between them. Of course, the digital health consumer has a choice so it is important to look at the relative merits of the platforms. Presented here are five cross platform studies:

1. A log metric comparison between the three platforms, examining relative use and user performance.
2. A comparison of the health content of the three platforms.
3. The impact of platform location on health information seeking behaviour.
4. Consumer characteristics of information seeking behaviour in a digital environment.
5. Characterising users according to types of health information sources used/ preferred.

Log metric comparison of use and user performance

Introduction – platform characteristics

Table 6.1 provides a summary of the key characteristics of each platform, to which we will refer in the following sections.

Table 6.1 A summary of key platform comparison

Delivery mechanism	Potential of service	Typical location	Main Navigation tool	Main Navigation Structure	Data capture
Kiosks		Public place	Touchscreen	Mainly menu	On screen and printout
Web	Text, Audio and video viewing	Work home	Mouse and keyboard	Menu and search engine	On screen, save to disk, printout
DiTV		Home	Remote control	Mainly menu	On screen
Broadband telephone (ADSL)		Work Home	Remote control and keyboard		On screen, printout

Kiosks are single information source points that potential users have to seek out or come across in their travels in order to use them. Recent developments (web-enabled kiosks etc.) mean that kiosks can now offer a more comprehensive and current information service. Kiosk information services generally comprise text and images only. However, video viewing is possible on both web-enabled and 'traditional' kiosks. Kiosks are also theoretically capable of interactivity. Information is presented in a multi-level menu structure, and there is also a search facility. Users navigate menus, usually via a touch sensitive screen. A keyboard, with integrated roller mouse is sometimes available. There is usually a printer attached, but the facility is not always available or working. Kiosk information services can either be distributed to kiosks via a dedicated telephone line or the information may be stored on a hard disk associated with the kiosk.

The World Wide Web offers a relatively cheap environment onto which information suppliers and services can be made available. The low start up costs mean that the web is populated by a vast array of competing and overlapping sites. Web services are also generally a text and image-based, although video viewing is possible. The web offers interactivity either in real time (chat rooms, online bookings) or via email. Users navigate between sites using search engines (e.g. Google), information directories and menus (e.g. Yahoo) or by jumping from one site to another (hyperlinks). Information within sites is usually presented in a multi-level menu structure, though many sites offer a single one click to information menu. Users navigate menus using a mouse and via a keyboard. Searching between sites and within sites is made prominent and is regarded as being standard, but not easy, for most web users. User search expressions are not particularly well constructed and once at a site most users seem to prefer to use online menus to determine where they go. The web is mainly used at home, work, or increasingly, from public locations such as Internet cafés or libraries. It is relatively easy to record the information found either by printing or saving to disk.

A DiTV information service is a 'multi-channel' or 'multi-modality' service environment provided under a single umbrella organisation to which the user subscribes to receive the service. Each information service offers a text and image or a video service accessible via the television screen. The service offers interactivity either in real time (e.g. video-link, online bookings) or with email. As with the other platforms, users navigate between and within information services via a multi level menu structure but unlike the web searching is rather difficult.

Users navigate menus, usually from a hand held remote control, but also less commonly from an optional keyboard. The remote is particularly important and can be used to generate alphabetical characters using a similar convention as mobile phones. Searching on DiTV is limited as most people use a hand held remote to key-in alphabetical characters. Topics, however, can be accessed via an on-screen-alphabetical listing. Printers are not normally linked to the TV, although they can be. DiTV information services are distributed to the users' television either by cable (Living Health), telephone link (Communicopia/NHS Direct Digital) or telephone satellite combination (Channel Health).

The architecture for DiTV and the web is similar in that a server is used to store pages, images etc. and clients or users make requests for information, which are interpreted by the server. Files are then sent from the server to the user. However, a DiTV information system is closed in that other information owners are not permitted to supply information, as they can do so easily on the web. Thus, information content and choice is much more limited than that offered on the Internet, especially so in the case of health. For a DiTV system, unlike the web, all users are known, as they are subscribers. For the Internet no one information provider will have an idea of the likely population of web users and there will be a very large number of information services. For a DiTV service, however, there is only one server distributing information to a known number of subscribers, and this means, in theory, it is easier to relate usage with users (and their characteristics). For the web there may be as many servers as there are information providers. Kiosks can be linked to a server hub and be updated and supplied with information by that hub. Alternatively the information can be placed and locked on to the kiosks hard disk and be updated locally.

Site architecture will also vary between platforms. To understand the impact of architecture on use it is necessary first to define both a page and a screen. A 'page' is defined as a self-standing information statement on a particular topic, while a 'screen' can be defined as either a series of pages or part of a page. For the purposes of transactional log analysis, page views are estimated by counting screen views. However a screen view does not necessarily correspond to a single page view. This is because a number of pages can be presented on a single screen or, conversely, a single page is spread over a number of screens. What this means is that counting screens does not give an accurate count of the number of pages. Three models of page-to-screen relationships can in fact be denoted:

- Multiple page-to-screen: In a multiple page information screen a number of information pages are stored on a single screen view.
- Page-to-screen unity: In an information unity model each screen is a single page. One page is linked to one screen.
- Divided page-to-screen: In a divided page information screen model, users' view a number of screens to view a single page.

Plainly, the most straightforward case is where there is page-to-screen unity. This was the case with the InTouch with Health kiosks. Here each topic is represented by a single page and screen view (albeit the user is often required to scroll a page to read all the text). Furthermore, all screen views are uniquely recorded. For web users (SurgeryDoor and NHS Direct Online) the situation is more complicated and sites may correspond to either a multiple or a divided page-to-screen model. Indeed it is not uncommon for a site to adopt different styles of architecture and page-to-screen models for different parts of the same site.

Both Kiosk and Internet users have a scroll function that provides the option to move down to further information. This is not the case for DiTV users. Instead of offering a scroll function, DiTV has the option to view another screen by loading another screen view. Hence, to view a similar amount of page information as Internet users, DiTV users have to view a greater number of screens. DiTV online information systems usually adopt a divided page-to-screen model and this results in the over reporting of usage. This was the case for Living Health, although Communicopia had a unity set up and this partly explains differences in used content between these two services.

Site architecture and page-to-screen relationships will impact on site or platform use comparisons. In a multiple page-to-screen, pages, as estimated by screen views, will be underestimated. In a divided page-to-screen model page views would be over estimated. To date there is no set formula to adjust for architecture differences between sites and platforms. The impact is predominately on use statistics though there will be an impact on content, particularly where content and use statistics are employed together.

Users

Reach is defined as those people who used the service as a proportion of those to whom it is exposed. In the case of DiTV this would be the number of users (households) as a percentage of the subscribers. For kiosks, the reach figure is rather more complicated to calculate. Thus for kiosks in GP surgeries, the population base could be the number of patients registered with that surgery. For kiosks in other public locations such as pharmacies, however, there is a problem. While there may be a record of number of individuals to whom goods were sold, there may be many other visitors who did not make a purchase. For hospitals and libraries also, it may be difficult to know how many potential users (i.e., visitors) there were. For the Internet there are also huge problems with establishing a base population.

Table 6.2, using a range of sources, compares reach with regards to the three digital information platforms and the likely audience of health information by the general population. It was estimated, albeit some time ago (Nammacher and Schmitt 1999), that 15% of the population have actively sought health information. This figure doubles to about 30% for Internet users and to 32% for DiTV users. Kiosks do not perform so well and it is estimated that approximately 17% of users exposed to kiosks in a surgery will use them.

Table 6.2 Percentage of the population seeking health information

Total population	15%	US study based on urban sample (Nammacher and Schmitt 1999)
Kiosk population	17%	Based on questionnaire results
Internet population	30%	US study based on urban sample (Nammacher and Schmitt 1999)
DiTV population	32%	Based on recorded logs of 45,000 potential users

Our kiosk figure is supported by an early study on kiosks by Jones and colleagues (Jones, Naven and Murray 1993). A random telephone survey undertaken five months after installation of twenty-five terminals sited in a variety of places in Clydebank in 1991 showed that 17% of the sample had used at least one of the terminals.

The comparison between Internet and DiTV reach figures is not straightforward. Estimates of reach for the use of health information over the total population and the Internet, is based on US users responding to a telephone question asking if they have 'ever' sourced health information. Reach figures for DiTV (Living Health) were based on actual use over a specific period, in this case over a four month period. This is a shorter period than 'ever'. Given that users are likely to return as and when they need the information we would expect the final reach figure for DiTV to be higher.

Table 6.3 provides a breakdown of the pattern of those returning to the NHS Direct Online and Living Health over a one-month period. It is not possible to discern repeat visitors from the kiosk logs, as users are anonymous. For NHS Direct Online 84% of users visited the site once only. For Living Health this figure was a little lower – 74%.

Table 6.3 Web v DiTV – return visits within a month

	NHS Direct Online	Living Health DiTV
Visit one day	84%	73.8%
Visited 2-5	12.4%	24.8%
Visited 6-15	2.3%	1.2%
Over 15 times	1.2%	0.2%
	100%	100%

(Excluding Robots)

It may be that web users were returning, but to another health site. There are a large number of health websites available for people to use. There are no competing health information services on the DiTV services we studied users have no other options available to them. The general low level of returns for both sites can be attributed to two factors: (1) user promiscuity; (2) the need for health information is not necessarily periodic or frequent.

Use

The number of pages viewed in a session is a hybrid metric, which tells us how active (or interested) people are when they engage with a system. Of course, it is not quite as straightforward as that, as it might also be a sign of the difficulty or laboriousness of navigating the system to find what is needed. We have two possible ways of presenting this data – just as an average or as a means of determining relative depths of site/service penetration.

Firstly, we can just take the average or mean, which will give us an idea of how intensively a system is being used. Used in this way the data can be especially effective in making comparisons between the use of different digital information platforms. Table 6.4 provides an illustration with a comparison being made between a kiosk, the Internet and a DiTV channel in the health field.

**Table 6.4 Estimates of the average number of pages viewed in a session –
comparison between digital platforms**

	NHS Direct Online Internet*	Living Health DiTV	InTouch with Health kiosks
Mean	12.7	23.6	7.7
Median	6	13	5
5%	8.4	19.2	6.4
Huber's M-estimator	6.6	14.6	5.4

* Excluding Robots

DiTV users viewed nearly three times as many pages as kiosk users and about twice as many pages compared to Internet users (Huber's estimator). Internet figures are not strictly comparable, as they do not include views to cached pages that are not recorded in the logs. The data suggest that kiosk users tend not to view as many pages as users of other platforms, while DiTV users generally view the most pages. The difference is largely a result of a greater proportion of kiosk users ending their search prematurely without having viewed many pages.

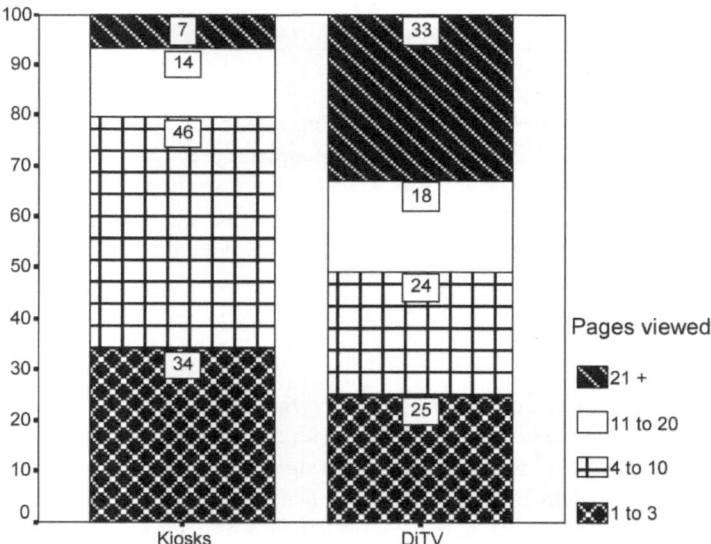

Figure 6.1 System page penetration – comparing kiosks with DiTV

Alternatively, the information can be presented as a distribution of sessions grouped by number of pages viewed – we call this site penetration. This is given in Figure 6.1 for kiosks and DiTV only. Clearly what constitutes positive use must imply that the information seeker navigates beyond the collection of initial menu screens to information pages. In broad terms, because of site architecture, users viewing only one to three pages were unlikely to have accessed an actual information page and can be termed 'bouncers'. By contrast, users viewing over 20 pages can be said to be heavy users or 'burrowers'. This group of users displays a good understanding of how to jump between pages and how to use the technology to find the information they seek.

Kiosk users viewed the least number of pages (5.4) and recorded the highest percentage (34%) of sessions which saw three pages or fewer being viewed. There are a number of reasons for this:

- *Time pressure*: Kiosk users may well be using the kiosk at a time just before or just after a doctor's appointment. Both may be pressurised periods and a user might terminate a session because their appointment had been called or as a result of having to get back quickly to work or the home. Surgeries are not the kind of places people 'hang-around'.
- *Prior experience*: It is thought that kiosk users may not penetrate the service as well users of other platforms as many will have had no prior experience of menu-based technology and will be using the service for the first time. The kiosk section of this book (Chapter 3), for example, found significant evidence of little experience among kiosk users and this may impact on use. Hence kiosk users may well give up after only having seen a couple of menu screens because they were not inclined to learn the new technology or master the navigational structure.
- *Service misuse*: Users might start to activate a session out of boredom while waiting in a service queue. This was observed at pharmacies.
- *Search disclosure*: Users might terminate their session early as they realised that they did not want to search for sensitive information in a public place; in other words they felt uncomfortable. Though this is thought to impact on the user's willingness to search on this platform.

The number of pages in a web session was 6.6. However, this figure is likely to be an under-estimate as a result of cached pages not being included in the calculations. Allowing for the fact that 30 to 40% of pages viewed by Internet users will be cached then web users would have viewed approximately 9 to 10 pages in a session.

DiTV users viewed the most pages in a session – 15. The penetration of a site was significantly greater for DiTV users. Looking at the percentage of users viewing 20 pages or more, only 7% of kiosk users viewed 21 pages or more, while 33% of DiTV users did so. There were factors other than purely interest ones that might explain this:

- *Penetration of information*: As mentioned above, DiTV users may have to delve further into the system to extract as much information as an Internet or kiosk user. This is because, as less information can fit on a DiTV screen as compared to a web or even a kiosk one, DiTV is a menu rich environment. However it should be noted that the average is calculated on the basis of accesses within the service and excludes page (menu screen) accesses made prior to arriving at the service.

- *Time pressure*: Internet and kiosk users may feel pressured to finish their session early, the former, because of the (telephone) cost of being on-line (unless they have a broadband connection) or the pressures that come from using the Internet for personal purposes at work; and the latter because of the social pressures of using the technology in a public place. There is little pressure on DiTV users. They are viewing the information at home at a time relatively convenient for themselves. However, there may be competing demands for the television in a household.
- *Prior experience*: DiTV users were relatively experienced with this type of information system – they would have used the remote device before for watching a standard television and probably for a video as well. This is not true for a large percentage of kiosk users, for whom the system was certainly new at the time.
- *Site architecture*: Both Kiosk and Internet users had a scroll option that enables them to scroll down to further information. This was not the case for DiTV users. Instead of offering users a scroll facility DiTV users could view another screen or 'turn a page'. Hence to view a similar amount of information DiTV users would have had to view a greater number of pages.
- *Search disclosure*: users were searching at a time and place convenient to themselves and could view sensitive health topics that they may find uncomfortable to view in a more socially open environment.

Session view time appears to be a worthy metric for comparing use between platforms as the session time metric is not degraded by caching. Longer sessions might indicate greater use, interest and, perhaps implicitly, satisfaction or at the very least a greater engagement with the information.

DiTV users spent just under half as much time again on a session as an Internet user and approximately four times as long as a kiosk user. People spent approximately three minutes on the website, four and half minutes on the DiTV channel and just over a minute on a kiosk session. The data suggest that kiosk users were rapid viewers while DiTV users spent a long time looking at their screens. Reasons have already been furnished why DiTV users have longer sessions and these include prior experience, time constraints, search disclosure (more on which follows) and site architecture. However, the fact that users cannot print, and therefore have to read every page carefully, possibly even making notes, has an impact here, too. Furthermore, the person's distance from the screen (typically further away) may also be important. Finally, the loading of additional pages and managing the changing of pages via the remote will also add to session time. Furthermore, Internet users will conduct shorter sessions than DiTV users as many Internet users will have viewed a number of health sites and some of these 'bouncer' sessions will be quite short.

The web (NHS Direct Online) recorded its highest use mid-week – on Wednesdays (19% of pages viewed) and on Thursdays (17%). DiTV also registered its highest use on Wednesdays and Thursdays (20% and 19% respectively), while kiosks notched-up their highest use on quite different days – Tuesdays (17%) and

Fridays (17%). DiTV attracted a higher percentage of weekend use than the other two platforms, which is not surprising as this is the only information platform found almost exclusively in people's homes.

Both DiTV and the Internet were available 24 hours a day, whereas kiosks were available only during the opening hours of the premises on which they were located (albeit some hospital locations are open 24 hours). Both DiTV and NHS Direct Online were used throughout the 24-hour period, although percentage use remained fairly small between about midnight to 8 am in the morning. The web peaked between about midday and 3pm while use at kiosks peaked in the afternoon about 4pm (shortly after children leave school). There was a noticeable evening peak in DiTV use between 7pm and 9pm – corresponding approximately to peak TV viewing time generally. This latter statistic show that DiTV users were not constrained in their search for health information by the viewing exigencies of other members of their families. Clearly, however, research of a more ethnographic nature is required to examine the dynamics of home viewing.

Conclusions

- It was estimated that about 15% of the general population actively search for health information at any given time. This rose to about 17%, not really a significant difference, for those who have access to a health information kiosk, but increased to 30% for those with access to a health information service on the Internet or DiTV.
- In terms of system penetration DiTV users were far less likely to view just one to three pages than kiosk users – only about 20 to 25% did as compared to about 34% of kiosk users.
- In terms of session time, DiTV users spent about half as much time again on a session as Internet user's did on a single site and approximately three and half times as long as kiosk users. The average Internet session will be shorter compared to a DiTV session as Internet users are likely to view a number of health sites and some of these 'bouncer' sessions will be short.
- DiTV attracted higher use on weekends compared to both the Internet and Kiosks. DiTV had a peak use in the evening compared to the Internet which peeks about lunchtime.

There were a number of significant differences between platforms. The most used platform appeared to be DiTV, followed by the Internet, with kiosks the least used. There appears to be many reasons for this. Some of these are system related, for example, the site architecture and the uni-site system of the DiTV as compared to the multi-site availability of the Internet accounts for much. Other reasons for the differences include: where the platform is situated, for the information requirements of the user, and how familiar the system is. These factors together explain differences in online behaviour, which in turn, explains the differences in: page and session view times, number of pages downloaded in a session, and the content of pages viewed.

Ease of use (and prior experience)

Perhaps the most telling statistic we have generated was that about twice as many kiosk users abandoned their searches after having just viewed menu (introductory and explanatory) screens as compared to DiTV users. This was as also true, but slightly less so, in the case of kiosks situated in information centres as it was for kiosks located in surgeries or hospitals. Furthermore, that session duration, an alternative metric for system penetration, on the kiosk was about a third of that compared to either the Internet or DiTV. One reason for this was ease of use, and the user's skills experience of the three platforms.

Thirty eight percent of kiosk users conducted sessions viewing three pages or fewer and they were highly unlikely to have viewed an information page. The users' previous experience has an impact on whether the user found an information page. Skilled employed workers were twice as likely to find an information page as those in non-skilled employment. It was found that previous skills experience with microwaves and computers also had a positive impact on kiosk use: that is, the number of pages viewed in a session was greater in locations with a high incidence of microwave ownership. This was additionally confirmed from interview data at various surgeries, in which issues related to kiosk use were explored. Some participants drew analogies from other systems to illustrate their comfort with the system: 'it is similar to using an ATM [cash point] machine'; 'similar systems are at the ticket office (railway stations)'.

The users' system experience, and the availability and convenience of the system were found important for Internet users. This was illustrated by a 20-30 year old female questionnaire respondent, who said: 'it is difficult to know whether I would have used other sources if the net was not around or whether my interest in health info (sic) developed in line with the availability on the net'. Similarly, as another respondent pointed out 'generally the Internet provides information that just wasn't available before to normal (i.e. non-medical) people'.

The Internet study found that those more experienced with using the Internet felt that they had obtained higher health outcomes. In particular, those visiting more than one health site recorded higher outcomes and dealt more realistically with problems of trust and authority compared to respondents just viewing a single site. The authors believe that the skills needed to use Internet based information systems are more diverse and complicated compared to a comparable DiTV service. Both are multiple service information environments. DiTV users navigate between sites in much the same way as they navigate within a service, that is with a remote and menus. Internet users navigate between sites and within sites using different search tools: search engines, and by using a mouse to click on menus and links. In addition Internet users have to critically compare and contrast the information found from a variety of competing health sites, for DiTV users generally only one health site option is offered.

The way that users discover a site is typically via browsing. For DiTV browsing between services is via the remote and requires similar skills to that needed to navigate within a service. Internet users browsed by using a search engine and through a menu-based service. The fact is that using a search engine, unless used well, is not particularly efficient at finding sites (in terms of relevance). And this was born out in the figures of how respondents said that they found sites. On the Internet about 30 to 40% of respondents first found a site by browsing, the comparable figure for DiTV was about 60 to 70%, just less than double the Internet figure.

Previous platform skill was found to be important for the effective use of the DiTV service. The NHS Direct Digital service on Kingston Interactive Television (KIT) offered users a mix of both a text and a video health information service. It was found that those with previous skills of DiTV in general were found to be more likely to report that they had used the service. The users' prior skill or experience of DiTV was estimated by their use of an existing video download service available on KIT. It was found that users who had rented a commercial video online were four times more likely to have viewed the NHS Direct Digital health text service compared to those who had not visited the existing video service. Further, users who had downloaded a commercial video were three times more likely to have viewed a free NHS Direct Digital health video.

The DiTV study also found that users applied their skills across platforms, skill transfer, if you like. It was found, for example, that those who were currently using an Internet service were more likely to have used the text DiTV service: 35% who had Internet access had used NHS Direct Digital compared to 27% who did not have an Internet connection. The relationship was the same for use of the video service: 23% of those with an Internet access had used the video clip service compared to 17% who did not have access. It should be stressed that Internet access here was access via the KIT telephone service.

Interestingly, the users' prior experience of the Internet also had an impact on kiosk use. Those who used and felt comfortable with IT were more likely to have used the kiosk: 21% of these computer literate users had done so compared to 6% of users who avoided computers. This was further confirmed by interview data. For those unfamiliar with information technology the kiosk might appear to be rather daunting: '... I am computer literate so I found using the system quite easy. Someone who isn't familiar with a computer might be intimidated by the technology'. This was reflected in interviews with GP patients, but only partially. A small minority of non-user respondents (six out of 40) mentioned the technology as a factor in their non-use. Typical of the comments this small group made was 'When I see a computer I just turn away'. Reference was made of inexperience or a lack of prior experience, explained in terms of age: 'We weren't brought up with these things [computers]. They don't mean anything to me'.

Turning our attention now to usability, Figure 6.2 compares how easy (or not) people found the kiosk (InTouch) and DiTV (NHS Direct Digital) system with regard to understanding the content, readability and menus. The platforms, kiosk and DiTV, were found to be similar in regard to ease of use in terms of understanding content and readability. There was a slight tendency for DiTV to perform better and 33% found DiTV easy to understand and read all the time compared to 30% of kiosk users who said so. About 9% said that the kiosk was at no time easy with regard to readability compared to about 5% who said this for DiTV users.

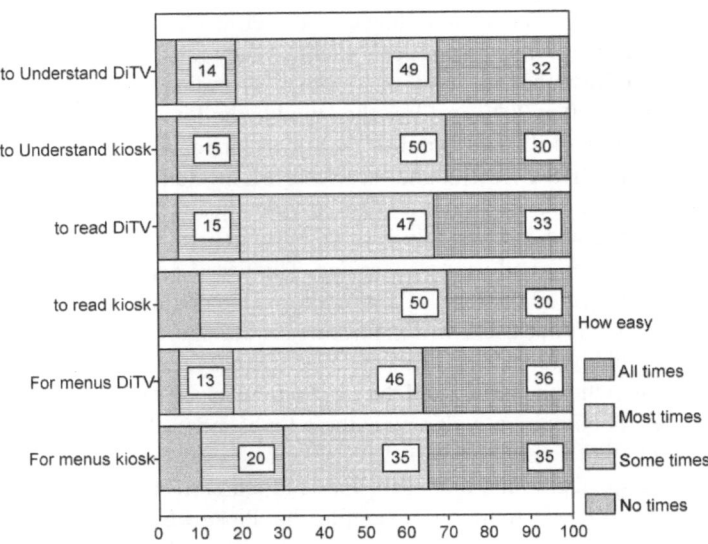

Figure 6.2 How easy the service was to use – kiosk vs. DiTV

However, there was more of a difference when it came to the menus (Figure 6.2). While 30% of kiosk users said the menus were at no time or only sometimes easy, this was only true for 18% of DiTV users. In addition kiosk users were more likely to report that menus were at no time easy – 10% reported this compared to 5% of DiTV users. The ease with which menus could be used did not relate to the kiosk touchscreen area, which was covered by a separate question.

Kiosk menus appeared to be a particular problem for users, and clearly some were not finding the menu structure easy to use. Kiosks present a particular problem for system designers in that the touchscreen areas have to be quite large and so not many menu items can be fitted on the screen. This results in a menu heavy system. One solution is to design kiosks with menus items that reflect the likely health related interest implied by the kiosks location.

Users were also asked how easy it was to navigate each information platform. Figure 6.3 reports the results and compares ease of navigation for a variety of health information services on a variety of platforms: a kiosk (InTouch with Health), the Internet (SurgeryDoor) and two DiTV services (Living Health on Telewest and NHS Direct Digital on Kingston Interactive Television).

In terms of ease of navigation it seemed that Living Health (DiTV-text based service) was thought to be the easiest to navigate, 82% of respondents found navigation easy either all the time or most of the time. Interestingly, not everything on television succeeds. For example, the DiTV service offering both text and videos (NHS Direct Digital) performed poorly and this suggests that users may have found the navigation between text and videos confusing. Internet navigation too was thought to be a problem and was rated by users to be harder than either kiosks or

DiTV. Twenty-three percent of Internet users found navigation only easy at times or not at all, compared to 20% of kiosk users and 17% of DiTV users. It seems that once a person became familiar with kiosk navigation was not all that difficult to undertake.

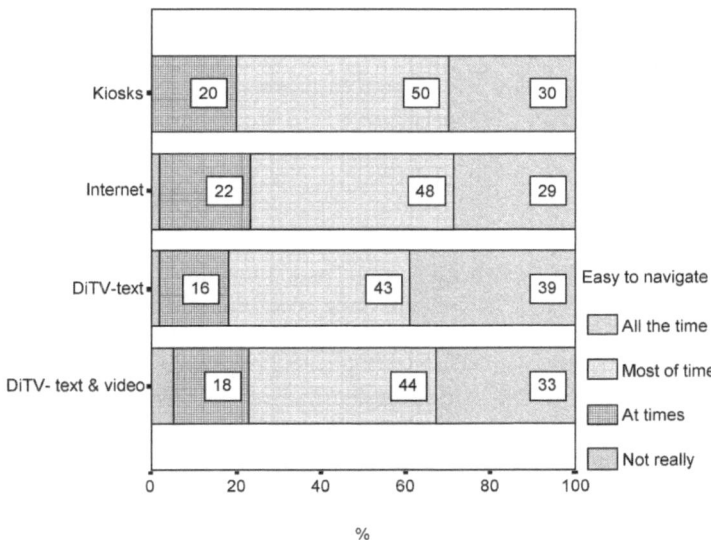

Figure 6.3 Ease of navigation for three platforms

There were indications in the usability studies with the Internet (SurgeryDoor and NHS Direct online) that navigating these systems and retrieving information may not have been particularly intuitive for some people, particularly if they were unused to electronic systems. In evaluating the usability of DiTV applications, Serco found that some subjects thought the 'Home' button on the information service referred to information about the home, rather than to a 'start' or 'title' page. Kiosk users may have been using an electronic information source for the first time, and not experienced in negotiating menu hierarchies etc. The 'prev screen' button on the kiosk, for example, was far from intuitive for non Internet users.

In multiple service information environments such as DiTV and the Internet, the user has opportunities to learn the necessary on-line searching skills to explore parts of the service, like a specialised health information service. This was not true of kiosk type information systems that were very much stand-alone and presented the database of just one subject, in this case health. The point being that the user has a greater reason to use the more comprehensive and general Internet and DiTV services. The greater use of health information on the Internet and DiTV as compared to the kiosk was in part a result of this prior platform experience.

Comparison of the health content of three digital platforms

Analysing digital content pages poses plenty of problems for researchers, especially when comparing content coverage of various related services. It is quite normal, even for digital services of the same organisation, to adopt different page-naming conventions for each service. This is more true about digital services run by different organisations. What all this means is that there is no easy way to compare topic and page use as revealed by access behaviour. This study sought to compare content offered by two kiosks services: NHS Direct Online and InTouch with Health kiosks, an Internet service and two DiTV services: NHS Direct Digital/Communicopia and Living Health.

Exposure

Logically, the greater the exposure a system has to the public, the greater will be its use and the more likely that its content, once accessed, will be used, be it simply to inform or to make health-related behaviour decisions or to seek further medical advice from a doctor. Hence, exposure will have an impact on what content is used. One difficulty faced was that not all of the five services were equally exposed. InTouch with Health logs were evaluated over a 24-month period compared to one month for NHS Direct kiosks, while NHS Direct Kiosks were evaluated across 120 outlets compared to 21 for InTouch kiosks. The Communicopia (NHS Direct Digital) service was available to 10,000 households while Living Health was available to nearly 40,000, and this is complicated by the fact that the logs for Living Health were recorded for just under twice as long: five months, as compared to three for NHS Direct Digital. For the Internet the number of potential outlets was unknown, but is likely to run into millions. The Internet is further complicated by the existence of many competing services.

To assess the impact of exposure on used content figures, differences in used content over time and across different levels of outlets were considered.

For the Internet and kiosks, the amount of 'used' (i.e. accessed) content increased month on month, but at a declining rate. The addition to used content from the first to the second month was 10% in the case of kiosks (InTouch) and about 5% for the Internet (SurgeryDoor). The big changes in the number of unique pages viewed occurred in the first three months. After four to five months, the addition of new pages viewed was minimal. From the first to second monthly period the percentage increase to used content was about 5%, however, this increase declined to about 1%, period on period, between period four and period five. Thus exposure will affect the analysis but the effect declines over time and was relatively minor after two months and negligible after about four to five months of exposure. Hence, for SurgeryDoor, in the six-month study, 93% of used content was attained in the first month. This suggests that users tend to re-visit the same pages and after about a two to three month research period the likelihood of a new subject being viewed was relatively small.

The NHS Direct Digital service, however, did not correspond to this pattern. In fact, in its case, the largest increase in used content occurred between periods two and three. However, there was no difference in used content between period three and four. This DiTV channel offered, for the first time, Internet like health information services on the television and this was clearly a new experience for virtually the whole audience.

Variations in exposure may also result from differences in the number of service outlets – clearly, the greater the number of possible outlets the greater the exposure. For kiosks, outlets are the actual number of kiosks available, for DiTV and Internet this is the number of locations (households or offices) that can receive the service. In the case of the particular study covered here logs were collected for 21 InTouch with Health kiosks and 120 NHS Direct Online kiosks. DiTV outlets were calculated by the estimated number of subscribers to the service for Living Health. This was nearly 40,000; for NHS Direct Digital it was about one quarter of this, 10,000. It was not possible to estimate the number of Internet outlets as an outlet can be any computer that can connect to the Internet.

To test this idea that variations in exposure may also result from differences in the number of service outlets a comparison was undertaken of random samples of the outcome of outlet use for SurgeryDoor and NHS Direct Digital. The comparison is between the topics viewed from taking say a 20% and 40% sample. Four samples were taken, a 20%, 40%, 60% and 80% random sample from both data sets. Then the percentage addition in topics viewed between each random sample was calculated and compared. The percentage change in used content for different quantities of use was then examined in order to answer the question: what is the increase in used content as use increases?

The data showed that the percentage increase in used content was only marginal with greater levels of use. There was only about a 4% increase in used content as randomly selected use was increased from 20 to 40%. Exposure was thus a factor in usage. However, the impact on used content was minimal so long as the period studied was greater than two to three months or where the number of outlets was large. That is, nearly all content that will be used was used at this point – by about month three.

Results

Table 6.5 details, for the various survey periods, the number of outlets or stations where users could access the services, the number of pages viewed, the number of unique pages viewed and the first and last access dates covered by this study.

To illustrate the potential of digital content analyses a number have been conducted on this data-set, and these analyses provide the structure for this section. The analyses conducted are as follows:

- Overall comparisons of used and unused content of digital health services operating in the same area
- A combined subject page group analysis
- Broad comparisons of content coverage between digital services
- Detailed comparisons of category coverage between digital services
- Relationship between use and content coverage

Table 6.5 Outlets, page views and unique pages viewed – five health information services

	No of outlets covered	No of page views	No. unique pages viewed (used content)	First date	Last date
InTouch kiosks	21	223,124	864	17-Mar-99	01-May-01
NHS Direct kiosks	120	170,615	537	1-July-01	31-July-01
NHS Direct Digital DiTV channel	10,000	85,131	454	17-Dec-01	01-May-02
Living Health DiTV channel	40,000	327,223	2,648	18-Jul-01	25-Oct-01
SurgeryDoor website	Unknown	1,037,185	2,341	01-Oct-01	29-Sep-02

In all, the five studies of the three different digital platforms covered almost two million page views (usage). About 5,000 unique health pages were viewed (used content). We believe that this makes this analysis one of the biggest of its kind. Used content views refer to pages that were accessed and, of course, information services may well have additional pages that have not been viewed (unused content). For example, InTouch with Health kiosks had approximately 1,100 viewable pages. However, for this study, only 864 pages or just over three quarter of these unique pages were actually viewed over the period and via the outlets included in this study.

Unused content may just be difficult to find (has poor digital visibility), in which case the analysis can point to areas where steps could be taken to make more prominent needed but not used data, or could concern subjects that users were not so interested in, and therefore highlight areas for pruning, although, of course, pages on rare conditions that may only be of use to a small minority of users may, nevertheless, be considered as fulfilling a valuable role; a case where use does not equal value.

There were large differences between services in regard to the amount of content that was used, with the Living Health channel (2648 content pages) having most content used and NHS Direct Digital the least (454 pages). A comparison between the two DiTV services shows that used content of the NHS Direct Digital service was approximately about a fifth or a little under 20% of that used on the Living Health service. This might reflect – correctly in this case – the fact that Living Health had more content. However, other factors could also have an impact – for example, site architecture, digital visibility and size of the population served. The Living Health service appeared to be closer in content coverage (as indicated by used content) to the SurgeryDoor website. In fact, although the Living Health service obtained less usage than SurgeryDoor, it did have a greater proportion of used content. The lower usage figure for the Living Health service can be explained by the fact that, unlike the SurgeryDoor, the service was not a national service (it was only available to

Telewest subscribers in Birmingham), and was only available for a relatively short period – a little under six months.

The used content for InTouch with Health and NHS Direct kiosks differed less. However, it should be noted that the InTouch with Health logs were collected over a longer period than was the case for NHS Direct Online kiosks (12 months compared to one month), while a greater number of outlets were included in the NHS Direct Online analysis (120 compared to 21).

To compare subject coverage of used content between platforms a random sample of pages used (excluding menu pages) was taken from each data set and to classify the used content of this sub group. This was done as it was not feasible to classify all 5000 used topic pages. A random sample of 0.01% of page view use was taken across the five services. This resulted in a selection of about 20% (972) of unique used content pages. To classify the pages, we adapted the National Library of Medicine topic categories used in the Medline Plus information service.[1] The used content pages were classified into 37 health categories (Figure 6.4 shows 24 of them which were more popular). The most popular pages proved those to be on wellness and lifestyle (13%), illustrating the consumer traits of the sites. This was followed by treatments and procedures (8%), miscellaneous (8%) and pregnancy and reproduction (7%). Use of pages from the just the top four categories accounted for about one third of all use.

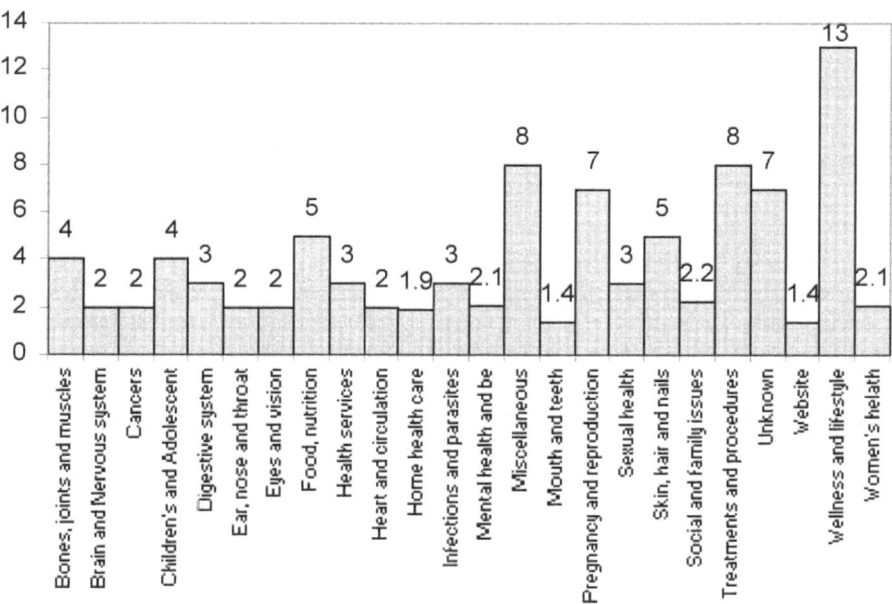

Figure 6.4 Cumulated health content – frequency distribution for 38 health categories (%)

---

1   See http://www.nlm.nih.gov/medlineplus/healthtopics.html.

The most under-used categories were ethnic minorities, non-specific symptoms, substance abuse and old age health. Each attracted less than half a percent of use and may reflect poor coverage on these topics on the digital services covered. The latter finding confirms that the Government were right to be concerned about getting information and health advice to the elderly and to other minority and possibly vulnerable groups.

Not all the online information services recorded used content for all of the 37 categories. Table 6.6 gives the number of topics covered by each service and the percentage of coverage. The best performing service in this respect was the Internet service SurgeryDoor. In all, 36 of the 37 topics were covered by this service and represented approximately 97% coverage. Used content on the DiTV service Living health covered 81% or 30 of the topics, while used content for the NHS Direct Digital accounted for 59% of the categories. There was not a lot of difference between the two kiosk services, both were estimated at about 65% – higher than NHS Direct Digital but lower than either SurgeryDoor or Living Health.

Table 6.6 Coverage distribution and ranks – digital platform comparisons

	Topic Coverage	% coverage	Standard Deviation Topic use
InTouch kiosk	23	62%	11.68
NHS Direct kiosk	24	65%	9.04
NHS Direct Digital	22	59%	2.58
Living Health	30	81%	11.07
SurgeryDoor	36	97%	31.47

Table 6.6 (Column 4) also gives an estimate of the variation of topic use between services. It gives an idea of the standardised variation of screens viewed for each service. This variation was greatest for SurgeryDoor (31), was about the same for InTouch, NHS Direct Online and Living Health (9 to 11) and was lowest for NHS Direct Digital (3). What this means is that the distribution differences of use over topics viewed was greatest for SurgeryDoor and least for NHS Direct Digital.

We now turn to a more detailed comparison of category coverage between services (Figure 6.5). Each of the 38 categories (Figure 6.4) was allocated into one of five broad topic groupings: Disorders and Conditions, Treatments and Procedures, Health and Wellness, Demographic groupings and Other. Figure 6.5 gives the use distribution of topics for each service.

There are quite big differences here. NHS Direct Digital attracted a greater proportion of use to pages related to Disorders and Conditions than the other services: 58% compared to about 40% to 45% for other services. This service also had relatively fewer pages used in the Treatments and Procedures (12%) and Health and Wellness (27%) areas. InTouch with Health kiosks showed a greater use of Health and Wellness pages (35%) and a relatively higher use of Treatments and Procedures (16%). Both SurgeryDoor and NHS Direct kiosks had a high 'Other' content use and both these services had a relatively low use of Treatment and Procedure pages. Living Health had the highest percentage regarding Treatments and Procedures, and 20% of page views related to this topic.

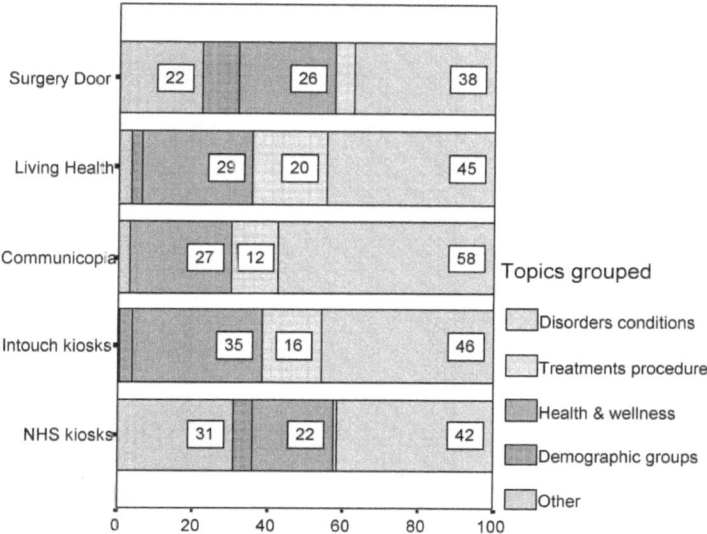

Figure 6.5 Topic use as a percentage within each service

An important factor impacting on the use of pages and topics was 'digital visibility' (Nicholas *et al* 2002). It describes the relationship between use of a service/page and its prominence in the site. For example, Health and Wellness pages were particularly prominent on the InTouch with Health kiosk menu. These topics were highly visible to kiosk users and were accessible within three prominent and clear menu screens. This was not the case with other menu options that required users to scroll through many option lists and turn pages, both more difficult to do on a touchscreen kiosk. This might partly explain the greater use of these pages on this system. However, another explanation is that kiosk users were more interested in general health, although this was not supported by usage of this topic as a percentage share on NHS Direct Online kiosks.

Figure 6.6 takes a different approach to topic coverage, this time giving a breakdown of use for each of the 38 categories by each digital service as a percentage of category use. It gives the percentage use for each health category. Living Health was particularly strong on pages related to Sexual Health, Kidney and Urinary, Endocrine Systems and Cancers. NHS kiosks had a greater presence in the areas of Genetic and Birth Defects, Injuries and Wounds, Non-Specific Symptoms and Skin, Hair and Nails. While InTouch with Health kiosks appear to have a greater used content of pages related to Bones, Joints and Muscles, Endocrine System, Kidney and Urinary and Wellness and Lifestyle.

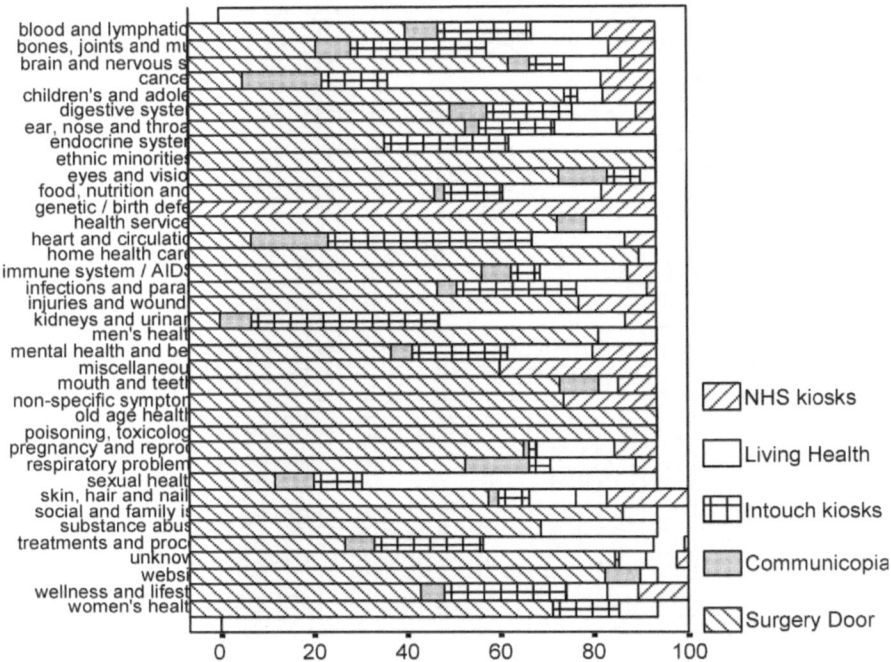

Figure 6.6 Category use and online service – digital platform comparisons*
* Percentage based on total number of pages use within each category.

Figure 6.7 examines nine health categories as a percentage of use for each system. The nine categories accounted for about 51% of all sampled used content. For kiosks, greater use of wellness and lifestyle pages was made seen for the InTouch kiosks (27%) as compared to NHS Kiosks (15%). NHS kiosks, however, showed a greater use of Skin, Hair and Nail pages (10%), while InTouch kiosks had considerably fewer views to this category (3%). NHS kiosks also performed well on providing information on Food, Nutrition and Diet (7%), compared to InTouch kiosks (5%). InTouch kiosks performed better, however, on providing information on Treatments and Procedures (16%) and Bones, Joints and Muscles (8%) compared to NHS Direct Online kiosks (respectively 1% and 5%).

In comparing the two DiTV services, NHS Direct Digital performed relatively well in Wellness and Lifestyle (15%) and the Digestive System (6%) compared to Living Health (respectively 7% and 3%). Living Health performed better in terms of providing information on Treatments and Procedures (20%), Sexual Health (11%), Pregnancy and Reproduction (8%) and Food Nutrition and Diet (7%) Compared to the NHS Direct Digital service (respectively 12%, 5%, 4%, 4%).

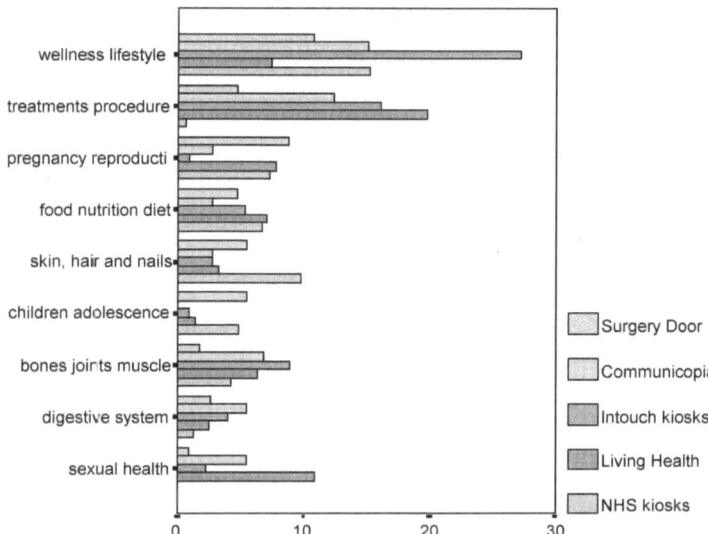

Figure 6.7 Use within service – focus on nine health categories

The only health category where the two DiTV services were ranked both first and second position was on the sexual health category. This suggests that users were particularly willing to investigate this topic on this platform. The authors have argued that the privacy afforded by this platform makes this a particularly good medium for viewing this type of topic (Nicholas *et al* 2003b). However this may also partially reflect topic menu prominence and topic page proliferation. However it does seem that users made good use of these pages.

Both kiosk systems were well used in regard to wellness and lifestyle information, and it appears that this platform is a good medium for this type of topic. This, in part, reflects the public nature of searching on this platform. Many users will avoid searching for sensitive information if they feel that their search process will be observed (search disclosure) and would be more likely to search for socially acceptable or less challenging topics.

We might naturally expect a greater use and more repeat use of services that had the most comprehensive content, and we sought to determine whether this was indeed the case. In comparing the two DiTV services it was apparent from the above that Living Health had more available pages and generally a greater page content compared to the NHS Direct Digital service. In all it was estimated that the content of Living Health was three times the size of the available content on the NHS Direct Digital service.

There were use differences between the two services. The most significant being reach, which is the percentage use made of a service by those people who potentially could access it (the population of subscribers). The reach figure for the NHS Direct Digital service was estimated at 20%, while for the Living Health service this figure was 30% – about a third higher.

The number of users returning to a service is also an important metric of use and this was also higher for the Living Health as compared to the NHS Direct Digital – 41% compared to 36.9%.

In a study comparing the two services it was found that respondents who had reportedly used Living Health service were just under twice as likely as non-users to say they would use medical information sources as an alternative to seeing the doctor (1.79 estimated odds). While 52% of Telewest subscribers who had not used Living Health had substituted information found for a visit to the doctor this was true of 69% of subscribers – approximately 40% more – who had used Living Health. The finding was also true for KIT subscribers using the NHS Direct Digital, but the result was only significant at the 10% level and the estimated odds were lower: 1.39 compared to 1.79. This suggested that the impact of the NHS Direct Digital service was lower on this outcome compared to the Living Health. Content differences between the services maybe one of the reasons explaining the lower impact made by NHS Direct Digital.

Content differences will be one reason that helps to explain outcome and use differences between services. Clearly the relationship implied here between content and use differences is circumstantial. Living Health had more content than NHS Direct Digital; Living Health was also found to have a higher reach figure, a greater number of returnees and a more likely outcome. However, use and outcomes will also be affected by digital visibility with regard to other services on the DiTV, by advertising, ease of use as well as the content on offer. Regarding the latter, the important question to ask is what is the impact on usage and outcome measures of a marginal increase in content? That is what is the optimum content that maximises usage and outcomes?

We have sought to examine the problems of making content comparisons between digital information services and platforms on the basis of pages viewed, and looked at both the procedures and at the type of comparisons that can be made. Online system architecture, the length of the monitoring period and the number of outlets was found to impact on such comparisons and these were discussed. A 0.01% sample of five data-sets was taken and data accrued classified and compared. Services were examined as to their use across health categories and differences found. InTouch with Health kiosks had a greater use of Wellness and Lifestyle pages, while NHS kiosks had relatively a greater use of Skin, Hair and Nail pages. Living Health had a greater use of Treatments and Procedures pages, and both the DiTV channels had a significant use of Sexual Health pages. These differences reflect coverage differences (availability), search disclosure and digital visibility. For example, Health and Wellness pages are particularly prominent on the InTouch with Health kiosk menu. These topics were highly visible to kiosk users and this might partly explain the greater use of these pages on this system. Also users seemed more willing to use pages related to Sexual Health in their own homes. Content differences and coverage have an impact on overall service usage and outcomes.

The impact of platform location on search behaviour (search disclosure)

People are understandably sensitive about matters to do with their health and confidentiality is an essential aspect of the patient-doctor dialogue. Clearly, these concerns extend to the use of health information systems and platforms, though this is a little researched topic; hence, the importance of what we have to say here. For the purposes of this discussion we propose a concept of 'search disclosure' to assist in the understanding of the variations in digital information health seeking behaviour as a result of the perceived degree of anonymity afforded at the point of searching and information consumption. The anonymity offered by certain digital health platforms in certain locations might be seen as an asset when communicating about highly sensitive topics, such as sexually transmitted diseases, or embarrassing topics, like incontinence.

Touchscreen kiosks

Kiosks, as they are available in public places will be moderated negatively by search-disclosure. That is, people experience discomfort when searching for private, confidential or embarrassing information using kiosks because they are situated in public areas. This factor may especially influence the use of a digital health platform such as a touchscreen kiosk in a pharmacy or doctor's surgery, where other people may be physically present.

Evidence of search disclosure was found in a comparison between kiosk use at four location types (information centres, pharmacies, hospitals and surgeries). Pharmacies performed poorly. They recorded the lowest number of pages viewed in a search session, under six on average, compared to about seven at other locations. Furthermore, they recorded the lowest average session duration time of less than 50 seconds. Kiosks located in hospitals and information centres recorded the longest average session duration time of approximately 80 seconds while surgeries recorded an average session view time of about one minute. Surgeries and pharmacies recorded the shortest average page view time of about eight seconds, while users at hospitals and information centres recorded average view times of about 10 seconds. In terms of overall use, estimated by the number of sessions per hour per kiosk, kiosks located in information centres performed well and recorded just over one user session per hour. Surgery kiosks were the most under-deployed and recorded on average around one session every two hours (0.5 users per hour). Pharmacies attracted just fewer than two sessions every three hours (0.66 users per hour.), while hospitals performed slightly better than this and recorded just over four sessions every five hours (0.8 users per hour). Surgeries also performed poorly according to the number of pages printed per hour per kiosk and surgery locations recorded just less than one page printed per day. Information centres again performed well with one page printed every two and a half hours. Pharmacies performed poorly with less than one page printed every four hours.

Surgeries appeared to perform the least well – especially according to the number of sessions conducted in an hour and the number of pages printed per hour. This may not be surprising. After all, surgeries are not the most relaxing of locations, and people are faced with time constraints and doubts before their appointments, not knowing how long they will have to wait beforehand. Also, locations with a large throughput of people, such as hospitals, will record higher levels of use. However, some of the variation in kiosk use between locations is thought to result from the anonymity offered by the location, with surgeries and pharmacies being the most visible of all locations and surgeries being the most personal.

Evidence of search-disclosure was uncovered in the questionnaire study of potential users' of a kiosk situated in a doctor's surgery in Scotland. Respondents who did not use the kiosk were asked whether the reason for non-use was anything to do with the fact that it was situated in a public place. Just under half of non-users (47%) said that this was, indeed, a factor. There was some evidence that older users were more likely to say that they did not like using the kiosk in public place: 56% of over 55 years agreed compared to only 32% of non-users aged 35 and under. The search-disclosure model predicts that potential users would be put off using the kiosk if issues around privacy were compromised. In fact, a little below 50% of those who were identified as non-kiosk users preferred not to use the system rather than conduct their information search in a public place.

This was further confirmed from interview data conducted in pharmacies in which various issues related to kiosk use were explored. Although interviewees were not asked specifically about the positioning of the kiosk in relation to their propensity to use it, some respondents raised the topic themselves, saying that use of the system for them would be dependent on the actual placement at the location. One user commented that 'If it is positioned in such a way that someone can see over your shoulder I would not want to use it', while another said that 'yes, I would use it anywhere as long as it is in an area that offers some amount of privacy'. One interviewee even said 'there is always the chance of running into someone I know there, I would feel uncomfortable for them to see me searching for information in a doctor's surgery'. Finally, one respondent highlighted the hazards of going ahead with a search interaction: 'I was trying to print some information and the machine stuck. I asked the pharmacist for help even though I was a bit embarrassed because I considered that particular information rather confidential, but I really needed it. She assisted me in printing all my pages'. These comments point to the existence of search disclosure because users were fearful of their search being seen.

Relative topic use at the various kiosk locations also provided some evidence of self-disclosure. Thus, in comparing the use of the kiosk page on depression, a clearly sensitive topic, between four kiosk locations – hospital, pharmacy, information centre and surgery – it was found that users were about 25% more likely to search for this topic at a hospital compared to either a surgery or an information centre.

Internet

Searching the Internet may offer users some anonymity, albeit depending on the location of the terminal. Typically use tends to be in environments where the user has their own personal space, where there is likely to be a degree of privacy and on someone's own machine. Clearly, the degree of privacy associated with PC-based

Internet behaviour can vary. Use of a PC to surf the web in an open-plan office may not offer the level of privacy that accessing the web via a PC at home does.

A study was conducted in which web logs were used to compare access to pages on depression (a possibly sensitive topic) and healthy eating (a less personal/sensitive topic) by hour of day. The aim was to find out if these potential differences in content sensitivity manifested itself in use patterns. The analysis was targeted at UK users only so as to restrict the analysis to a single time zone. Only commercial registered domain names were included. Unfortunately, these domains are also used by IP providers and thus this group does not consist wholly of commercial organisations but will include home users linking to the Internet via IP providers with a '.com' or '.co.uk' address, for example www.demon.co.uk. Thus, the analysis cannot be said to be wholly confined to commercial organisations. Of course, search disclosure is one of many effects on information seeking and is difficult to isolate. In fact, the diurnal patterns may also reflect other factors associated with these two groups of users: users of depression pages and users of healthy eating pages. A similar analysis was repeated with DiTV (Figure 6.9) giving perhaps a wider insight into diurnal patterns between these platforms as well as within platforms. If there are specific influences related to use of depression pages other than search disclosure and wanting to find a 'quiet' time to search this topic, then this should show up in a comparison between the Internet and DiTV. However, it does not look as though there was. The diurnal patterns of online searching for information about depression followed the same general trend in each case but seemed to be accentuated at certain periods of the day.

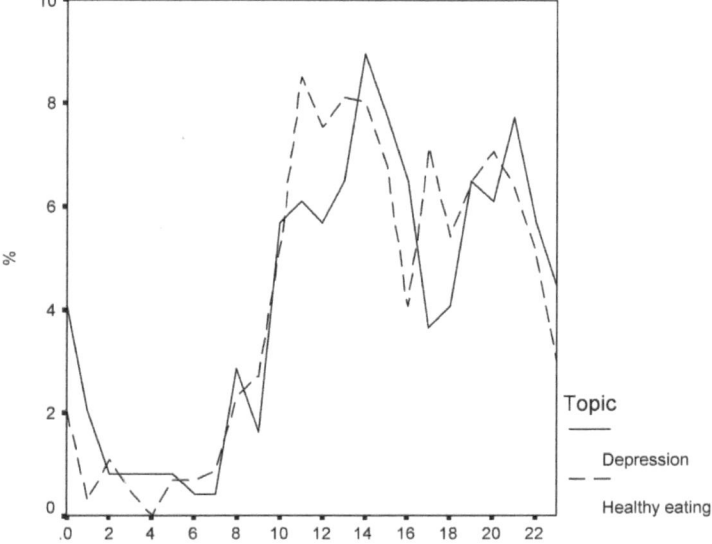

Figure 6.8 SurgeryDoor – percentage share of use over hour of day for pages related to depression and healthy eating*

* SurgeryDoor Dec 2001 to Nov 2002 UK and commercial domain registered use.

Figure 6.8 compares use of pages on depression and healthy eating on the SurgeryDoor health website over the course of a day, divided by time of day. It was posited that depression was a more sensitive search subject and that some users at least would seek a more private period to search for this information.

There was greater use of Depression pages at periods that could be described as more private: in the evening from about 6pm to about 2am and at about 1pm as people went to lunch. Users may have been waiting till after 6pm when, again, the office may have been less busy. The use after 8pm and 9pm might include that by evening workers, and may be augmented by users accessing the Internet from home linking into the site from 'dot com' ISPs. What is apparent is that the differences at certain times of the day were considerable. Approximately 25% more views were made to Healthy Eating pages as compared to the share made to Depression pages between 10am and 12am and between 2pm to 5pm. The views to Depression pages increased by about a third in the period coming up to the lunch break, between 12am and 1pm. Views to this page peaked at 1pm then fell back sharply after the lunchtime break. By 3pm views to Depression pages were about 50% of its lunchtime value. However, use subsequently climbed after 5pm. Here there is some evidence that users indeed preferred to search for certain pages, in this case Depression, when the office was less crowded: during the lunchtime break and in the period after work. As indicated search disclosure may only be one factor impacting on use here; in fact, users in each case might well have different demographic and health interest profiles. However, this is indicative evidence that users may indeed choose their own time to search for sensitive topics, but further research is needed to clarify causality.

A questionnaire of NHS Direct Online users asked where they searched from and a comparison between home and work use was made. It was noticeable that the only health sections, where the percentage of home views exceeded the percentage of work views, were 'Conditions and Treatments' and Listen Here, a facility offering a health information audio clip. Some users seemed to prefer to search for Conditions and Treatments in the more private environment of home. This section includes much more sensitive health topics compared to sections such as the Healthy Living, Health in the News or Healthcare Guide sections. This is further suggestive evidence that people may want to view some pages in a more private home environment.

Qualitative research confirmed the home environment as being one that offered privacy and anonymity. In an analysis of NHS Direct Online users' responses to questions on why the Internet was the chosen medium for procuring health information, anonymity, alongside the convenience of having information provided in one's own home, were mentioned as positive Internet attributes. It was interesting that, despite not being prompted (i.e., by multiple-choice answers) a large majority of the 42 respondents – 26 (62%), mentioned privacy or anonymity. In some cases it was found, by follow-up email queries, that 'convenience' was interchangeable with 'anonymity'. This was also clear from the juxtaposition of the two ideas in the messages of some respondents. For example, one remarked that 'It is extremely convenient to use my own PC in the privacy of my home', while another described the Internet as 'A readily available (24*7 at home) and anonymous source of information'. Apart from the linkage of the home with privacy, those who mentioned anything concerned with anonymity or confidentiality did so in somewhat general terms (i.e., such as simply stating that one could look up information privately). One person did confirm that this was for information he felt 'unable to ask doctors about', and another said that the advantages included having no direct contact with health professional.

The importance of searching in a home 'Internet' based environment was further highlighted by the qualitative study on kiosk mentioned above. One user compared their kiosk search to their Internet search and indicated a preference for the Internet over kiosk in terms of convenience and privacy. In terms of convenience their comment was: 'I can sit at home, whenever I like, and surf around' while for privacy their related comment was: 'its one thing standing there in front of everyone at a doctor's surgery, and another sitting comfortably at home, in the privacy of your own house, looking up your condition with no-one peering over your shoulder'.

DiTV

DiTV does perhaps offer users of digital information system the greatest level of privacy and security. Although, in the main, television sets are situated in public areas of the home (although many people might have them in their bedroom too), users can choose to a secure time to use the service. DiTV users are searching in their own home and on a medium with which they are very familiar.

DiTV transaction logs were examined and a comparison was also made of the use of the pages about Depression and Healthy Living on the Living Health channel over the course of a day, divided by time of day (Figure 6.9).

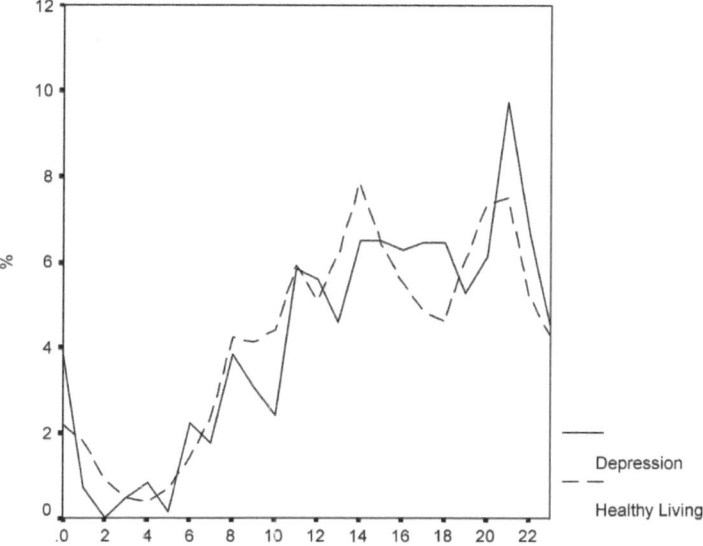

**Figure 6.9 Percentage share of use over hour of day for pages
related to depression and healthy living (Living Health)**

The profile of use for Depression pages and Healthy Living pages was quite different. There was an increased incidence of use of Depression pages after 6pm. The peak use of Depression pages was at 9pm. Use at this time was about 20% more compared to use of Healthy Living pages. Note that the pattern of page use on a DiTV system was very different from the pattern of page use of an Internet information service. The recorded swing from the lunchtime peak in use to the fall off in use in the afternoon was much greater on the Internet. There was a much steadier build up in use on DiTV peaking at about midday.

Interview data with the Living Health viewers also indicated, significantly, that time of access was a factor in privacy and usage. Although only a minority of respondents specifically mentioned privacy, those who did, said they generally looked for health information 'when the kids are in bed'. One respondent said: 'In the morning everyone is out [at work and school] so I can look at anything I want to on the box. I don't really want my 11 year old asking me what "period pains" are'.

The use of sensitive pages was compared between DiTV and other digital platforms. The purpose was to analyse page usage between platforms to see if there was any variation in use of sensitive pages. It was posited that there would be less usage on the more open and less private kiosk platform compared to either the web or DiTV. However, there are considerable difficulties in making such comparisons. Kiosk pages, for example, tended to cover one topic per page whereas web pages were often grouped so a number of topics were covered by a single 'web' page, while DiTV topics tended to be spread over a number of pages. However, a comparison proved possible in the case of HIV topic pages on Kiosk and DiTV. Results from this comparison supported the search disclosure model. For the kiosks the sensitive HIV topic received just 7 out of 223,124 page views and accounted for just 0.0003% of all kiosk content page views. This can be compared to the views to an HIV page on the Living Health DiTV information service.[2] Here 395 out of 328,894 page views were recorded, accounting for 0.1% of all content page views. Clearly users were more willing to view an HIV page on a DiTV platform compared to a kiosk. Part of this difference must be accounted for by the anonymity offered by a DiTV service that can be accessed from home compared to a public touchscreen kiosk.

It was decided also to look at a broad sweep of page views and Table 6.7 lists the top 15 pages viewed on each platform. The willingness of DiTV users in the privacy of their own home to view pages of a private nature can be seen more clearly here, and the sexual nature of topics searched for (column 1) is plain although curiosity viewing may also play a part here.[3] Furthermore, web topics were more sensitive or personal than touchscreen kiosk topics.

---

2   This comparison is between use of an HIV labelled page on both platforms. Living Health also had additional HIV related pages including HIVAIDS, HIVAsia, HIVVaccine and hepatitusHIV however these were not included in this analysis.

3   Curiosity viewing was thought to play a part in the record hits to sex information pages on the DiTV platform. However the information was comprehensive and this may just as well reflect a real demand for this information.

Table 6.7 Health topics viewed by digital platform in rank order

Top 15 pages viewed on Living Health (DiTV)	Top 15 pages viewed on the NHS Direct Online Website*	Top 15 pages viewed on InTouch with Health kiosks
Orgasmproblems	Anthrax	Good eating
Impotence	Depression	Alcohol
Prematureejaculation	Haemorrhoids	Exercise
Keepyrsexlifeingoodsha	Thrush	Weight
NoContent	Hypertension	Cancer prevention
NHSDirectinVision	back_pain	Smoking
Dyspareunia	joint_pain	Backpain – strain
SexualInfections	urinary_tract_inf	Brazil
GaySex	chlamydia_infecti	Stress
SexualHealthHelp	influenza	Asthma in childhood
Thrushandcystitis	accidents	Enuresis
Preventingprostatecanc	body_mass	China
Flatulence	dizziness	Chickenpox
Practisingsafersex	diabetes	Abnormal heart rhythms
Injurytreatmentprincip	pregnancy_childbi	– atrial
		Abnormal heart rhythms
		– ventricular
Accounts for 7.9% of all information pages	Accounts for 16.1% of all information pages	Accounts for 26.3% of all information pages

* NHS pages viewed based on logs from the NHS DO site for October 2001.

The idea that people might be more willing to use DiTV to look for information which they did not want to discuss with other people was further examined in a questionnaire study of NHS Direct Digital DiTV users. Respondents were asked if respondents looked for information on their DiTV service that they did not want to discuss with their doctor.

A significant proportion, (27%), said that they would use the service to look for information that they would not want to discuss with their doctor; an indication that users were attracted to the service for its apparent anonymity and the low search-disclosure factor. Of course, we are talking here about self-disclosure, in that it says something about the willingness or otherwise of a person to talk about a private matter with their doctor. However, it also says something about the willingness of users to use on-line methods, in this case DiTV, to search for private information.

Conclusion

In conclusion there does seem to be a tendency for users to moderate their online search behaviours as a function of the anonymity afforded at the point of search and information consumption. Under the proposed search disclosure model, touchscreen kiosks were hypothesised to invoke different patterns of health topic search behaviour from either the Internet or DiTV because kiosks because they offered less search anonymity. There was evidence to support this: users were attracted to both an Internet and DiTV platform because of the privacy and anonymity that they offered. Differences were also found between work and home Internet content search behaviours.

Characteristics of information seeking behaviour in a digital environment

Provided with an unparalleled range of choice when it comes to digital health information and advice it is inevitable that people will behave in a different way than if they were offered a limited choice or no choice at all. The characteristic behaviour that arises as a result of being given digital choice is one of bouncing, in which users seldom penetrate a site to any depth, tend to visit a number of sites for any given information need and seldom return to sites they once visited. They tend to 'feed' for information horizontally, and whether they search a site of not depends heavily on 'digital visibility', which in turn creates the conditions for 'bouncing'. This phenomenon is investigated more detail and across services and platforms in this section.

Site penetration

A typical website, like that of a newspaper or health service, might contain hundreds, if not thousands, of pages. However, research shows that during a visit people are unlikely to view more than a very few of them. For example, during the 12-month period October 2001 to September 2002, SurgeryDoor health website was visited by 381,704 separate IP addresses and 3,680,453 pages were viewed (excluding declared robots). The log data show how much use has been made of the site, and the extent of site penetration. It also shows how active or busy (or, possibly, confused in the case of sessions where little is viewed) they were when online. Approximately three quarters of all visits featured three or fewer page views (and 43% viewed only one page), 20% saw between four to 10 pages, and 6% saw 10 pages. Of course, site architecture and the caching of pages to the user's machine create problems when it comes to estimating the number of pages viewed by a user on the Internet.

Figure 6.10 provides more detail on the brevity and shallowness of the user's visit for two health information websites, by showing how many of the pages viewed were actually information pages. It shows the distribution of pages viewed by single session one-page users only. What is of interest is whether users arrived at an information page. To determine this pages have been classified into three groups: an information page, a menu page and the home directory, or main menu. Users accessing only the latter two did not access any significant information from the site, other than the negative information (i.e. that from the menu lists, it is clear that the site was not relevant or useful to them). These users can be thought of as the stereotypical 'bouncers' – they have bounced in and out of the site without having accessed an information page.

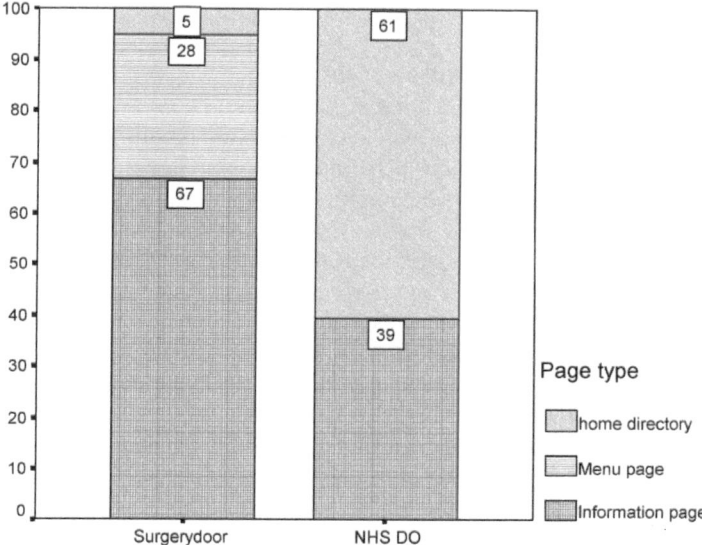

Figure 6.10 The distribution of pages viewed by single session one-page users only

Turning our attention more closely to these 'bouncers', 61% of NHS Direct single session one-page users (accounting for 8.5% of all session accesses) and 33% of SurgeryDoor users (13.9% of all session accesses) viewed the opening menu/home directory screen and left without accessing any further pages.

Clearly, there is a big difference between the two sites and the likely explanation is the 'digital visibility' of each service. For the web this visibility is partly defined by sites' 'visibility' on search engine directories such as Yahoo, and its positioning on the list of sites returned by search engines in response to a user entered search query. The NHS positioning on the returns was poor at the time of the study, as discovered by an examination of the referrer logs. It was found that nine of the top 20 search terms[4] used incorporated NHS in the search expression. This indicates that the most popular way of linking to the NHS Direct Online website via a search engine was by typing NHS as part or all of the search expression. In the main users did not find the NHS by typing in their medical condition/problem but found it by first realising that there was a NHS site. Hence, many users only found the site by including 'NHS' rather than a medical term within their search expression. Searchers who did not include NHS in their search expression were unlikely to be offered the NHS site within the first two or three pages of 'hits' returned by a search engine. Thus, fewer users arrived at the NHS site via a search engine since this was further down the returned search engine list. People used this list to bounce from site to site; hence NHS Direct Online attracted less bouncer hits compared to their commercial competitors (SurgeryDoor). Furthermore, when users arrived (those who included

---

4   The top 20 accounted for 60% of all terms used to find the main server site.

NHS in their search term) they were 'more' likely to arrive at a home directory page rather than a content page.

This was additionally confirmed as SurgeryDoor was proportionally found to have more users who accessed the Internet from home. These users are thought to be more likely to use an Internet IP service provider to find (health) sites. SurgeryDoor had more home users because the NHS Site had poor digital visibility on search engine returns and people use the list returned by search engines to bounce between sites. The NHS was just too far down that list for people to bounce between sites.

One implication of the bouncing/flicking kind of information seeking behaviour is that the home and individual page landed at play a very important role and are crucial as to whether or not someone decides to go on and view pages within the site or not. We have some research to show how important this is. Again, it all relates to digital visibility. While evaluating the logs of the NHS Direct Digital health channel on Kingston Interactive Television it became clear that the channel was losing viewers over the four-month study period. Furthermore, the decline was not gradual, but was characterised by a number of big and abrupt falls coinciding with a number of changes to its positioning on the KIT service. At each change the service became more remote from the home page and consequently less visible. It transpired that the major impact was on new customers. New users were not coming through because of the increasing difficulty of finding the service. However, those people who had found the service when it was in a more visible location showed their tenacity by making more extensive use of the channel when they arrived.

Considering the evidence the positioning of services within an electronic environment, be they pages on the web, DiTV channels or on stand-alone computer terminals, is a vital component of usage. Content may still be king – but if that content cannot be accessed its quality, relevance and presentation are as good as wasted.

Promiscuity

Promiscuity results from consumers being provided with good access and wide choice. In information seeking terms it manifests itself in two ways. Firstly, people visit a (large) number of sites to find what they want. Secondly, and this is related, they do not often return to sites they once visited.

An online questionnaire hosted on the SurgeryDoor website for the month of November 2000 was used to determine the number of health sites visited. In total 1068 users answered the questionnaire, which represented 5% of the 21,118 visitors (as denoted by unique IP addresses) to the site in November 2000. It showed that vast majority of people (71%) said they visited two or more sites, 29% visited three to five sites and 11% visited five or more. Clearly those who used just one site were heavily in the minority. And, of course, this is likely to be an underestimation of the number of sites visited, as users were unlikely to remember sites, which they do not find useful or visited long ago and since have not returned.

A questionnaire study of health channel (NHS Direct Digital) viewers on the Kingston Interactive Television Service pointed to the general information seeking behaviour that results in people searching a number of sites in pursuit of information.

Viewers of the service were asked their reasons for using it. Browsing for health information proved by far to be the most popular reason over two thirds (68%) of users reported browsing as a reason for use (Figure 6.11).

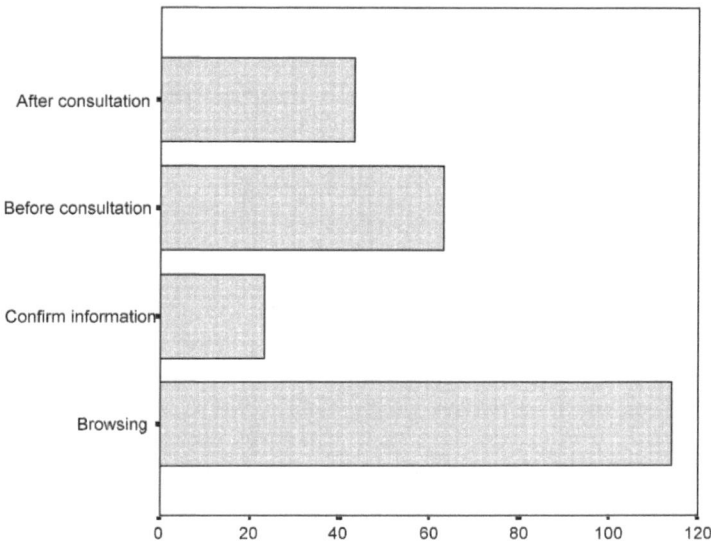

Figure 6.11 For what purpose did you use the service?

This result was further backed-up by a study of users of a digital interactive television programme on pregnancy, called Bush babies, on the Channel Health service on Sky TV. Sixty-eight percent of Bush Babies respondents had just found it by browsing while 14% saw an on screen promotion, and about 5% saw an advertisement.

There is evidence from the SurgeryDoor study to indicate that the younger the user the more likely they were to exhibit promiscuous information seeking behaviour. Forty-six percent of those aged under 34 visited three or more sites compare to 41% of those aged 35 to 54 and 22% of those aged 55 and over. Those aged 55 and over were more likely to visit just one site.

The same survey provides another explanation of why so many sites were being visited. Respondents were asked to rate SurgeryDoor in regard to breadth and depth of content and trust in the information. The number of health sites visited was found to be correlated to a scoring over the three attributes derived by factor analysis. Importantly, a relationship was found between the respondent's score in regard to content and the number of health sites visited. As the number of health websites visited increased so the user's rating of content depth, breadth and trust declined. This suggests that users who visit a number of sites were not as worried about content attributes of an individual site as these attributes were maximised by visiting a number of sites. Alternatively, they realised that all sites lacked the content attributes they required and that content attributes can only be maximised by visiting many sites. What we might be witnessing is the kind of remote-flicking channel behaviour that children exhibit while watching television.

By comparing information seeking behaviour on different digital platforms we can get some further insights into promiscuity. Here we take the case of health information channels on digital interactive television, where there is not so much choice and for which there are no search engines to stimulate bouncing. Instead users are forced to move around pre-selected menus and individual pages. In such circumstances, the question that needs to be posed is whether a frenetic form of behaviour still manifests itself. In other words, would DiTV users flick between pages in way that Internet users flick between Internet sites? Research showed that, indeed, this was the case. Thirty-three percent of DiTV users viewed 21 pages or more in a search session and 50% viewed 11 pages or more. This is high volume use and is far in excess of that expected (compared to other platforms) and users must be viewing more pages than they necessarily need in order to discover what they need.

Coming back to a site constitutes conscious and directed use – as good an approximation of this as you are likely to get from web logs. A service with a high percentage of returnees can be regarded as having a 'brand' following, the goal of all service providers. This makes return visits a powerful performance – and, possibly, quality – indicator. The industry calls this 'site stickiness'. Loyalty or repeat behaviour, however appears not to be a trait of the digital information consumer. A study of the SurgeryDoor website (Nicholas *et al*, 2003c), which allowed for the workings of proxy servers and floating IP addresses, found that over a relatively long period of 12 month two-thirds of visitors never returned, with 33% visiting the site two to five times. Plainly it is difficult to develop repeat behaviour in these circumstances.

Conclusion

It would be useful to try and explain the kind of information seeking behaviour that has been sketched above. As already suggested, what we are probably seeing is what happens when people are presented with massive and increasing choice, which they have to make themselves, and quickly. The traditional library-driven user of the not so distant past relied on the library for (limited) choice, and for a stamp of quality or authority. The assumption was that if it was in the library it was good and, anyway, the choice was largely made for the consumer because the intermediary conducted the search. Today most people search for themselves, often from non-library or evaluated information environments, most obviously seen in the health field. In consequence they are forced to make the evaluations once made by librarians, and with so much choice and new products coming on stream, they have to make many, many evaluations. They generally do this with the help of a search engine, on the basis of long-experience with searching the web, practice in making constant comparisons and a process of trial and error. The phrase 'we are all librarians now' is a particularly apt one.

It appears to be common knowledge that this has happened, but few previously have accrued the data to show what has actually occurred as a result, and the logs and associated questionnaires show us clearly. People's information seeking behaviour in these circumstances can best described from the logs as one of flicking, bouncing or surfing. These people can also be viewed as consumer 'checkers' or 'evaluators'. Evaluation is largely undertaken by making comparisons, and is a key element of digital literacy. To stay afloat in the ever-expanding digital environment you need to evaluate, and evaluate well. Web provides huge opportunity to suck it and see and this of course is a form of evaluation. Evaluation is not only made on the basis of content, but also on the basis of authority, access, design, currency and interactivity, to name only the most important.

Information professionals viewing such behaviour should not be mislead into believing that this is a dumbed-down form of information searching and retrieval – that people cannot make up their minds or that they are obtaining just a thin veneer of information. One is minded of the father watching his young daughter who is using the remote to flick from one television channel to another. A slightly irritated father asks his daughter why she cannot make up her mind and she answers that she is not attempting to do so, but is watching all the channels. She, like our bouncers, is gathering information horizontally, not vertically. The single authoritative source, which is always consulted and deeply mined, seems to be a thing of the past. Loyalty might be a thing of the past.

Characterising users according to types of health information sources used/ preferred

This section sets out to identify information user groups, based on the preferences for information sources derived from a questionnaire of Telewest DiTV respondents. Although, clearly, this study only considered users of a cable network it asked them about all the sources they used. Thus it identifies groups beyond the DiTV health environment.

Figure 6.12 ranks health information sources by their importance to Telewest viewers. The two most important sources of information were plainly oral – their own doctor and the practice nurse. Seventy-nine percent said that their doctor was a very important source for health information. The NHS Direct telephone line and friends and family were also important, and, respectively, 37% and 26% said these were very important sources. Perhaps, surprisingly for digital TV owners, who might be expected both to be high consumers of digital (i.e. electronic) information, and had the means to afford Internet access, the web was the least important source of information. Fifty eight percent of users cited this source as either not at all important or not very important. A relatively large percentage of respondents did cite television and Telewest in particular as a source of health information. While only 16% cited television as very important, a significant 53% cited it as fairly important. Telewest was cited by 28% as a very important health information source (the NHS Direct Digital service) and by 48% as a fairly important source – and this is barely three months after the introduction of the service, but, clearly, very much to the front of people's thoughts.

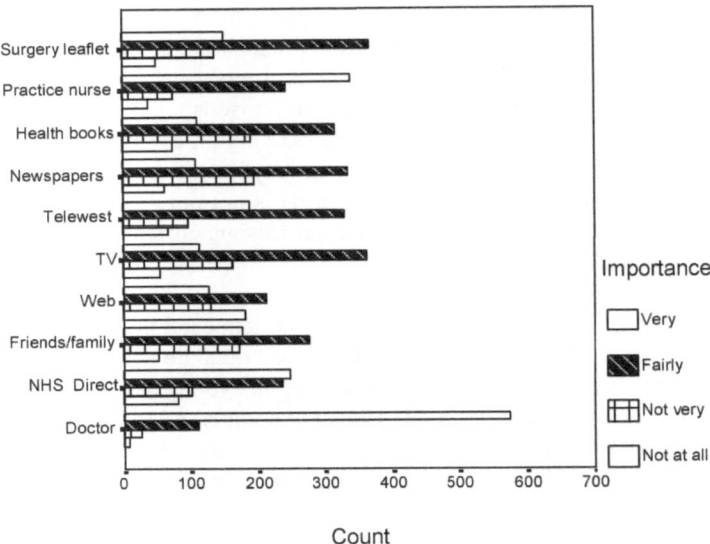

Count

Figure 6.12 Telewest viewers – importance of various sources of
health information

It was decided to see whether respondents could be grouped by their rating of health information sources. Respondents had the option to say how important each of ten information sources were. By using factor analysis the combination of sources used could be defined. Factor analysis identifies groupings of variables. Variables within the group are highly correlated while the resulting combinations are un-correlated and independent. The procedure identified four groups according to their selection of information sources. The four combinations accounted for 52% of the variance (Table 6.8) hence the groupings cover about half the respondents and about half do not fit so well in these four groups. The results should be read within context of the profile of users using each of the platforms.

Group one can be described as being formed by those people obtaining health information from traditional media sources – mainly from health books (.680) and publications (.675) but also from television (.450). They rely on traditional sources, but actively seek information, and so can be personified as 'Active traditional information users'. Group two people rely much more on in-house sources – leaflets in the doctor's surgery (.627), and oral information from the practice nurse (.663) or doctor (.491) for health information. They are also users of traditional sources, but they did not actively seek health information but let health professionals feed them with it. We have labelled them 'Passive traditional information seekers'. Group three people use 'electronic information' and identify themselves by their use of Telewest and Living Health (.830) and the NHS Direct telephone line (.527), and also, but to a lesser extent, television (.380), for health information. These people can be called 'Active new information users'. They use electronic sources, but not in a social way. The last group consists of a quite different kind of electronic user. These people use the web (.392) but also rely on friends and family (.561) and can be termed 'web opinion communicators'. They form opinions about health, albeit about alternative health, and they are active communicating and discussing these opinions.

Table 6.8 Types of user identified by information sources used

	Group 1: Active Traditional information users	Group 2: Passive traditional information users	Group 3: Active new information system users	Group 4: Web opinion communicators
Surgery leaflet	-	.627	-	-
Practice nurse	-	.663	-	-
Health books	.680	-	-	-
Papers/magazines	.675	-	-	-
Telewest/Living Health	-	-	.830	-
TV	.450	-	.380	-
Web	-	-	-	.392
Friends & Family	-	-	-	.561
NHS Direct	-	-	.527	-
Doctor	-	.491	-	-

* Principal axis factoring, Varimax rotation, KMO=0.85. Factor scores 0.4 and greater are given.

The factor analysis generates values for each respondent based on their combined use of information sources. We have identified four combinations or information types. A high value score on a combination identifies that that respondent is likely to use a particular combination of information sources and hence is a particular type of user. By using the scores as the dependent term in a multiple linear regression model we can then see what characteristics of the user, if any, were likely to identify that type of information source used. Table 6.9 reports the results of four regression models.

Table 6.9 presents the results of four regression models corresponding to the four identified information types: the active traditional information user; the passive traditional user; active new information system users and lastly web opinion communicators. The characteristics of users are given on the left and the significant coefficients, related to each type of information user, are given in the table. Four types of user characteristics were included, those related to the users (gender, age, visits to the doctor), the household area in which they lived, (incidence of high earners in the area, microwave ownership etc), their health topic interest and other details, for example, if the user was responsible for the health of another. This does not represent all the characteristics that are likely to determine information type, for example there is no variable covering educational qualification of user. Furthermore, household area information related by post code details only gives approximate figures for the area. However, it was felt that the data does give an indication of the likely characteristics of each information user type. The following looks at the significant characteristics of each type of information user.

Table 6.9 Regression Models: identifying possible identifiers of information user types

	Information types			
	Group 1: Active Traditional information users	Group 2: Passive traditional information users	Group 3: Active new information system users	Group 4: Web opinion communicators
Age	-0.40*** (0.09)	-	-	-0.09*** (0.02)
Gender	-	-	-0.19* (0.8)	0.10+ (.06)
Interest in Health info.	-0.21** (0.07)	-	-0.65*** (0.18)	-
Interest in Medical news	0.29*** (0.06)	-	0.14* (0.06)	-
Interest in Alternative health	0.19***(0.06)	-	-	-
Interest in Treatments	-	0.11+ (0.06)	-	-
Interest in General Health	-	0.31*** (0.07)	-	0.09+ (0.06)
Interest in Complementary Medicine	-	0.12* (0.06)	-	0.15*** (0.04)
Interest in Diet	0.10+ (0.06)	-0.12+ (0.06)	-	-
Interest in Health responsibility for another	-	-	0.27** (0.10)	-
Interest in Prescription Drugs	-	-	0.12** (0.05)	-0.13*** (0.04)
A particular condition	-	-	0.21** (0.06)	-
How often have you visited the doctor	-	0.17** (0.06)	-	-
Watches ITV	-	-	0.17*** (0.05)	-
Earning 20,000+	-	-0.10* (0.04)	-	-
Incidence of Microwave ownership	-	-	-	0.19** (.07)
R (R2)	0.52 (0.27)	0.39 (0.14)	0.45 (0.20)	0.41 (0.17)

Levels of Significance (t-test statistic): + P<0.10, *P<0.05, ** p<0.01, *** p<0.001.

Active Traditional information user

This user seeks health information but tends to use traditional sources such as health books, newspapers and the television. The regression co-efficient for age (-.40) and a general interest in health information (-.21) were negative, suggesting that this type of user was, surprisingly, young (one might have expected younger people to use electronic sources to a greater extent) and did not have an interest in health information. Furthermore, coefficients were positive suggesting that these users had an interest in medical news (.29), dieting (.10) and alternative health topics (.19). This combination suggests a person who has an interest in being healthy and who keeps up to date with health topics by reading traditional media. They probably feel that their current sources meet their needs and that they have sufficient information and hence they do not need to search electronic sources such as DiTV or the web, although they are freely available to them.

Passive traditional information user

These users are likely to rely on health professionals and information in their doctor's surgery for their health information. They tend to be less well off and were likely to earn less than £20,000 (-.10). Furthermore, they were not interested in dieting (-.12), and may be unwell or have children as they were more regular visitors to the doctor (.17) and expressed an interest in both treatment (.11) and general health (.31). These people may not be active readers of traditional media that include health information, but have not as yet taken up digital sources – although, by definition, they plainly have access to digital TV health information. However, they recognised the importance of health information but relied on the doctor and surgery environment for this. There was some evidence (see below) that these users were more likely to be women under the age of 55. The income variable may also be an indication of an educational variable and these users may be slow to take up health information. The fact though that they were regular surgery visitors suggested that these users could be encouraged to take up such services at this point. These people may well benefit the most by being exposed to better health information. There is some evidence in our data that passive traditional information users are drawn from lower income groups (less than £20,000).

Active new information system users

These people use electronic health information sources they use their television – especially digital television, and the NHS Direct telephone line as health information sources. The variables identified as possible explanatory characteristics were that the user is more likely to be male (-.19); may have a health responsibility for another (.27); an interest in health information (.65) and in a particular condition (.21), medical news (.14) and prescription drugs (.12); and a high incidence of watching ITV (.17). This pointed to a user who is possible male or who has a minor long-term condition and who has recognised the importance of health information. Their interest in prescription drugs, a particular condition and medical news suggests that they have more than a general or passing interest in health topics. The high use of ITV suggests a high degree of TV watching and channel investigation and they may well have found the digital DiTV health service, Living Health, by surfing the channels. These users were already interested in accessing health information and had actively taken up the DiTV service as a source of information and are benefiting from the service.

Web opinion communicators

The fourth group also used electronic sources but the web rather than DiTV, and further communicated with friends and family about their health information. The variables identified as being important to this group were: that users were likely to be aged 35 and under (-.09), were more likely to be female (.10), were likely to have an interest in general health (.09) and complementary medicine (.15) but had a low interest in prescription drugs (.13) and had a higher incidence of microwave ownership (.19). These users gained an interest in health information via complementary medicine and currently were ambivalent towards tradition drug based treatments. Hence they are likely to be quite opinionated about this. They were young and possible regarded this interest as fashionable. These views were likely, however, to change as they get older when they perhaps have more contact with health services. Their current interest in complementary medicine was fuelling and engaging their interest in health information.

Focus on age and gender

Banks (2001) cites research indicating that men do not go early enough to the doctor, avoid the doctor altogether and are generally reluctant to talk about health. In fact, according to our research, men appear to come late to digital health information, but do use it. The study of the users of the Living Health and NHS Direct online showed that there is a relationship between use and age and gender. A higher proportion of younger respondents tended to be women while older respondents tended to be male and this is true for both DiTV and for the web based health information sources. For example, just below two-thirds of respondents between 16 and 55 were women, however, only about a quarter of respondents were female in the 56 to 75 age group. These data fit with results from other research by the present writers (Nicholas *et al*, 2001a), which showed that older health information kiosk users tended to be male, and younger ones female.

The breakdown of age and gender relationship across the four types of information users identified showed that women under the age of 55 scored particularly highly in both acquiring health information from traditional media sources with men registering low scores. Traditional media sources might not offer sufficient detailed information and hence may well be not particularly useful and this might explain the particularly low score by the over 55's, males and females.

Young men aged 35 and under in particular appeared, from their low scores, not to acquire information from a surgery environment (doctor, practice nurse, surgery leaflet etc.). In fact, men of all age groups performed badly at acquiring health information from this source. However, later in life men do make more use of this information source– possibly forced to by circumstances. Women under the age of 55 performed well at acquiring information from this source.

Men over the age of 35 were more likely than younger men to acquire health information, either from the DiTV or the NHS Direct telephone line. This was particularly true for men over the age of 55 who scored particularly high in this regard. In age groups, 36 to 55 and 56 and over, men were heavier users of health information compared to women. Though men 35 and under performed poorly. All this points to a real take up of health information by men 36 and over and suggests that these digital sources were particularly effective in targeting men.

There is some evidence that men aged 35 and under will use the web and family/friends to acquire health information. However, women in this age group tended to be far keener users of this type of information source. However, given the apparent unwillingness of men in this age group to acquire information from either DiTV sources or the surgery environment, the use of health web information was promising. The apparent low take up of health information by older users may reflect poor access to web-based technology at home and problems with using the technology.

Conclusions

The two most important sources of information for respondents were their own doctor and the practice nurse. Seventy-nine percent of users said that their doctor was a very important source for health information. Four groups of people were identified on the basis of their health information sources: the passive traditional media users, who do not actively seek health information but let health professionals feed them with it; active new information system users, who used electronic DiTV and NHS Direct telephone sources, but not in a very sociable way; and, finally, the web opinion communicators who search the web but also rely on friends and family for information. These four groups account for about half the variance of the data hence the study gives an additional view on potential user types however it should not be read as giving definitive groupings. About half of users do not fit well in these four groups.

There is some evidence that links can be made between these groups and personal characteristics. A tentative linkage, from the evidence presented in this study, is that:

- The active traditional media information user is young, interested in diets, and feel they are up to date with general health issues, and probably do not have any specific or pressing health information needs. They may not be currently using new digital sources for health.
- The passive traditional user is economically disadvantaged, unaware of other information sources but has an identified need for health information. They are currently more likely to visit the surgery for health information.
- Active new information system users, who are more likely to be men or have an identified health condition. Television maybe a focal point for this type of user and their interest in both health information and TV as led them to find and use the Living health service on DiTV.

- Web opinion communicators are younger people, interested in general health, more likely to be women, and have developed an interest in general health via an interest in complementary medicine. They are fuelling this interest by talking to friends and family and by looking on the Internet.

Chapter 7

Barriers and Inequalities

One of the UK Government's main concerns was to reduce the barriers and inequalities associated with health provision and there was a feeling amongst their health policy makers that digital information services might help to reduce the barriers and inequalities. We wished to determine whether there was any evidence to indicate this was happening. In this respect we needed to discover: 1) what were the barriers to the general public accessing electronic health information systems, and how they could be overcome; 2) whether health inequalities actually arose as a result of widespread digital information provision. In the case of barriers, this was especially important as the target audience – the nation – would inevitably include many groups and communities who had little or no familiarity with digital information services of any kind, never mind employing them to directly help with their health, and there were plainly big dangers in second guessing their difficulties. In the case of inequalities there was a danger that in the attempt to minimise inequalities through the widespread provision of health information, the very opposite would occur with the information rich becoming even richer and the information poor, poorer.

Barriers

Firstly, there were the information seeking barriers created by the digital platforms themselves, and in this respect we have already identified the problems caused by 'search disclosure' and 'digital visibility', so we shall only briefly go over these two barriers. Secondly, there were the human barriers, which included cultural factors, confidence or proficiency with ICT, mis-conceptions about the services and systems, and lack of engagement by health professionals.

Search disclosure

'Search disclosure' describes what appears to be a major barrier to using health information systems in public places, and especially where the potential user might come into contact with people they know. Investigations have shown that different patterns of use were exhibited depending on both location types (medical/non-medical; public/private), and that kiosks performed poorly in doctors' surgeries. This points to a reluctance to use such a system in the glare of other patients -often a substantial number – in a waiting room or, indeed, even in the less confined space of a supermarket or pharmacy. 'Search disclosure' suggests that instead of simply replicating the same content and uploading it onto each platform (in other words just broadcasting it), it may be advisable to tailor content to specific circumstances.

Having, perhaps, less – but more focused – information on the system may make it more navigable, and avoid the problem of users inadvertently accessing a page about, for example, sexual disease, whilst in a supermarket where passers-by may be able to see them. Kiosks in public places could either restrict themselves to more general health information or, at least, have information about sensitive topics more deeply buried in the menu hierarchy – although this may lead to the problems of digital visibility mentioned below.

The phenomenon of 'search disclosure' strongly suggests that health information may be more effectively delivered via a system available in one's own home – DiTV or the Internet, for example. It could be argued that, therefore, material one might prefer not to access in a public place could be deposited on this medium. However further research is needed to investigate the problems related of children's access of this material.

Digital visibility

Digital visibility – the positioning of digital information so it can be easily and quickly spotted – has been shown to be a significant factor in accessing particular health pages and services. When the link to a health information service on a DiTV system was moved further down the hierarchy – in other words, when more links had to be activated in order to access it – use dropped significantly. Also, more than one third of kiosk users appeared to have failed to arrive at an information page, because of the (numerous) levels it is necessary to negotiate. The use of several hierarchical levels, then, represents a barrier to information access it may be difficult to overcome where digital services are very comprehensive or encyclopaedic in nature. People will, of course, use what information they can see, rather than what they need, and this has enormous implications for health professionals, as well as for the users themselves.

Following on from this, the Government seems to be right to consider kiosk locations such as supermarkets and libraries, where members of the public can access health information both anonymously and without the need to seek a medical appointment. This raises questions about the purpose of kiosks, and whether the menu structure should be tailored differently for the various locations. In a medical setting they might be regarded as an adjunct to a consultation with the doctor, in which case they might be utilised by staff in tandem with patients and with a menu structure to reflect this. In non-medical locations, the role would be more that of an alternative to or substitute for an appointment – again pointing to a possible variation in content and again the menu structure should offer easy access to such information.

There are, of course, pedagogical barriers with regard to the provision of health information – be it in electronic or hardcopy form. Interviews with medical professionals indicated that they often make judgements about patients' competencies to understand and handle information. This leads to the professionals' differential actions with regard to information provision and recommendation. We have argued in this book that, as people have such varied information needs, and abilities to comprehend information, it may be advisable to provide 'vertical' layers of pages. These would offer information on each topic at different depths or levels of detail, in addition to the 'lateral' arrangement of material organised by topic. This same solution should apply also to people with different reading and reading comprehension levels. Clearly, the designers of any system which did this would have to be cognisant of digital visibility issues, and consider how the information could be displayed in the fewest hierarchical levels, perhaps with the informational levels 'side-by-side' on the menu option e.g. 'treatment of kidney disease: basic information; more detailed information; advanced information' – where each option was an active link.

Cultural barriers

Cultural barrier factors related to the use of electronic health systems also apply to information produced in any format. Principal amongst these factors is the view that the health professional is the keeper of information, and tells patients all they need to know. Significantly, patients who adopted this view – predominantly, but not exclusively, the elderly and lower socio economically grouped women – appeared to be happy to simply absorb information related to them by their GP or nurse. A second cultural factor also prevalent amongst elderly and lower socio economic patients was a reluctance to personally seek information simply because it has not been a practice or habit, in any sphere. The trend towards digital; information-seeking, stimulated by the explosion in amount of information available, has not affected everyone, and a major task facing health professionals is how to engage patients in this respect.

Low confidence and proficiency with ICT

Confidence with, and a (perceived) lack of competence, in using information technology presented a greater barrier for kiosk users and to a certain extent Internet users. Only DiTV users were found to engage with the system with little or no problems. This barrier may, in part in the case of kiosks, be addressed by the active engagement of health professionals in showing patients the system and helping them understand how to use it. However, it has to be said such help was generally missing from the environments investigated. The problem also shows, once again, the importance of channelling information to people's own homes, on a DiTV environment. Users appear to have generally a higher confidence level engaging with this platform as a result of previous experiment with and learned skills in navigating and retrieving information.

Public's misconceptions about nature of digital services

Another barrier, related to the lack of engagement by health professionals, is that of misconceptions about the nature of the service. Findings showed that many people in the health environment where a touchscreen kiosk was located either simply did not notice it; thought it was for a professional user group, or had other misconceptions. Essential, therefore, is the need – wherever the location – to advertise the presence, purpose and availability of the kiosk. For Internet users misconceptions related to the abundance of both information and the number of competing health sites. This resulted in a questioning of the information.

It is worth considering multi-function kiosks in that the health-related information may be used if this is bundled in with information of other kinds – general community information for example. For one thing that way there would be more reason to use the kiosk system, and for another, people would be exposed to the possibility of accessing health information whilst undertaking other information retrieval tasks, and might do so spontaneously. However this must be balanced against the inevitable addition of hierarchical levels and increased complexity of the menu structure. The role of such kiosk needs further investigation.

Lack of interest/engagement by health staff

There was a marked reluctance on the part of doctors to engage with their patients with regard to the use of electronic health information systems – most specifically the touchscreen kiosk, and thus were not undertaking the positive engagement this book has highlighted as being so necessary. Indeed, our studies have shown that where doctors did engage, use of the system was higher. The instant seeking of professional help by the majority of patients interviewed for the study, and the continuing trust in their advice, appears to suggest that many would certainly use the information service if recommended by their GP. It would be even more effective for the doctor or nurse to actually use the kiosk with the patient although, of course, time constraints may preclude this. What may be possible instead would be for the doctor to be equipped with a CD-ROM version of the kiosk in the surgery which could be used either at the end of a consultation or actually as part of it. Patients might then see the benefits of the information and be encouraged to undertake independent use.

The findings have clear implications for the training of health professionals. Firstly, although nurses appeared to be very involved with patients' information needs, GPs were less so. With the burgeoning availability of information, and with a general acceptance that information can improve health, as emphasised most notably in the report by Wanless (2002) it is essential that medical staff really engage their patients, and include information as part of their consultations. Secondly, it appears inevitable that patients will shop around ever more for their information. We have described these information seekers as promiscuous users. It might be incumbent upon future health professionals to help patients understand how to evaluate different sources. Certainly, there seems to be already much more of a climate of negotiated care, and patients will be ever more informed by a wide variety of information sources.

Inequalities

Socio-economic factors, age, health/disabilities, education and ethnicity may all lead to inequalities.

Socio-economic inequalities

DiTV, appeared to be used by lower socio-economic groupings. For example, people from postcode areas with a low incidence of £20,000+ earners were about twice as likely to use the Living Health and NHS Direct Digital services, and those from middle and lower social classes were two to three times more likely to have viewed the programme Bush Babies on Channel Health. This does not hold for other platforms, however. There is suggestive evidence that the Internet was more likely to be used by educated and relatively well off groupings. In fact, the skills needed to manage and use health information on the Internet – evaluating information from a variety of disparate sources, navigating through a huge number of pages – suggest a more educated user. With regard to kiosk use, where a neighbourhood housing a kiosk had a high incidence of mortgages, generally there were a lower number of kiosk users; these users might well have had their own Internet access. Those high income users that did use the service knew how to use it as session time was longer in areas where average earnings were above £20,000, indicating a more profitable use.

Age

Elderly people have been shown to be low Internet and kiosk users. Even when availing themselves of the opportunity to use systems, their usage was restricted – they viewed fewer web sources of health information and opened fewer kiosk pages. The latter is of some cause for concern because many elderly people clearly did not reach an information page. Questionnaire returns suggested that elderly people did not consider themselves to be competent in using new technology, and this impacted on their use of both kiosks and DiTV. For example, older NHS Direct Digital users, particularly women aged over 55, said in questionnaire returns that they found the service difficult to use, however the percentages saying this were a lot smaller compared to those older users using the kiosk.

There were other factors exacerbating age inequalities. A reluctance to obtain and use information from any sort was found, both from interviews with elderly people and from health professionals who dealt with them. This appeared to be partly because they were not used to living in an 'information age', in which it was common for younger people to seek out their own information. This was partly due to deference to their GPs, and partly due to a kind of fatalism with regard to the technology.

Finally, with regard to the elderly, there was some evidence that 'search disclosure' factors came into play to a greater extent than with younger people. Older respondents were more likely to say that they did not like using the kiosk in public place: 56% of over 55 year olds in a questionnaire agreed this was a factor in their non-use, as compared to 32% of those non-users aged 35 and under. However the over 55's might well have more serious health conditions.

Health/disabilities

There is suggestive evidence that a person's health status created inequalities, with concerns expressed by health professionals that kiosks built for 'standing' use did not serve people who may be too frail to stand for the period of time necessary to profitably use the kiosk (as might well occur in medical locations). Wheelchair-bound patients would also be debarred, and there is no provision currently for those with visual impairments (i.e. audio-pages or screen readers). Web-enabled kiosks, perhaps, discriminate even more against this group, as the websites to which they give access cannot be reconfigured, as they can on a dedicated terminal, for large font size. The main contents list on InTouch with Health's own website (SurgeryDoor), shown to be too small for some users in a usability study, appears even smaller on the web-kiosk. The kiosk was not usable by people with other physical disabilities either. Unlike computer 'mice', which can be adapted for disabled use, the touchscreen mechanism does not appear to readily lend itself to suitable modification for disabled people.

Education

Health professionals were concerned that many patients were unable to understand information relating to their condition. At one fieldwork site nurses who made a point of referring patients to the kiosk declined to do so in cases where they felt that the information would be too difficult to understand. They included native English speakers in their health information 'rationing'.

   Also related to education is ICT competence. A, perhaps, surprising degree of antipathy towards computers was shown and not only by elderly respondents. Forty two percent of kiosk respondents said that they actually avoided computers. Those who used and felt comfortable with ICT were more likely to have used a kiosk: 21% of these computer literate users had done so compared to 6% of users who avoided computers.

   There was evidence that successful use of the Internet for health information required an approximate graduate level of education. The skills needed to manage and use health information on the Internet include the evaluation of an array of sources, and to extract information from lengthy hit-lists. Users need to navigate within sites, navigate between sites using a search engine and to critically contrast and compare information.

Ethnicity

Research at a kiosk site with a high ethnic patient group elicited some differences between UK and non-UK born users. Only 12% of the former, between 16 to 35 years of age, reported the system not easy to use, whereas 44% of non-UK born users did so. Focus group interviews with regard to a DiTV video-on-demand service revealed a reluctance of ethnic males to seek health information, for fear of appearing vulnerable.

Conclusion

There is a good deal of evidence to support the belief that the best platform for delivering health information to the population at large is DiTV, as it appears to reach a broader audience. The application of DiTV for delivery of health information should be easier in the near future as in September 2005, the British Government confirmed that digital switchover will take place between 2008 and 2012. This means that by 2012 the analogue terrestrial transmissions network will be entirely switched off will be replaced with all-digital terrestrial network.[1] DiTV is followed by the Internet, excellent for the expert patient, and then – some way behind – kiosks, embellished with local content.

We have a number of recommendations in regard to inequalities and barriers:

- Kiosks should be targeted at locations with low ratios of owner- occupiers in the population, and in areas poorly served by either the Internet or DiTV. Information centres, libraries and surgeries, within the designated information areas, are the preferred locations.
- Installed kiosks should be backed up with adequate marketing and integrated to local health routines and procedures. Without this kiosks in surgeries are very ineffective.
- The menu structure and content of the kiosks should be customised to reflect the specific information needs of users at kiosk locations. Kiosks, are unusual in that they can be firmly linked to a community and as a result customisation can proceed more effectively.
- Research to investigate multi subject kiosks (i.e. such as those containing community information) and the role and impact of kiosk menu structure.
- Health professionals need to work in tandem with users with regard to the meeting of their information needs, and be aware of the information available on NHS Direct Online that can help particular patients. Perhaps one way to foster a patient and profession partnership in the digital environment would be a pilot scheme specifically targeting the development of an email facility between professionals and those patients aged over 60.
- With patient self-help groups so successful and popular, NHS Direct Online should move to hosting links and references related to support groups.
- NHS Direct Online should approve and acknowledge the role played by other health information sites by listing these on the 'home page' of its site, as it does for individual topics. This is based on the argument that users – the end-user checkers – generally do this anyway so it is advisable to attempt to influence this form of information seeking behaviour for the better.
- DiTV health services must learn the lessons taught to us by digital visibility, and should be piloted in their development by continuous deep log analysis to make sure the system is ever alert to the dynamic behaviour of the digital health consumer. In particular, care needs to be taken with regard to the positioning of services and nomenclature. Using terms derived from the Internet 'Home

---

1   http://www.digitaltelevision.gov.uk/.

page' etc.) may not be appropriate in the short term, where a significant proportion of DiTV users may not have experience with the Internet.

- A review of the use of video information on digital platforms is needed, especially as the new NHS Online Digital Television service has chosen not to host them.

Chapter 8

Conclusions

Overall, three digital health platforms and ten major health services were evaluated in considerable detail. As a consequence the online behaviour of about 868,500 digital health consumers, who made 8,531,000 views to digital health related pages of various kinds, were put under the microscope. In addition 18 questionnaire surveys were undertaken, canvassing the views of a total of 10,413 users and non-users and, finally, just over 350 people participated in formal or informal interviews, or focus group discussions. Another 350 were observed in kiosk locations, using, looking at or, frankly, ignoring kiosks. We can truly say that this has been the biggest evaluation of the health information consumer ever, digital or otherwise. A massive evidence base has been accumulated to provide policy makers and health professionals with the information they need to help them develop effective services and help keep in track those that are already running.

The assemblage of such a vast bank of robust evidence, replacing anecdote, hype, and the wisdom of PowerPoint presentations is the study's major achievement. Another major achievement has been the development of a methodology that enables health information managers and policy makers (not just researchers) to keep close track on the progress of digital health platforms and services, and, importantly, from a consumer's perspective. Much innovative methodological work has been undertaken, positioning the health field at the forefront of digital service evaluation, and only some of it has been demonstrated in the book itself because of size constraints. Those who are practically interested in deep log analysis methodology can find more details in Nicholas *et al* (2000).

Undoubtedly one of the most important findings has been the extent to which the various digital information platforms and services differed in terms of the kind of use they attracted, the people who used them and the purposes to which they were put. Any strategy for providing the general public with digital health information must take cognisance of this. It is certainly not a case of one size fits for all.

The kiosk strand of the study enabled comparisons to be made between the same digital health information service in a number of different environments – geographical and institutional, for instance. Thus usage comparisons have been made, for instance, between Penzance and Oxford and surgeries and supermarkets. In regard to the latter the book is probably the first of its kind to examine in detail, and on a national scale, usage of health information systems outside of health environments, which is increasingly where the public get there health information from these days, and as our findings show there is a large variation in behavioural patterns and types of user.

And then there were the surprises, an inevitable outcome of rolling a digital service out to a huge, relatively unknown and unsuspecting audience. This, of course, underlines the need for ongoing evaluations of the kind undertaken here; the kind of evaluation that checks what people actually do before drawing up questions on why they did so or what they thought of it; informed questioning, if you like. The biggest surprise of all was surely the very high take-up of the health kiosks by children, for a whole range of reasons (good and bad, it must be added). But not far behind must be the huge impact that positioning of data has on information seeking in the digital environment, the impact of where the consumer searches from on what they search (which we have called 'search disclosure'), and the lack of integration, of kiosks particularly, but all digital consumer platforms really into the routines of health practices and professionals (surely big opportunities are being lost here?)

Trust and authority are important issues in the health field. All platforms enjoyed a degree of trust and mistrust. What was most apparent was the way that users handled their mistrust on each platform. This was most apparent when comparing the Internet and DiTV. For DiTV users there was only one service and users looked for labels, such as the NHS label, to accredit the information found. This was not so true for the Internet. Users managed their trust of a health site by viewing and comparing information from a number of sites. For kiosk users trust maybe more related to the location of the kiosk. One reason why a Safeway kiosk might have double the blank sessions (those where only three pages or fewer were viewed) compared to, say, health information centres was that users were more likely to trust the kiosk content in a health environment and hence engaged more fully with the kiosk.

The role of kiosks in providing health information was limited by a relatively poor take-up amongst the general public (although aggregated data are more impressive) and the limited static menu and content. Kiosks were also associated with limited health outcomes. Kiosks in health settings were not really integrated into the routines of the surgery or hospital, and this must surely represent a big opportunity lost. Most of our findings relate to the use of the InTouch with Health standard kiosk, a kiosk that has been superseded by a web-enabled version and which looks much more promising on many fronts.

Internet users did use the platform for health information. Positive outcomes were associated with more experienced and educated use of the Internet. The Internet had particular problems around trust, authority, an ability to find sites and to critically review content that stems, in part, from the unorganised, but abundant, array of available information sites. However, health users utilised the Internet for a variety of services and purposes; many actively visited a number of health websites and participated in online activity such as support groups. There was evidence that some Internet health use related to personality and life style choice, such as that related to alternative medicine and to check on health information for a friend or relative. However, those currently suffering, those with a long term condition and those seeking general health information did use the Internet.

DiTV viewers used the platform for health information and this use was associated with positive outcomes. The extent of use maybe limited by the services menu prominence, other limiting features are the inability to print out information, something overlooked by system designers. The transactional services services explored the potential of DiTV as a two-way medium where the user becomes an information sender as well as receiver, and a dialogue established. Such applications represent more advanced forms of interactivity and require a different mindset on the part of users who engage in a customised activity geared to addressing their specific problems rather than ones of a more general nature. The applications tested in the pilot study included visual interpersonal communication with an NHS nurse, online appointments booking with one's GP, and the maintenance of personal medical details online, in this instance personal immunisation records. In addition, one consortium tested a small-scale email support service for a specific group – pregnant women.

Both the Internet and DiTV performed well according to all the use metrics. However, suggestive evidence indicated that these platforms target different types of users. DiTV appeared more likely to attract users from lower socio-economic groupings and those who did not like addressing diverse and, possibly conflicting, information sources (choice in these circumstances not being welcomed). Internet users appeared to be slightly more educated, come from a higher income group and seem to prefer to hunt or flick from one site to another viewing an amount of contradictory information as a consequence (they appear to revel in the choice available). These are, however tendencies, and both digital platforms were used by all income and socio-economic groups.

The take up of kiosks from the potential population has been comparatively poor: about 17% compared to about 30% for DiTV and the Internet. This is partly a result of poor prior experience with kiosks and ICT. In addition users shunned kiosks as they offered little in terms of privacy to the searcher ('search disclosure') compared to either DiTV or the Internet – something that has been shown to be very important.

Finally, despite the fact that much of the evidence provided in this book is the product of research investigations undertaken a few years ago, none of it has lost its potency or value. There are two reasons for this. Firstly, a project of this duration, depth and power is unlikely to be conducted ever again, or certainly not for many years. The evidence we have presented is the evidence we shall all have to work with for the next five years at the very least. This is because the project was born in the Department of Health at a time when there was the resource and willingness to conduct projects of this type, and on this scale. What is described here is the high watermark of digital health information consumer services, provided on a national scale. The money that funded this project over a period of nearly five years now funds research into the hospital super bug (MRSA) – something which currently has much more political capital than health information systems for the consumer. Secondly, all digital roll outs, whatever their nature or no matter their size, require benchmarking and this study clearly provides that, for all following studies. It also provides what is probably the key evaluation of the digital transition, that of the early leaders.

As a postscript there are no longer any NHS kiosks and the exciting digital health television services described in the book have been replaced by a television service that is noted for its mediocrity and anonymity. However, the other services continue to prosper.

Bibliography and Further Reading

Albert, T. and Chadwick, S. (1992), 'How readable are practice leaflets?', *British Medical Journal* 305, 1266-7.

Ankem, K. (2006), 'Factors influencing information needs among cancer patients: A meta-analysis', *Library and Information Science Research* 28:1, 7-23.

Arthur, A.M. (1995), 'Written patient information: a review of the literature', *Journal of Advanced Nursing* 21, 1081-6.

Bacon, E.S. (1999), *A description of an Internet self -help group for widows with dependent children*. Hampton University, 51p [Volume 37/05 of Masters Abstracts of Dissertations Abstracts International].

Baker, L., Wagner, T.H., Singer, S. and Bundorf, M.K. (2003), 'Use of the Internet and e-mail for health care information: results from a national survey', *The Journal of the American Medical Association* 289:18, 2400-6.

Balint, M., Hunt, J., Joyce, D., Marinker, M. and Woodstock, J. (1970), *Treatment or diagnosis: a study of repeat prescription in general practice* (London: Tavistock).

Banks, I. (2001), 'No man's land: men, illness, and the NHS', *British Medical Journal* 323, 1058-60.

Beresford, B. and Slopper, T. (2000), *The information needs of chronically ill or physically disabled children and adolescents* (York: York University, Social Policy Research Unit). <http://www.york.ac.uk/inst/spru/pubs/rworks/may2000.pdf> accessed 18 February 2004.

BHIA (British Healthcare Internet Association) (1996), Quality standards for medical publishing on the web. Online: <http://www.bhia.org/reference/documents/recommend_webquality.htm> accessed 18 February 2004.

Blake, M. (1998), 'Internet access for older people', *Aslib Proceedings* 50:10, 308-15.

BMA (British Medical Association) (2000), *Health Which? And NHS Direct - BMA Comment* (London: BMA Press) <http://web.bma.org.uk/pressrel.nsf/a4a6effeb2d171b8802568590051feb8/3b29a1270768f118802569350032e09c?OpenDocument> accessed 18 February 2004.

BMA (British Medical Association) (2001), *Crisis in Care: A GP Dossier: overworked family doctors speaking out for patients* (London: BMA).

Boudioni, M. (2003), 'Availability and use of information touchscreen kiosks (to facilitate social inclusion)', *Aslib Proceedings* 55:5/6, 320-33.

Bristol Inquiry Unit (2000), *The inquiry into the management of care of children receiving complex heart surgery at the Bristol Royal Infirmary Unit, Final Report*. Available at: <http://www.bristol-nquiry.org.uk/final_report/index.htm> accessed 18 February 2004.

Brooks, R.G. and Menachemi, N. (2006), 'Physicians' Use of Email With Patients: Factors Influencing Electronic Communication and Adherence to Best Practices', *Journal of Medical Internet Research* 8:1, e2 <http://www.jmir.org/2006/1/e2/> accessed 14 August 2006.

Brotherton, J.M., Clarke, S.J. and Quine, S. (2002), 'Use of the Internet by oncology patients: its effect on the doctor-patient relationship', *Medical Journal of Australia* 177:7, 395.

Car, J. and Sheikh, A. (2004), 'Email consultations in health care: 2—acceptability and safe application', *British Medical Journal* 329:7463, 439-42.

Carvel, J. (2000), 'Doctors attack 'consumerist' NHS initiatives', *The Guardian* 27.06.00, p.9.

Chapman, P. (1998), 'Developing "This Is The North East"' *Aslib Proceedings* 50:9, 255-63.

Chen, X. and Siu, L.L. (2001), 'Impact of the media and the Internet on oncology: survey of cancer patients and oncologists in Canada', *Journal of Clinical Oncology* 19:23, 4291-7.

Clark, M., Ghandour, G., Miller, N.H., Taylor, C.B., Bandura, A. and DeBusk, R.F. (1997), 'Development and evaluation of a computer-based system for dietary management of hyperlipidemia', *Journal of the American Dietetic Association* 97:2, 146-50.

Cline, R.J. and Haynes K.M. (2001), 'Consumer health information seeking on the Internet: the state of the art', *Health Education Research* 16:6, 671-92.

Coulter, A., Entwistle, V. and Gilbert, D. (1999), 'Sharing decisions with patients: is the information good enough?' *British Medical Journal* 318:7179, 318-22.

Cox, B. (2002), 'The impact of the Internet on the GP-patient relationship', *Informatics in Primary Care* 10:2, 95-9.

Craft, P.S., Burns, C.M., Smith, W.T. and Broom, D.H. (2005), 'Knowledge of treatment intent among patients with advanced cancer: a longitudinal study', *European Journal of Cancer Care*, 14:5, 417-25.

Cumbo, A., Agre, P., Dougherty, J., Callery, M., Tetzlaff, L., Pirone, J. and Tallia, R. (2002), 'Online cancer patient education: evaluating usability and content', *Cancer Practice* 10:3, 155-61.

Cummings, J.N., Sproull, L. and Kiesler, S.B. (2002), 'Beyond hearing: where real-world and online support meet', *Group Dynamics: Theory, Research and Practice* 6:1, 78-88.

Cyber Dialogue (2000), Cyber Dialogue releases Cybercitizen Health 2000 [press release]. Online: <http://www.cyberdialogue.com> accessed 18 February 2004.

Davison, K.P., Pennebaker, J.W. and Dickerson, S.S. (2000), 'Who talks? The social psychology of illness support groups', *American Psychologist* 55:2, 205-17.

Department of Health (1997), *The New NHS, Modern, Dependable, White Paper* (London: Department of Health).

Dervin, B. (1983), 'An overview of Sense-Making research: Concepts, methods and results to date', Paper presented at the *International Communication Association Annual Meeting, Dallas Texas May 26-30th*.

Dervin, B., Harpring, J. and Foreman-Wernet, L. (1999), 'In moments of concern: A Sense-Making study of pregnant, drug-addicted women and their information needs', *The Electronic Journal of Communication* 9: 2,3&4, (Private access URL available from Jayme Harpring at partners@nettally.com.

Ekman, A., Hall, P. and Litton, J. (2005), 'Can we trust cancer information on the Internet? – A comparison of interactive cancer risk sites', *Cancer Causes and Control* 16:6, 765-72.

Esquivel, A., Meric-Bernstam, F. and Bernstam, E.V. (2006), 'Accuracy and self correction of information received from an internet breast cancer list: content analysis', *British Medial Journal* 332:7547, 939-42.

Eysenbach, G. (2000), 'Towards ethical guidelines for dealing with unsolicited patient emails and giving teleadvice in the absence of a pre-existing patient-physician relationship - systematic review and expert survey', *Journal of Medical Internet Research* 2:1, e1. <http://www.jmir.org/2000/1/e1/> accessed 14 August 2006.

Eysenbach, G. and Diepgen, T.L. (1999), 'Patients looking for information on the Internet and seeking teleadvice: Motivation, expectations, and misconceptions as expressed in e-mails sent to physicians', *Archives of Dermatology* 135:2, 151-6.

Ferguson, T. (1997), 'Health care in cyberspace: patients lead a revolution', *The Futurist* 31:6, 29-33.

Ferguson, T. (2002), 'From patients to end users', *British Medical Journal* 324:555-6.

Ferriman, A. (2001), 'Poll shows public still has trust in doctors', *British Medical Journal* 322:7288, 694.

Finn J. (1999), 'An exploration of helping processes in an online self-help group focusing on issues of disability', *Health & Social Work* 24:3, 220-31.

Fox, S. and Rainie, L. (2000), 'The online health care revolution: how the Web helps Americans take better care of themselves'. Online: <http://www.pewinternet.org/reports/pdfs/PIP_Health_Report.pdf> accessed 18 February 2004.

Friedewald, V.E. Jr. (2000), 'The Internet's influence on the doctor-patient relationship', *Health Management Technology Online* 21:11, 79-80.

Gann, R. (1998), 'Empowering the patient and public through information technology' in Lenaghan (ed.), *Rethinking IT and Health* (London: Institute for Public Policy Research), 123-38.

Gann, R. and Sadler, M. (2001), 'Letter: Quality of information on NHS Direct Online' *British Medical Journal* 322:7279, 175.

Gillam, S. and Levenson, R. (1999), 'Editorial: Linkworkers in primary care: an untapped resource', *British Medical Journal* 319, 1215.

Goldsmith, D.M. and Safran, C. (1999), 'Using the web to reduce postoperative pain following ambulatory surgery', *Proceedings of the American Medical Informatics Association*, pp. 780-784.

Graber, M., Roller, C. and Kaeble, B. (1999), 'Readability levels of patient education material on the World Wide Web', *Journal of Family Practice* 48:1, 58-61.

Greenfield, S., Kaplan, S. and Ware, J.E. (1985), 'Expanding patient involvement in care: effects on patient outcomes', *Annals of Internal Medicine* 102:4, 520-8.

Greenfield, S., Kaplan, S.H., Ware, J.E., Yano, E.M. and Grank, H.J.L. (1988), 'Patients' participation in medical care: Effects on blood sugar control and quality of life in diabetes', *Journal of General Internal Medicine* 3:5, 448-57.

Griffin, J.P. and Griffin, J.R. (1996), 'Informing the patient', *Journal of the Royal College of Physicians*, 30:2, 107-11.

Griffiths, K.M. and Christensen, H. (2000), 'Quality of web-based information on treatment of depression: cross-sectional survey', *British Medical Journal* 321:7275, 1511-5.

Harrison, J. and Cooke, M. (2000), 'Study of early warning of accident and emergency departments by ambulance services', *Journal of Accident and Emergency Medicine* 16:5, 339-41.

Hart, A., Henwood, F. and Wyatt, S. (2004), 'The role of the Internet in patient-practitioner relationships: findings from a qualitative research study', Journal of Medical Internet Research 6:3, e36. <http://www.jmir.org/2004/3/e36/> accessed 4 September 2006.

Hernández-Borges, A.A. et al. (1999), 'Can Examination of WWW Usage Statistics and other Indirect Quality Indicators Help to Distinguish the Relative Quality of Medical websites?', *Journal of Medical Internet Research* 1:1, e1. <http://www.jmir.org/1999/1/e1/index.htm accessed 18 February 2004.

Hesse, B.W. et al. (2006), 'Trust and sources of health information: the impact of the internet and its implications for health care providers: findings from the first Health Information National Trends Survey', *Archive of Internal Medicine* 165:22, 2618–24.

Hjortdahl, P., Nylenna, M. and Aasland, O.G. (1999), '[Internet and the physician-patient relationship--from 'thank you' to 'why'?] Tidsskr Nor Laegeforen 119:29, 4339-4341. [Article in Norwegian - summary by PubMed at: <http://www.ncbi.nlm.nih.gov/entrez/query.fcgi?cmd=Retrieve&db=PubMed&list_uids=10667133&dopt=Abstract> accessed 18 February 2004.

HONF (Health on the Net Foundation) (1997), HON code of conduct for medical and health websites. <http://www.hon.ch/HONcode/Conduct.html> accessed 18 February 2004.

HONF (Health on the Net Foundation) (1999a), *HON's Fourth Survey on the Use of the Internet for Medical & Health Purposes* <http://www.hon.ch/Survey/ResumeApr99.html> accessed 18 February 2004.

HONF (Health on the Net Foundation) (1999b), *5th HON Survey on the Evolution of Internet Use for Health Purposes* <http://www.hon.ch/Survey/ResultsSummary_oct_nov99.html> accessed 18 February 2004.

HONF (Health on the Net Foundation) (2001), *Survey: Evolution of Internet use for health purposes* <http://www.hon.ch/Survey/FebMar2001/survey.html#shortcomings> accessed 18 February 2004.

HONF (Health on the Net Foundation) (2005), *Analysis of 9th HON Survey of Health and Medical Internet Users Winter 2004-2005* <http://www.hon.ch/Survey/Survey2005/res.html> accessed 14 September 2006.

Hoot, J.L. and Hayslip, B. (1983), 'Microcomputers and the elderly: new directions for self-sufficiency and lifelong learning', *Educational Gerontology* 9:5/6, 493-9.

Impicciatore, P., Pandolfini, C., Casella, N. and Bonati, M. (1997), 'Reliability of health information for the public on the World Wide Web: systematic survey of advice on managing fever in children at home', *British Medical Journal* 314:7098, 1875-81.

Internet magazine (2000), 'Getting quality health advice online', *Internet Magazine* No. 6 [Dialogweb file 148: full text].

Jadad, A.R. and Gagliardi, A. (1998), 'Rating health information on the Internet. Navigating to knowledge or to Babel?', *Journal of the American Medical Association* 279:8, 611-14.

Jamali, H. R., Nicholas, D., and Huntington, P. (2005), 'The use and users of scholarly e-journals: a review of log analysis studies', *Aslib Proceedings* 57:6, 554-71.

James, C., James, N., Davies, D., Harvey, P. and Tweedle, S. (1999), 'Preferences for different sources of information about cancer', *Patient Education and Counselling* 37:3, 273-82.

Jones, D. and Gill, P. (1998b), 'Refugees and primary care: tackling the inequalities', *British Medical Journal* 317, 1444-6.

Jones, D. and Gill, P. (1998a), 'Editorial: breaking down language barriers', *British Medical Journal*, 316, 1476-80.

Jones, R., Navim, L.M. and Murray, K.J. (1993), 'Use of a community based touchscreen public-access health information system', *Health Bulletin* 51, 34-42.

Kai, J. (1996), 'Parents' difficulties and information needs in coping with acute illness in their pre-school children: a qualitative study', *British Medical Journal* 313, 987-90.

Katzen, C.S. and Dicker, A.P. (2001), 'A survey to evaluate patients' perspective concerning e-mail in an oncology practice', *International Journal of Radiation Oncology, Biology, Physics* 51:3 (Suppl. 1),101.

Kenny, T., Wilson, R.G., Purves, I.N., Clark, J., Newton, L.D., Newton, D.P. and Moseley, D.V. (1998), 'A PIL for every ill? Patient information leaflets (PILs): a review of past, present and future use', *Family Practice* 5:5, 417-79.

Kim, P., Eng, T., Deering, M. and Maxfield, A. (1999), 'Published criteria for evaluating health related websites: review' *British Medical Journal* 318, 647-649.

Kitching, J.B. (1990), 'Patient information leaflets - the state of the art', *Journal of the Royal Society of Medicine* 83, 298-300.

Klemm, P., Bunnell, D., Cullen, M., Soneji, R., Gibbons, P. and Holecek, A. (2003), 'Online cancer support groups: a review of the research literature' *CIN: Computers, Informatics, Nursing* 21:3, 136-42.

Klemm, P., Hurst, M., Dearholt, S., Trone, S. (1999), 'Cyber Solace: Gender Differences on Internet Cancer Support Groups', *Computers in Nursing* 17:2, 65-72.

Lattimer, V., Sassi, F., George, S., Moore, M., Turnbull, J. and Mullee, M. (2000), 'Cost analysis of nurse telephone consultation in out of hours primary care: evidence from a randomised controlled trial', *British Medical Journal* 320, 1053-7.

Ley, P. (1982) 'Satisfaction compliance and communication', *British Journal of Clinical Psychology* 21, 241-54.

Leydon, G.M., Boulton, M., Moynihan, C., Jones, A., Mossman, J., Boudioni, M. and McPherson, K. (2000), 'Cancer patients' information needs and information seeking behaviour: in depth interview study, *British Medical Journal* 320, 909-13.

Lindberg, A.B. (1998), 'Testimony of Dr Donald Lindberg, Director of the National Library of Medicine, to the House Appropriations Sub-Committee on Labour, HHS and Education, (published online 18 March 1998) <http://www.nlm.nih.gov/pubs/staffpubs/od/budget99.html> accessed 18 February 2004.

London, J. (1999), 'Lay public use of healthcare websites', in Davidson, P.L. (Ed.), *The Handbook of Healthcare Information Systems* (Boca Raton: CRC Press).

M2 Presswire (2000), *UK-specific health website aims to capture a fifth of online health market M2 Presswire news release* (Lexis-Nexis Universe UK News database).

Mair, F. and Whitten, P. (2000), 'Systematic review of studies of patient satisfaction with telemedicine', *British Medical Journal* 320:7248, 1517-20.

Mann, C. and Stewart, F. (2000), *Internet communication and qualitative research* (London: Sage Publications).

Marsh, B. (2000), 'GP tells sick not to call "dangerous NHS helpline"', *Daily Mail* 22.02.00, p41

Marwick, C. (1999), 'Cyberinformation for seniors', *Journal of the American Medical Association* 281:16, 1474-7.

Mayberry, J.F. and Mayberry, M.K. (1996), 'Effective instructions for patients', *Journal of the Royal College of Physicians* 30:3, 205-8.

McIntosh, J. (1977), *Communication and awareness in a cancer ward* (London: Croom Helm).

McCray, A.T. (2005), 'Promoting Health Literacy', *Journal of the American Medical Informatics Association* 12:2, 152-63.

McNicol, S. and Nankivell, C. (2002), 'Creating access to the National Electronic Library for Health Birminham: University of Central England' <http://www.cie.uce.ac.uk/cirt/publications/NELH.pdf> accessed 18 February 2004.

Menou, M. (2000), 'Impact of the Internet: some conceptual and methodological issues or how to hit a moving target behind the smoke screen' in Nicholas, D. and Rowlands, I. *The Internet: its impact and evaluation* (London: Aslib).

Meredith, P., Emberton, M. and Wood, C. (1995), 'New directions in information for patients', *British Medical Journal* 311, 4-5.

Morahan-Martin, J.M. (2004), 'How internet users find, evaluate, and use online health information: a cross-cultural review', *CyberPsychology & Behavior* 7:5, 497-510.

Mulligan, J. (2000), Policy comment: what do the public think? Healthcare UK Winter. Available from: URL: <http://194.66.253.160/pdf/PUBLIC.PDF. accessed 18 February 2004.

Mumford, M.E. (1997), 'A descriptive study of the readability of patient information leaflets designed by nurses', *Journal of Advanced Nursing* 26, 985-91.

Munro, J., Nicholl, J., O'Cathain, A., and Knowles, E. (2000) *Evaluation of NHS Direct first wave sites. Second interim report to the Department of Health.* <http://www.shef.ac.uk/scharr/mcru/reports/nhsd2.pdf> accessed 18 February 2004.

Nammacher, M., Schmitt, K. (1999), 'Consumer use of the Internet for health information: a population survey', in *Proceedings of the 1999 AMIA Annual Symposium.* <http://www.amia.org/pubs/symposia/D005008.PDF> accessed 13 September 2006.

Nicholas, D., Huntington, P., Gunter, B., Russell, C. and Withey, R. (2003a), 'The British and their use of the web for health information and advice: a survey', *Aslib Proceedings* 55: 5/6, 261-76.

Nicholas, D., Huntington, P., Williams, P. (2003b), 'Delivering health information digitally: a comparison between the Web and Touch Screen Kiosk', *Journal of Medical Systems* 27:1, 13-34

Nicholas, D., Huntington, P., Williams, P. and Gunter, B. (2003c), 'Broadband nursing: an appraisal of pilot interactive consumer health services: case study In-vision', *Journal of Documentation* 59:3, 341-58.

Nicholas, D., Huntington, P., Williams, P. and Gunter, B (2002), 'Digital visibility: menu prominence and its impact on use of the NHS Direct information channel on Kingston Interactive Television', *Aslib Proceedings* 54:4, 213-221.

Nicholas, D., Huntington, P., Williams, P. and Blackburn, P. (2001d), 'Digital health information and health outcomes', *Journal of Information Science* 27:4, 265-276.

Nicholas, D., Huntington, P. and Williams, P. (2001), 'Health kiosk use: a national comparative study', *Aslib Proceedings* 53:4,130-40.

Nicholas, D., Williams, P. and Huntingdon, P. (2001), 'Healthy Email: NHS Direct Online Interactive Enquiry Service Evaluation of the Pilot stage', London: City University. Unpublished report submitted to NHS Direct Online operational team.

Nicholas, D., Huntington, P., Lievesley N. and Wasti A. (2000), 'Evaluating consumer Web site logs: case study The Times/Sunday Times Web site', *Journal of Information Science* 26:6, 399-411.

Nicholas, D., Huntington, P., Williams, P., Lievesley, N. and Withey, R. (1999), 'Developing and testing methods to determine the use of web sites: case study newspapers', *Aslib Proceedings* 51:5, 144-54.

Nielsen, J. (1994), 'Report from a 1994 Web usability study', <http://www.useit.com/papers/1994_web_usability_report.html> accessed 23 April 2001.

O'Cathain, A., Munro, J.F., Nicholl, J.P. and Knowles, E. (2000), 'How helpful is NHS Direct? Postal survey of callers', *British Medical Journal* 320, 1035.

Owen, J., Yarbrough, E.J., Vaga, A. and Tucker, D.C. (2003), 'Investigation of the effects of gender and preparation on quality of communication in Internet support groups', *Computers in Health Behavior* 19:3, 259-75.

Pastore, M. (2001), *Online Health Consumers More Proactive About Healthcare* <http://www.clickz.com/stats/markets/healthcare/article.php/10101_755471> accessed 18 February 2004.

Patt, M., Houston, T.K., Jenckes, M.W., Sands, D.Z. and Ford, D.E. (2003), 'Doctors who are using e-mail with their patients: a qualitative exploration', *Journal of Medical Internet Research* 5:2, e9. <http://www.jmir.org/2003/2/e9/> accessed 18 February 2004.

Pearson, J., Jones, R., Cawsey, A., Mcgregor, S., Barrett, A., Gilmour, H., Atkinson, J. and McEwen, J. (1999), The Accessibility of Information Systems for Patients: Use of Touchscreen Information Systems by 345 Patients with Cancer in Scotland. American Medical Informatics Association Annual Symposium 1999: Session 66 - Consumer Health Informatics II <http://www.amia.org/pubs/symposia/D005289. htm (Accessed 23/04/2001).

Pergament, D., Pergament, E., Wonderlick, A. and Fiddler, M. (1999), 'At the crossroads: the intersection of the Internet and clinical oncology', *Oncology* (Huntingt) 13:4, 577-583.

Pinder, R. (1990), *The Management of Chronic Illness* (Basingstoke: MacMillan).

Poensgen, A., Larsson, S. (2001), *Patients, physicians and the Internet: myth, reality and implications* (Boston MA: Boston Consulting Group) <http://www.medical-communities.de/pdf/bcg2001.pdf> accessed 18 February 2004.

Pointon, T. (1996), 'Telephone interpreting service is available', *British Medical Journal* 312, 53.

Potts, H. and Wyatt, J. (2002), 'Survey of Doctors' Experience of Patients Using the Internet', *Journal of Medical Internet Research* 4:1:e5. <http://www.jmir. org/2002/1/e5/index.htm> accessed 18 February 2004.

Quick, B.G. (1999), *The role of support groups on the Internet for those suffering from chronic kidney disease.* University of the Pacific [Volume 37/05 of Masters Abstracts of Dissertations Abstracts International].

Reeves, P.M. (2000), 'Coping in cyberspace: the impact of Internet use on the ability of HIV-positive individuals to deal with their illness', *Journal of Health Communication* 5(Supp1), 47-59.

Rimer, B.K., Lyons, E.J., Ribis, K.M., Bowling, M., Golin, C.E., Forlenza, M.J. and Meier, A. (2005), 'How New Subscribers Use Cancer-Related Online Mailing Lists', *Journal of Medical Internet Research* 7:3, e32. available at < http://www. jmir.org/2005/3/e32/> accessed 3 September 2006.

Rodgers, S. and Chen, Q. (2005), 'Internet community group participation: Psychosocial benefits for women with breast cancer', *Journal of Computer-Mediated Communication, 10:*4, article 5. available at <http://jcmc.indiana.edu/vol10/issue4/rodgers.html> accessed 14 August 2006.

Rumbelow, H. (1999), 'Doctors usurped by the Internet', *The Times* 6/11/1999.

Salman, P., Sharma, N., Valori, R. and Bellenger, N. (1994), 'Patients intentions in primary care: relationship to physical and psychological symptoms, and their perception by general practitioners', *Social Science and Medicine* 38, 585-92.

Serxner, S. (2000), 'How readability of patient materials affects outcomes', *Journal of Vascular Nursing,* 18:3, 97-101.

Shepperd, S. and Charnock, D. (2002), 'Against Internet exceptionalism', *British Medical Journal* 324:7337, 556-557.

Shum, C.M., Humphreys, A., Wheeler, D., Cochrane, M.A., Skoda, S. and Clement, S. (2000), 'Practice nurse-led management of patients with minor medical conditions: a randomised controlled trial', *British Medical Journal* 320, 1038-43.

Simon, P. (2001), 'The strange online death and possible rebirth of brand theory and practice', *Aslib Proceedings* 53:7, 245-9.

Smith, R. (2000), Doctors and nurses: a new dance? British Medical Journal 320 p7241. Available at: <http://bmj.com/cgi/content/full/320/7241/0/a?view=full&p mid=10764394.

Smith S. (1998), *Readability Testing Health Information Pre-natal Education newsletter* <http://www.beginningsguides.net/sitemap.htm> accessed 18 February 2004.

Stewart, R., McWhinney, I.R. and Buck, C. (1979), 'The doctor-patient relationship and its effect on outcome', *Journal of the Royal College of General Practitioners* 29:199, 77-82.

Strom, L., Pettersson, R. and Andersson, G. (2000), 'A controlled trial of self-help treatment of recurrent headache conducted via the Internet', *Journal of Consulting and Clinical Psychology* 68:4, 722-7.

Tassone, P., Georgalas, C., Patel, N.N., Appleby, E. and Kotecha, B. (2004), 'Do otolaryngology out-patients use the internet prior to attending their appointment?', *Journal of Laryngology & Otology* 118:1, 34-8.

Tate, D.F., Wing, R.R. and Winett, R.A. (2001), 'Using internet technology to deliver a behavioral weight loss program', *Journal of the American Medical Association* 285:9, 1172-7.

Travis, D. (2000), *What drives repeat visitors to your website?* <http://www.system-concepts.com/articles/forrester.html> accessed 18 February 2004.

Tucker, D. (2000), *Women's health information on the Internet: a patient satisfaction survey. Advances in Clinical Knowledge Management Workshop 3.* <http://www.ucl.ac.uk/kmc/kmc2/News/ACKM/ackm3/tucker.html> accessed 18 February 2004.

Wanless, D. (2002), *Securing Our Future Health: Taking a Long-Term View: Final Report* (London: HMGO) <http://www.hm-treasury.gov.uk/Consultations_and_Legislation/wanless/consult_wanless_final.cfm?> accessed 24 December 2003.

White M. and Dorman, S. (2000), Online Support for Caregivers: Analysis of an Internet Alzheimer Mailgroup. Computers in Nursing 18:4, 168-179.

White, M. and Dorman, S. (2001), 'Receiving social support online: implications for health education', *Health Education Research: Theory & Practice* 16:6, 693-707.

Williams, P., Jamali, H.R. and Nicholas, D. (2006), 'Using ICT with people with special education needs: what the literature tells us', *Aslib Proceedings*, 58:4, 330-45.

Williams, P., Madle, G., Weinberg, J., Kostova, P. and Mani-Saada, J. (2004), 'Information for the public about disease: usability issues in the development of the National Electronic Library for Communicable Diseases', *Aslib Proceedings* 56:2, 99-103.

Williams, P., Nicholas, D. and Huntington, P. (2003), 'Non-use of health information kiosks examined in an information needs context', *Health information and Libraries Journal* 20:2, 95-103.

Williams, P., Nicholas, D., Huntington, P. and Gunter, B. (2002), 'Doc dot com: reviewing the literature in digital health information', *Aslib Proceedings* 54:2, 127-41.

Williams, P., Nicholas, D., Huntington, P. and McClean F. (2002), Surfing for health: user evaluation of a health information web site Part 1: literature review', *Health Information and Libraries Journal* 19:2, 98-108.

Williams, P., Nicholas, D., Huntington, P. and McClean, F. (2002), 'Surfing for health: user evaluation of a health information web site Part 2 – fieldwork', *Health Information and Libraries Journal* 19:2, 214-25.

Williams, P., Nicholas, D. and Huntington, P. (2001), 'Walk in to (digital) health information: the introduction of a digital health information system at an NHS Walk-in Centre', *CD and Online Notes* 14:2, 4-7.

Williams, P. and Nicholas, D. (2001), 'Navigating the news Net: how news consumers read the electronic version of a daily newspaper', *Libri* 51:1, 8-16.

Williams, P. and Nicholas, D. (1998), 'The Internet, a regional newspaper and an attempt to provide "value added" information', *Aslib Proceedings* 50:9, 255-63.

Williamson, K., Bow, A. and Wale, K. (1997), 'Older people and the Internet', *Link-Up* March, 9-12.

Wilson, S.M. (1999), 'Impact of the Internet on Primary Care Staff in Glasgow', *Journal of Medical Internet Research*, 1:2, e7. <http://www.jmir.org/1999/2/e7/> accessed 18 February 2004.

Xie, B., Dilts, D.M. and Shor, M. (2006), 'The physician-patient relationship: the impact of patient-obtained medical information', *Health Economics* 15:8, 813-33.

Zrebiec, J.F. and Jacobson, A.M. (2001), 'What attracts patients with diabetes to an Internet support group? A 21-month longitudinal website study', *Diabetic Medicine* 18:2, 154-8.

Further Readings

2004

Huntington, P., Nicholas, D., Gunter, B., Russell, C., Withey, R. and Polydoratou, P. 'Consumer trust in health information on the web', *Aslib Proceedings* 56:6, 373-82.

Huntington, P., Nicholas, D., Holmwood, J. and Polydoratou, P. 'The general public's use of (and attitudes towards) interactive, personal digital health information and advisory services', *Journal of Documentation* 60:3, 245-65.

Nicholas, D., Huntington, P. and Williams, P. 'The characteristics of users and non-users of a kiosk information system', *Aslib Proceedings* 56:1, 48-61.

Nicholas, D., Huntington, P., Williams, P. and Dobrowolski, T. 'Re-appraising information seeking behaviour in a digital environment: bouncers, checkers, returnees and the like', *Journal of Documentation* 60:1, 24-39.

Nicholas, D., Huntington, P., Williams, P. and Gunter, B. 'Pregnancy Information and advice on Sky Television', *Informatics in Primary Care* 12:4, 215-26.

Williams, P., Madle, G., Weinberg, J., Kostova, P. and Mani-Saada, J. 'Information for the public about disease: usability issues in the development of the National Electronic Library for Communicable Diseases', *Aslib Proceedings* 56:2, 99-03.

2003

Gunter, B, Nicholas, D., Huntington, P., and Williams, P. 'Digital interactive television: health information platform for the future', *Aslib Proceedings* 55:5/6, 346-56.

Huntington, P., Nicholas, D., Huntington, P., Williams, P. and Gunter, B. 'An evaluation of a health video on demand service available to the public via interactive digital television', Libri 53:4, 266-81.

Huntington, P., Nicholas, D. and Williams, P. 'Comparing the use of two DiTV transmission services: same service, different outcomes', *Aslib Proceedings* 55:1/2, 52-63.

Huntington, P., Nicholas, D. and Williams, P. 'Characterising and profiling health web users and site types: going beyond hits', *Aslib Proceedings* 55:5/6, 277-89.

Nicholas, D., Huntington, P. and Homewood, J. 'Assessing used content across 5 digital health information services using transaction log files', *Journal of Information Science* 29:6, 499-517.

Nicholas, D., Huntington, P., Williams, P. and Gunter, B. Broadband nursing: an appraisal of pilot interactive consumer health services: case study In-vision', *Journal of Documentation* 59:3, 341-58.

Nicholas, D., Huntington, P., Gunter, B. and Williams, P. 'Comparing the use of health information and advice in Birmingham and Hull: a case study of digital health information delivered via the television', *Journal of Informatics in Primary Care* 11:2, 75-87.

Nicholas, D., Huntington, P., Gunter, B., Russell, C. and Withey, R. 'The British and their use of the web for health information and advice: a survey', *Aslib Proceedings* 55 :5/6, 261-76.

Nicholas, D., Huntington, P. and Williams, P. 'Delivering health information digitally: a comparison between the web and Touch Screen Kiosk', *Journal of Medical Systems* 27:1, 13-34.

Nicholas, D., Dobrowolski, T., Withey, R., Russell, C., Huntington, P. and Williams, P. 'Digital information consumers, players and purchasers: information seeking in the new digital interactive environment', *Aslib Proceedings* 55:1/2, 23-31.

Nicholas, D., Huntington, P., Williams, P. and Gunter, B. 'An evaluation of the health applications :and implications) of digital interactive television; case study the Living Health Channel', *Journal of Information Science* 29:3, 181-92.

Nicholas, D., Huntington, P., Williams, P. and Gunter, B. 'Health information and health benefits: a case study of digital interactive television information users', in Wilson, D., Barrulas, M.J., (eds) *The new review of information behaviour research; studies of information seeking in context Volume 4* (London: Taylor Graham) pp.177-94.

Nicholas, D. and Huntington, P. 'Micro-mining and segmented log file analysis: a method for enriching the data yield from Internet log files', *Journal of Information Science* 29:5, 391-04.

Nicholas, D., Huntington, P. and Williams, P. 'Perceptions of the authority of health information: case study Digital Interactive Television and the Internet', *Health information and Libraries Journal* 20:4, 215-24.

Nicholas, D., Huntington, P., Williams, P. and Gunter, B. 'Search-disclosure': understanding digital information platform preference and location in a health environment', *Journal of Documentation* 59:5, 523-39.

Nicholas, D., Huntington, P. and Williams, P. 'Three years of digital consumer health information: a longitudinal study the touchscreen health kiosk', *Information Processing and Management* 39:3, 479-502.

Williams, P., Nicholas, D., Huntington, P. and Gunter, B. 'Home electronic health information for the consumer: user evaluation of a DiTV video-on-demand service', *Aslib Proceedings* 55:1/2, 64-74.

Williams, P., Nicholas, D. and Huntington, P. 'Non-use of health information kiosks examined in an information needs context', *Health information and Libraries Journal* 20:2, 95-03.

Williams, P., Huntington, P. and Nicholas, D. 'Health information on the Internet: a qualitative study of NHS Direct Online users', *Aslib Proceedings* 55:5/6, 304-12.

2002

Gunter, B, Nicholas, D, Huntingdon, P. and Williams, P. 'Online versus offline research: implications for evaluating digital media', *Aslib Proceedings,* 54:4, 229-39.

Huntington, P., Williams, P. and Nicholas, D. 'Age and gender user differences of a touchscreen kiosk: a case study of kiosk transaction log files', *Journal of Informatics in Primary Care* 10:1, 3-9.

Huntington, P., Nicholas, D., Williams, P. and Gunter, B. 'Comparing two digital consumer health television services using transactional log analysis' *Informatics in Primary Care* 10:3, 147-59.

Huntington, P., Nicholas, D., Williams, P. and Gunter, B. 'Characterising the health information consumer: an examination of the health information sources used by digital television users'. *Libri* 52:1, 16-27.

Nicholas, D., Williams, P., Huntington, P. and Gunter, B. 'Broadband nursing: how have the public reacted to being able to talk to an on-screen nurse for advice?' Library and Information Update, Chartered Institute of Library and Information Professionals Magazine 1:4, 50-1.

Nicholas, D., Huntington, P., Williams, P. and Gunter, B. and Monopoli, M. 'The characteristics of users and non-users of a digital interactive television health service: case study the Living Health Channel', *Journal of Informatics in Primary Care* 10:2, 73-84.

Nicholas, D., Gunter, B., Withey R, Huntington, P. and Williams, P. 'The digital information consumer: what we know about the newly information enfranchised general public', *Library and Information Update: the magazine of the Chartered Institute of Library and Information Professionals Magazine* 1:1, 32-4.

Nicholas, D., Huntington, P., Williams, P. and Gunter, B. 'Digital visibility: menu prominence and its impact on use of the NHS Direct information channel on Kingston Interactive Television', *Aslib Proceedings* 54:4, 213-21.

Nicholas, D., Gunter, B., Williams, P. and Huntington, P. 'DiTV – A healthy future', *usableiTV* 2, 13-17.

Nicholas, D., Huntington, P. and Williams, P. 'Evaluating metrics for comparing the use of web sites: case study two consumer health web sites', *Journal of Information Science* 28:1, 63-75.

Nicholas, D., Huntington, P., and Williams P. 'An evaluation of the use of NHS touchscreen health kiosks: a national impact study', *Aslib Proceedings* 54:6, 372-84.

Nicholas, D., Huntington, P. and Williams, P. 'The impact of location on the use of digital information systems: case study health information kiosks', *Journal of Documentation* 58:3, 284-301.

Nicholas, D., Huntington, P., Williams, P. and Jordan, M. 'NHS Direct Online: its users and their concerns', *Journal of Information Science* 28:4, 305-19.

Thompson D, Williams, P., Nicholas, D. and Huntington, P., 'Accessibility and usability of a digital TV health information database', *Aslib Proceedings* 54:5, 294-08.

Williams, P., Nicholas, D., Huntington, P. and Gunter, B. 'Doc dot com: reviewing the literature in digital health information', *Aslib Proceedings* 54 :2, 127-41.

Williams, P., Nicholas, D., Huntington, P. and McClean, F. 'Surfing for health: user evaluation of a health information web site Part 1: literature review', *Health Information and Libraries Journal* 19:2, 98-08.

Williams, P., Nicholas, D., Huntington, P. and McClean, F. 'Surfing for health: user evaluation of a health information web site Part 2 – fieldwork', *Health Information and Libraries Journal* 19:2, 214-25.

2001

Gunter B Huntington, P., Williams, P. and Nicholas D. 'Health advice on the TV: Early Opinions of Users', *CD and Online Notes* 14:9, 4-8.

Gunter, B, Nicholas, D., Williams, P. and Huntington P. 'Is DiTV good for you?', *Library Association Record* 103:9, 558-9.

Nicholas, D., Huntington, P. and Williams, P. 'Comparing web and Touch Screen Transaction Log Files', *Journal of Medical Internet Research* 2001, 3:2, e18 <http://www.jmir.org/2001/2/e18/> accessed 14 August 2003.

Nicholas, D., Huntington, P., Williams, P. and Gunter, B. 'Delivering consumer health information digitally: platform comparisons', *International Online Conference*, Olympia December 2001 (Oxford: Learned Information Limited) pp. 145-53.

Nicholas, D., Huntington, P., Williams, P. and Chahal, P. 'Determinants of health kiosk use and usefulness: case study of a kiosk which serves a multi-cultural population', *Libri* 51:1, 102-113.

Nicholas, D., Huntington, P., Williams, P. and Blackburn, P. 'Digital health information and health outcomes', *Journal of Information Science* 27:4, 265-76.

Nicholas, D., Huntington, P. and Williams, P. 'Establishing metrics for the evaluation of touchscreen kiosks', *Journal of Information Science* 27:2, 61-72.

Nicholas, D., Huntington, P., Williams, P. and Vickery, P. 'Health Information: an evaluation of the use of touchscreen kiosks in two hospitals', *Health Information and Libraries Journal* 18:4, 213-9.

Nicholas, D., Williams, P. and Huntington, P. 'Health information kiosk use in health organisations: the views of the health professionals', *Aslib Proceedings* 53:9, 312-330.

Nicholas, D., Huntington, P. and Williams, P. 'Health kiosk use: a national comparative study', *Aslib Proceedings* 53:4, 130-40.

Nicholas, D., Huntington, P. and Williams P. 'Searching intention and information outcome: a case study of digital health information', *Libri* 51:3, 157-66.

Nicholas, D., Huntington, P. and Williams, P. 'When titans clash: digital health information providers and the Health Service square up to each other', *Managing Information* 8:4, 50-7.

Williams, P., Nicholas, D. and Huntington P. 'Walk in to (digital) health information: The introduction of a digital health information system at an NHS Walk-in Centre', *Online & CD Notes* 14:2, 4-7.

2000

Nicholas, D., Williams, P. and Huntington P. 'Digital health information: case study, the information kiosk', *Aslib Proceedings* 52:9, 315-30.

Nicholas, D., Huntington, P. and Williams P. 'Digital health information provision for the consumer: Analysis on the use of web kiosks as a means of delivering health information', *He@lth on the Net* 17, 9-11.

Nicholas, D., Williams, P., Huntington, P. and Blackburn P. 'Get your medical info here', *Library Association Record* 102:12, 694-5.

Williams, P., Huntington, P. and Nicholas D. 'Remote health information for the patient: a touchscreen kiosk in action', *Managing Information* 7:9, 72-5.

Williams, P., Huntington, P. and Nicholas D. 'Women on the web: why the Internet may still be a male dominated information system', *Online and CD Notes* 13:9, 5-9.

Index

Figures are indicated by bold page numbers, tables by italic numbers.